THE HANDBOOK OF
CANCER
IMMUNOLOGY

THE HANDBOOK OF CANCER IMMUNOLOGY

Volume 2
Cellular Escape from Immune Destruction

THE HANDBOOK OF
CANCER
IMMUNOLOGY

Edited by
Harold Waters
**Smithsonian Science
Information Exchange**

Garland STPM Press
New York & London

15   14   13   12   11   10   9   8   7   6   5   4   3   2   1

Library of Congress Cataloging in Publication Data
Main entry under title:

Cellular escape from immune destruction.

(The Handbook of cancer immunology; v. 2)
Includes bibliographies and index.
1.   Tumors—Immunological aspects.   2.   Tumor
antigens.   3.   Immune response—Regulation.
4.   Immune complexes.   5.   Immunological tolerance.
6.   Immunosuppresion.   I.   Waters, Harold, 1942–
II.   Series: [DNLM: 1.   Antigens, Neoplasm—Handbooks.
2.   T-Lymphocytes—Handbooks.   3.   Macrophages—Physi-
ology—Handbooks.   4.   Immunity, Cellular—Handbooks.
5.   Antigen-Antibody complex—Handbooks.   6.   Antibodies,
Neoplasm—Handbooks.   QZ200 H235 v. 2]
RC268.3.H35   vol. 2   [QR188.6] 616.9′94′07908s

ISBN 0-8240-7001-1   [616.9′94′079]   77–18080

Printed in the United States of America

CONTENTS

PREFACE

For the longest time immunologists concentrated on characterizing the attack of antibodies against passively helpless antigens. Now it appears clear that not all antigen systems are as helpless as at first assumed. True, red blood cells, bacteria, and bovine serum albumin don't exactly fight back much, but some nucleated cells do, especially those with actively ruffled borders.

The concept of cellular escape from immune destruction advances the increasingly attractive promise that immunology has more to offer cancer research than just hope as another therapeutic modality. There are currently a sleeve-full of well documented tricks employed by tumors and tumor cells to avoid immune destruction and sometimes detection as well. Here major consideration is given to the role of tumor specific transplantation antigens, serum blocking factors, immunologic eclipse, antigenic modulation, suppressor T cells, macrophage function in anergic organisms, anti-inflammatory effects of cancer, the relationship of cancer to autoimmunity, and overall regulation of the immune response by tumors.

Special consideration is given to active, antigenic modulation through antigen capping, internalization, shedding, and complexing. The consequences of oncogenic virion genomes coding for cell surface and "self-surface" components as related to cell differentiation are also discussed. The relatively neglected topic of intracellular expression of thymus-leukemia and other cell surface antigens is pursued here in detail with the point being drawn that immunoelectron microscopy is an essential tool for demonstrating expression of these antigens on organelles. The functional presence of H-2 antigens within cells remains controversial, as do their cell surface and extracellular roles.

Some tumors are capable of affecting immune impairment directly by producing suppressive substances. Others appear to carry viruses that are immunosuppressive to tumor hosts. Still others are indirectly suppressive, possibly throwing out various immune smoke screens and generating non-malignant regulatory cells that serve to embarrass normal immune responses.

The controversy over the anatomical and functional characterization of lymphoid cell subpopulations continues. The spectrum and limits of these cellular subpopulations are not yet clear; the roles of macrophages, B cells, T cells, null cells and killer cells have not yet been crystallized.

For example, we may well be dealing with a broad spectrum of cells having at one end killer cells progressing through, say, T_2 cells, T_1 cells, t cells, tb cells, b cells, B_1 cells, and B_2 cells to plasma cells. Macrophages from the various organ systems and truly uncommitted lymphoid (null) cells might then fit into the scheme at right angles, with macrophages interacting directly with T and B cells. True null cells probably represent a small proportion of adult lymphoid cells and might be expected to feed in at the tb, or "bi-cell," level. It is unlikely that T cells, after their meaningful experience of traversing the thymus, ever cease being T cells, although it would not be surprising to find large numbers of them at any given time resting and for the moment receptorless as t cells.

Since these are largely functional distinctions between morphologically similar cells and since the lymphoid system represents the body's SWAT squad and fire department, we might expect a certain amount of running back and forth along the spectrum of lymphoid cell subpopulations depending on the needs and circumstances of the moment. We might also expect to find important functional keys in the ratios of these subpopulations to one another, especially with regard to regulatory and suppressor cell subpopulations.

—Harold Waters
Washington, D. C.
February 1978

CHAPTER 1

MECHANISMS BY WHICH TUMORS ESCAPE IMMUNE DESTRUCTION

Eugenia Hawrylko

Memorial Sloan-Kettering
Cancer Center
New York, New York   10021

The mechanisms by which tumors avoid immune destruction in hosts with competent immune systems have been subdivided into those in which either the tumor, serum factors, lymphoid cells, or macrophages play a primary role, although frequently all of these are interrelated. Major consideration is given to the role of: tumor-specific transplantation antigens; serum blocking or inhibiting factors such as antibodies, antigen-antibody complexes, and antigens; immunologic eclipse and suppressor T cells or factors which suppress lymphocyte function; and macrophage function in anergic tumor bearers.

INTRODUCTION

The concept that the host has a cellular form of immunity which provides a natural defense against the development of malignant cells was proposed by Paul Ehrlich in 1909 (76). It was not until the 1950s, however, that methylcholanthrene-induced murine sarcomas were shown to have tumor-specific transplantation antigens (TSTA), which were capable of eliciting immune responses in their autochthonous hosts (92,214). This posed the paradox: Why, in the presence of a competent immune system, do syngeneic tumors bearing TSTA provoke an immune response which promotes their continued survival, or "escape," whereas allogeneic tumors or transplanted organs, which have greater antigenic differences compared to their host, are effectively rejected?

The concept of tumor "escape" has in the past implied that the successful growth of a tumor represents a failure of the immune system. This derives from the concept of immunosurveillance, whose main support is based on the association of immunological deficiency with increased risk for tumor development (246). This subject has been extensively covered elsewhere (246) and will not be considered here. Rather, it has become apparent, in experimental animal models, that the successful growth of a tumor may be a function or result of the immune response to that tumor. This is well known: as "enhancement" in systems using allografts (147) and as "facilitation" in syngeneic systems (23).

It should be borne in mind that the paradox is not new, only newly applied to malignant growth. During the preantibiotic era, when problems of pathogenic microbes were a scourge to mankind, immunity to the classic extracellular pathogen, *Diplococcus pneumoniae*, was shown to be dependent on opsonizing antibodies; yet some hosts succumbed in the face of high titers (182). It was not until the advent of antibiotic therapy that successful elimination of the pathogen could be consistently predicted. In this case, the antibiotic restricted proliferation of the bacteria until such time as the immune response was primed and able to cope with infection (182). By analogy, the more antigenic leukemias, against which serum antibodies may play a significant role in immunity, have been responding to regimens in which tumoricidal drugs have been employed (140).

Perhaps of more relevance to the usual type of tumor escape is the hosts' response to facultative intracellular parasites such as *Mycobacteria*, *Brucella*, and *Listera*, in which a cell-mediated mechanism produces protection whereas antibodies, although sometimes present, do not (180). Mice given a massive dose of BCG intravenously would not express a delayed-type hypersensitivity (DTH) reaction 20 days later (60). Their spleen cells, however, would be capable of transferring DTH to normal recipients. If the recipients were X-irradiated prior to transfer, no DTH reaction was elicited, indicating that another cell type was required in addition to the immunologically committed lymphocyte, namely, the circulating monocyte (177). This cell can become the activated macrophage which is ultimately responsible for the death of the facultative intracellular parasite. How these mechanisms may relate to tumor escape is dealt with in Section V of this chapter.

One approach to dealing with the paradoxical growth of tumors in hosts with competent immune systems involved the use of the in vitro colony inhibition assay to show that mice bearing progressing Moloney virus-induced sarcomas (125) and rabbits bearing progressing Shope papillomas (124) had lymph node or peripheral blood lymphocytes which were cytotoxic in vitro against cultured syngeneic tumor cells. Shortly thereafter, the microcytotoxicity variant of this technique was used to detect cytotoxic lymphocytes in animals bearing both spontaneous and chemically induced tumors (129, 134). Although hosts with either progressing or regressing tumors possessed lymphocytes capable of in vitro cytotoxicity, factors in the sera of those with progressing tumors blocked that cytotoxicity (124, 125, 129). These demonstrations stimulated numerous in vitro studies of serum-blocking factors which have been well covered in reviews, emphasizing either the role of antibody and antigen-antibody complexes (22, 133) or antigen (4).

The explanation of the mechanisms by which syngeneic or autochthonous tumors flourish in the presence of the hosts' immune response bears very much on fundamental questions of immunoregulation of cell-mediated and humoral mechanisms, both of which are implicated in the hosts' response to tumors (4, 22, 133). Although the immune system is characterized by the well-integrated role of its various components vis-à-vis their protagonists, be they microbes, neoplastic, or foreign cells, the selective overview that follows focuses in turn on the several discernible factors that influence the continued survival of neoplastic tissues in hosts with apparently competent immune responses.

ROLE OF THE TUMOR IN ESCAPE

Nature of Tumor Antigens

The most obvious characteristic of a tumor is excessive multiplication by its "growth fraction," consisting of those cells in the population which are actively involved in DNA synthesis (235). In the case of solid tumors, such cells freed from contact inhibition invade adjacent territory. The role of the surface properties of tumor cells, such as their adhesive forces, shapes, movements, cell junctions, and intercellular communications, have been covered in a recent survey (9); they will not be discussed here, for at this time they do not bear an obvious relationship to the immune responsiveness of the host.

The other critical characteristic is the presence of tumor-specific transplantation antigens (TSTA) which can provoke tumor rejection by either a humoral and/or a cell-mediated response in the syngeneic or authochthonous host. These antigens have generally been described by the classic transplantation techniques, involving: (1) immunization by implantation and subsequent excision of living tumor cells (92, 214); (2) immunization with lethally irradiated tumor cells; or (3) immunization with a subthreshold dose of living tumor cells. Such studies, performed mainly in animal systems, have demonstrated essentially two types of TSTA:

1. *Individually distinct antigens on spontaneous or chemically induced tumors.* For example, the TSTAs produced by the chemical carcinogen, 3-methylcholanthrene, have been shown to have unique specificities, none of which cross-react with each other (e.g., 163). These are thought to result from somatic mutation or derepression of normal cellular genes (212). Support for this point of view comes from experiments such as those in which BALB/c 3T3 cells were cloned *in vitro* (27). Methylcholanthrene was then applied to progeny cells, which were subsequently cultured in diffusion chambers implanted intraperitoneally in syngeneic mice (27). The tumors that subsequently developed were shown to have individually distinct antigenic determinants even though they had derived from the same ancestral cell (27). This implied that the antigenic diversity of the chemically induced tumors did not preexist in the normal tissue but was in some way caused by the carcinogen treatment.

2. *Common antigens on tumors induced by individual strains of oncogenic viruses and presumably coded for by viral DNA or RNA present in the cells (221).* In contrast to the individually specific spontaneous or carcinogen-induced TSTA, it has been shown in experimental animal models that murine tumors induced by the same virus, whether in the same individual, in different individuals of a species, or in different species, have the same TSTA (115, 234). Tumors induced by different viruses, even within the same strain of inbred mice, carry distinct TSTA whose antigens do not cross-react (115). Interestingly *in vitro* experiments showed that lymphocytes from

human melanoma patients were specifically cytotoxic for the histological type of the patient's tumor, that is, melanoma patients' lymphocytes reacted against their own tumor and melanoma tumors from other patients but not against breast carcinoma or normal cells (131). Such results imply that human tumors may have either virally induced origins or that these reactions are detecting organ-specific antigens.

TSTA of the tumors induced by DNA viruses such as polyoma, SV40, and the adenoviruses could be distinguished from the antigens of the viruses themselves, for the tumors lacked infectious virus (174). With the oncogenic RNA viruses it was more difficult to distinguish the TSTA from viral antigens because most tumor cells produced infectious virus (174). There is evidence that the viral antigens are related to the viral structural proteins (11). For example, the Gross strain of the murine leukemia virus (MuLV-G) expresses its viral-envelope antigen at the budding site (11). The most abundant internal virion-group-specific antigen, p30, has been identified on the cell surface of oncornavirus-infected cells in several species (164). In the immune response of rats to an MuLV-G induced lymphoma, both cytotoxic antibody and cell-mediated cytotoxicity were directed toward virus-coded antigens, principally p30 (164). Sera from rats with progressively growing lymphomas containing p30 inhibited this cell-mediated cytotoxicity (164). Several variants of the envelope glycoprotein of murine leukemia virus, gp69/71, have been expressed on lymphoid cells in mice that are not producing detectable amounts of MuLV (e.g., 198). Membranes prepared from tumor cells infected with surface budding influenza virus were much more immunogenic than membranes from noninfected tumor cells in protecting mice from syngeneic challenge (103). More importantly, mice could be protected against Friend-virus-induced leukemia by inoculation with the major viral glycoprotein, gp71, or its antiserum (143).

A new concept of the possible role of viral antigens in antitumor responses has been developed. Like the T-cell-helper effect (152, 160), H-2 compatibility has been shown to be required for the T-cell-mediated in vivo lysis of target cells infected with lymphocytic choriomeningitis (LCM) (70, 277) or ectromelia virus (98), or trinitrophenyl-modified lymphocytes (228), as well as for the in vivo T cell effector activity in LCM (71), listeriosis (278), and ectromelia (40). Such T-cell-mediated lysis requires that the killer and target cells are syngeneic at the H-2K and/or H-2D loci (228). This H-2 restriction is also operative in the cytotoxic T cell response of syngeneic and semisyngeneic mice to cultured cell lines derived from tumors induced in vivo by Friend murine erythroleukemia virus (FV) (41). Evidence has been produced that H-2 molecules bind to virus molecules on the surface of infected cells, forming an immunogenic complex recognizable by immune T cells (223). The details of this mechanism remain to be worked out, especially the explanation of how allogeneic interactions fit into this scheme.

The TSTA are to be distinguished from tumor-associated transplantation antigens (TATA), which are not antigenic in the tumor-bearing host and are often of fetal origin (14, 59, 258). The expression of genes which were appropriately expressed during embryogenesis and are reexpressed in tumors results in the formation of so-called oncofetal antigens (e.g., see reviews in Refs. 2, 248). This finding has resulted in the concept that tumors may represent a disorder of the mechanisms of differentiation (59). The first reexpressed fetal antigen to be described was the α-fetoprotein, an abnormal protein synthesized by a chemically induced murine hepatoma which was antigenically identical to an α-globulin present in embryonic and neonatal mouse serum but absent from the adult mouse (1). Within one year a similar material was found in the serum of patients with primary hepatomas (249). Shortly thereafter, carcinoembryonic antigens (CEA) were found in human fetal gut and human colonic carcinomas (105, 242). Although the putatively embryonic tumor antigens are detectable under in vitro conditions using lymph node cells from syngeneic multiparous mice (14, 49, 127), immunity to these antigens is frequently inadequate for in vivo tumor rejection (14, 258). Therefore, this area has received relatively little attention from immunologists because it had been thought that embryonic antigens on tumors which elicited in vitro lymphocytotoxicity but not tumor transplantation resistance did not add significantly to tumor immunity (14). Potential importance of tumor-embryo cross-reactivity was stressed by Medawar and Hunt (184) and Coggin and Anderson (59), who indicated that immunization with fetal tissues could prolong survival of mice (184) or hamsters (58) challenged with chemically (184) or virally (58) induced tumors. The concept of viral induction of embryonic antigens has been raised with regard to virus-specific transplantation antigens, since fetal cells can immunize against polyoma-, SV40- and adenovirus-induced tumors. The existence of cross-reactions between antiviral tumor antibodies and fetal cells has been described (59). Thus it is not clear if they are truly embryonic antigens or are caused perhaps by an endogenous virus. For a detailed consideration of this question the reader is referred to References 59, and 248. The issue is further complicated by the demonstration that α-fetoproteins can suppress both humoral and cell-mediated responses (189, 190, 206, 207).

TSTA can elicit both humoral and cell-mediated responses (4, 133). Antibodies can react with tumor surface antigens, fix complement and lyze tumor cells (47) or interact with an as yet unidentified nonimmunized effector cell in antibody dependent cell-mediated cytotoxicity

(181). Sensitized lymphocytes or macrophages can interact with surface antigens and either destroy or inhibit tumor proliferation (6).

Mechanisms of Tumor-Mediated Escape

CELL SURFACE ANTIGENS. How do cell surface antigens contribute to the escape of tumors from the immune response?

Antigen density has been correlated with the sensitivity of tumor cells to cytotoxic antibodies (89, 188), but it fluctuated during the cell cycle such that maximal cytotoxicity was confined to the G_1 phase of cell growth (51, 204, 229). However, complement activation by the antibody-coated cells remained constant (175). A recent study, however, found that differences in antigen concentration were not a sufficient explanation for the variation in the sensitivity to antibody and complement-mediated lysis since two guinea pig hepatomas which bind similar numbers of antibody and C_1 molecules showed different susceptibilities to cytotoxic lysis (199).

Another of the simpler concepts held that antigenic determinants were masked by surface sialomucins which permitted them to escape interaction with the immune system (222). This provided the rationale for use of *Vibrio cholerae* neuraminidase to split off sialic acid residues in order to increase immunogenicity for therapeutic purposes (63, 64, 222), a maneuver which has had variable success (141, 230).

Recent studies, however, using methylcholanthrene-induced rat mammary carcinomas showed a direct relationship between the presence of a glycocalyx and immunogenicity (159). The highly immunogenic, non-metastasizing mammary tumor cells had acid mucopolysaccharide coats on their surfaces which could not be removed by neuraminidase, whereas the non-immunogenic, spontaneously metastasizing cells lacked such coats. The absence of glycocalyx from the metastasizing tumor cell surface seemed to result from its dissociation from plasma membranes for solubilized cell surface antigens were readily found by immunodiffusion assays in the blood of rats bearing metastasizing tumors, while there was no detectable tumor cell surface antigen in the blood of the hosts bearing non-metastasizing tumors (159).

A comparison of 6 spontaneously metastasizing and 4 non-metastasizing rat mammary carcinomas showed that the plasma membrane marker enzyme levels were significantly lower in all the metastasizing tumors (57). Enzyme activity decreased in direct proportion to the rate of metastasis, and increased in proportion to the immunogenicity of the tumors (57). Thus, the loss of glycocalyx and shedding of cell surface antigens by spontaneously metastasizing mammary tumor cells correlated with the loss of activity of plasma membrane marker enzymes.

PARTICULATE VS. SOLUBLE ANTIGENS. Soluble antigens are poorly immunogenic unless injected with adjuvant (95). Rats could not be immunized with solubilized preparations from syngeneic aminoazo-dye-induced hepatoma tumor cells (18), whereas the membrane fractions were immunogenic and could elicit tumor specific antibody (215). Tumor cell nuclei or soluble cytoplasmic proteins were lacking in this latter capacity (215). The crucial test, resistance to tumor cell challenge, could not be elicited with any of the subcellular fractions injected by a variety of routes either alone or in mixture with bacterial adjuvants (215). This stands in contrast to the immunity which is so readily induced by inoculation of intact cells attenuated by either irradiation or treatment with cytotoxic drugs or the concomitant immunity elicited by the concurrent growth of the autologous tumor (69, 101, 261).

In an allogeneic system, direct comparison of the ability of soluble or membrane transplantation antigen preparations from EL-4 or C57BL/6 spleen cells to inhibit *in vitro* specific cytotoxicity of sensitized spleen or T lymphocytes toward ^{51}Cr-EL-4 cells indicated that, given equal amounts of total protein, the membrane preparations were more inhibitory than the soluble EL-4 antigens (44). However, other studies which employed serologically active particulate membrane fractions in reciprocal experiments where both experimental and control extracts were tested against each of two killer populations, with reactivity towards one or the other targets, found that the inhibition of lymphocyte-mediated cytolysis was nonspecific, possibly due to mechanical interference by the membrane fractions (259). Neither was there evidence that soluble antigen preparations (extracted by papain or 3M KCl) from tumor target cells bind specifically to killer lymphocytes (259). Additional studies led to the conclusion that both the serologically active particulate and soluble tumor antigen preparations failed to inhibit lymphocyte-mediated cytolysis or bind to killer lymphocytes in an immunologically specific manner (259).

SOLUBLE ANTIGENS. Circulating soluble TSTA have been found by radioimmunoassays in the sera of rats bearing chemically induced sarcomas (e.g., 254). Immediately after intramuscular inoculation serum levels were elevated, presumably due to autolysis of the injected cells (254). They subsequently dropped, only to rise again between 10 and 16 days (254). If, however, the tumors were surgically amputated, the levels of TSTA in the serum fell within several days (254). Similar patterns of TSTA activity were found in the sera of mice bearing a spontaneous DBA/2 strain lymphoma in subcutaneous sites (273). If the tumor bearers received 500 rads total body irradiation prior to the intramuscular tumor implantation, circulating TSTA were not detectable in their sera

(254). This led to the proposal that a local immune reaction was required to produce detectable quantities of soluble TSTA in the sera of tumor bearers (254) with the further stipulation that this occurred in vivo only in those tumors that do not shed their antigens spontaneously at a high rate (3).

The role of spontaneously shed soluble TSTA was investigated in vitro using two methylcholanthrene-induced rat fibrosarcomas, the highly immunogenic, poorly metastatic MC-1 and the non-immunogenic, highly metastatic MC-3 (62). Culture supernatants of the MC-3, but not the MC-1 cells, could neutralize the specific cytotoxic action of lymphocytes taken from lymph nodes draining their respective tumors, indicating that MC-1 cells did not spontaneously release tumor antigens. Yet sera from mice bearing either tumor specifically inhibited their respective immune lymph node cells. Since it had been shown previously that MC-1 TSTA probably reached the serum after autolysis or as a consequence of immune attack, rather than by spontaneous shedding (254), it was proposed that the spontaneous shedding of MC-3 sarcoma antigen assisted metastatic spread by preempting the effector limb of cell-mediated immunity (62). Since the serum of both tumor bearers had similar inhibiting effects on their respective immune lymph node cells, it was suggested that the biologically important role of TSTA was in the microenvironment in which tumor cells lodged rather than in the blood (62).

Other support for the inhibition of cell-mediated immunity by soluble tumor antigens comes from the work of Baldwin et al. (13), who by means of indirect membrane immunofluorescence showed that sera from tumor bearing rats had specific antigen in excess in association with specific immune complexes. Similarly, sensitized lymphocytes from patients afflicted with colon carcinomas were specifically inhibited after incubation with tumor membrane preparations (16), again suggesting that cell-mediated immunity might be inhibited in vivo by circulating antigen.

Another attractive explanation for tumor escape in the immunocompetent host proposed that antigen released during the early stages of tumor growth was carried via the afferent lymphatics to the regional lymph nodes, where it resulted in a normal immune response with production of specifically reactive immunoblasts that were subsequently discharged into the lymph and eventually reached the blood stream (7). If tumor growth was not retarded at this point, more tumor antigen impinged on the node, where it reacted with newly formed immunoblasts and immobilized them so that instead of being released into the efferent lymph they settled in the medulla of the lymph node and transformed into plasma cells (7). This transformation has been shown (33), and high concentrations of antigen can inhibit normal traffic of cells through a node (116) at least transiently for a few days (53). Such "lymph node paralysis" can exist while nodes distant to the tumor respond normally to other antigens. Following excision of the primary tumor, the percentage of immunoblasts in the thoracic lymph duct can increase within one day (7).

A difficulty with this proposition is the demonstration by many, especially in human cancer patients, that specifically cytotoxic lymphocytes exist in the tumor patients' peripheral circulation (e.g., 133). There is, however, controversy over whether there is a relationship between the detection of cytotoxic peripheral blood or lymph node lymphocytes and stage of disease. Some studies have found patients with superficial or early cancers to be more likely to have cytotoxic lymphocytes than patients with advanced cancer (e.g., 29, 203), whereas others have found that specific lymphocyte cytotoxicity does not vary with the extent of disease (e.g., 15, 135). This question is dealt with in greater detail below in the section on The Role of Lymphoid Cells.

The findings that soluble antigen impaired the function of stimulated lymphocytes and was detectable in the sera, lymph, and urine of tumor-bearing rats (253) have a parallel in the clinical studies of Currie and collaborators (61, 65, 67). In a series of patients with malignant melanoma, lymphocytes cytotoxic for autologous tumor cells were detectable in only 15% of such patients and only in those with minimal tumor burden (67), unlike the studies by the Hellstroms in which virtually all their patients had specifically cytotoxic lymphocytes (130). If, however, the lymphocytes were repeatedly washed, it was found that after 6 washes maximal cytotoxicity was obtained (65). Thus, in a series of 14 melanoma patients of which only 3 had demonstrated cytotoxic autologous lymphocytes prior to washing, after extensive washing the remaining 11 were also shown to be reactive (61). Furthermore, the activity of the latter group was inhibited by the addition of autologous sera, whereas the addition of autologous sera to the lymphocytes from the 3 patients whose unwashed lymphocytes were cytotoxic, caused no inhibition (61). The inhibitory activity of the autologous sera on autologous lymphocyte cytoxicity correlated with the stage of disease and was specific for the tumor type (61).

TUMOR ANGIOGENESIS FACTOR. Continued escape or growth of a solid tumor ultimately faces restriction imposed by diffusion of essential gases, nutrients and wastes and depends on connection of capillary blood vessels which originate not from tumor tissue but from the host (8, 268). It was first demonstrated in 1968 that tumors stimulated capillary growth via a humoral mediator (111). Neovascularization was induced in host tissues separated from the tumor by Millipore filters with a pore size of 0.45 μ. It has since been shown that tumor cells release a diffusible factor, subsequently named tumor angiogenesis factor (TAF), which is mitogenic for capillary endothelial cells (94). TAF resembles a nondialyzable ribonucleoprotein of approximately 100,000 molecular weight found in the tumor cell nucleus in association with nonhistone proteins. It has also been isolated both from tumor cytoplasm and material which diffuses out of intact tumor cells. The relationship of this factor and the immune response is not clear. It may be that vascularization is a prerequisite for the expression of tumor immunogenicity if this is mediated by contact with blood-borne lymphocytes. If, however, a tumor spontaneously sheds antigens these may reach afferent lymphatics which can set up an immune response before vascularization. The reader is referred to a review by Folkman (93) for further information on this especial consideration of the role of the tumor in escape.

ROLE OF SERUM IN TUMOR ESCAPE

Antibody, Antigen-Antibody Complexes, Antigen

The important finding that factors in the sera of hosts bearing progressing tumors blocked the in vitro cytotoxicity of their lymphocytes towards their autochthonous tumors (124, 125, 129) seemed a good explanation for the failure of immunotherapeutic procedures in animals with tumors exceeding certain size limitations (e.g.. 19, 24, 28). During the past several years much effort has been expended to define the nature of serum blocking factors, for they might be of diagnostic or prognostic value in evaluating the status of tumor bearers, or provide some clues to the underlying mechanism(s) of tumor escape. Initial reports indicated that blocking was due to antibody since it could be absorbed by incubation with suspensions of target cells, separated with 7 S globulin fractions on Sephadex fractionation and was inhibited by antibody to IgG (125). The rapid loss of serum blocking activity within 3 days after rats were rendered tumor free was one of the earliest pieces of evidence which made it unlikely that blocking was due to antibody (17). The neutralization of the activity of tumor bearer serum by the addition of serum from immune animals suggested blocking was due to antigen-antibody complexes. Subsequent reports supported this premise (232). Blocking factors in serum from mice bearing Moloney virus-induced sarcomas were absorbed onto viable Moloney sarcoma cells and following elution with low pH buffer (glycine, HCl pH 3) separated into high and low molecular weight components which individually lacked in vitro blocking activity. Fractionation was achieved by ultrafiltration first through a membrane retaining molecules above 100,000 molecular weight (which would include immunoglobulins) and then the filtrate was passed through a second membrane retaining molecules above 10,000 molecular weight. Tests on these fractions showed that individually they were devoid of lymphocyte-blocking activity, but this function was restored when they were recombined in their original proportions. Blocking factors have also been eluted from human tumors and again low and high molecular weight fractions individually failed to block the cytotoxic action of patients' lymphocytes, but in a 1:1 mixture of the two, the blocking activity was restored (233). In tests where the two fractions were added separately to plated tumor cells, treatment with "low molecular weight" followed by "high molecular weight" fractions did not protect the tumor cells against lymphocyte cytotoxicity. If the sequence were reversed, treating tumor cells with "high molecular weight" fractions first, then blocking occurred. The "high" and "low" molecular weight fractions could therefore contain specific antibody and tumor antigen respectively, although neither has thus far been characterized. A study using human blocking sera indicated that blocking was mainly associated with IgG_1 and IgG_3 fractions (146). It should be pointed out that these studies of blocking did not define where biologically significant blocking activity occurred, whether it be at the level of the tumor cell or the immunologically committed lymphocyte since target cell, effectors and serum were incubated together.

In contrast to the bulk of the early studies of the Hellstroms, in which sera from tumor bearers were usually added to the target cells (e.g., 124, 125, 129), Baldwin et al. studied separately the effects of tumor bearer serum on either the lymphocytes or the tumor cells (16, 21, 22). These types of studies led to a distinction between "blocking," in which interactions with serum involve binding to tumor surface antigens, and "inhibition," in which interactions take place with sensitized lymphoid cells (22). Such distinctions tend to imply that these are the primary loci of activity in the immune response, although they exclude other components such as the macrophage, whose involvement has gained increasing attention (see The Role of the Macrophage below).

Direct proof that tumor-specific antigen-antibody complexes could block lymphocyte-mediated cytotoxicity when incubated with target tumor cells has been presented (20). A solubilized antigen from an extranuclear membrane fraction obtained from a transplanted rat hepatoma was prepared by homogenization and papain digestion. Mixtures of various proportions of postexcision sera (known to contain specific antibody) and this solubilized tumor antigen were tested for blocking activity. No blocking occurred with mixtures containing a very high or low proportion of antigen. Blocking activity was only observed with intermediate mixtures, thus indicating that antigen-antibody complexes made at equiva-

lence were capable of blocking lymphocyte cytotoxicity. Somewhat analogous studies in the Moloney sarcoma virus system have shown that
depending on the antibody concentration, the same serum can block or
augment the cytotoxic effect of lymphocytes on tumor cells when added
to the target cells (236).

In contrast, sera from rats bearing a transplantable hepatoma or a
solubilized hepatoma specific antigen preparation inhibited the
cytotoxicity of immune lymph node cells for plated hepatoma cells when
the sera was incubated with effector cells, rather than target cells as described above (21). Sera from hepatoma-immune rats, however, which
had been shown to "block" at the level of the target cell, failed to "inhibit" lymphocyte cytotoxicity when preincubated with the effector cells
(21). Sera from mice bearing spontaneous or either chemically or virally
induced syngeneic murine tumors have also been reported to significantly abrogate the specific cytotoxic effect of peritoneal cells when incubated with those effector cells (275). The same sera were much less efficient in protecting against the cytotoxicity of sensitized peritoneal cells
when incubated with the target cells (275).

Additional support for a role for tumor antigens in sera as inhibitors
came from the already-mentioned work of Currie and Basham (see Section
II), who demonstrated in a microcytotoxicity assay that lymphocytes from
human cancer patients had greatly enhanced specific cytotoxic effects if
they were extensively washed, and that sera from tumor bearing patients
added to well-washed lymphocytes inhibited in vitro cytotoxicity (65).
On the basis of these data and experiments on the release of soluble-tumor
antigens into the supernatants from cultured rat sarcomas (62) (see above),
it was postulated that antigenic determinants are constantly being shed
from the surface of a tumor. These leak into the extracellular fluid and
serum where they are complexed with antibody. Further tumor growth
results in a condition of antigen excess, such that antigen-antibody complexes act as inhibitors of antitumor-cell-mediated immune reactions by
preempting the effector limb of cell-mediated immunity (62).

The characterization of the serum factors which are blocking or inhibiting in vitro is dependent on the techniques used for their purification
and identification. Considerable time and effort have been spent on meth-
odological studies. The complexity of the situation is highlighted by the
report that BALB/c and BALB/cfC3H mice possessed serum factors which
specifically blocked spleen cell activity against isologous mammary-
tumor virus (MTV) induced mammary tumors (34, 35, 39) but fractionation by Sephadex G-200 gel filtration was required to reveal that such sera
also contained a mixture of specific factors with different functional activities (38). In vitro blocking activity was localized to 7 S fractions whereas
antibodies in 19 S fractions increased spleen cell cytotoxicity, recruited

previously inactive spleen cells to specific cytotoxic activity, and functioned as complement-fixing antibodies (38).

Kinetics of the Appearance of Serum Factors

The difficulties involved in devising suitable methodologies for detection of serum antigen, antibody, or antigen-antibody complexes resulted in the fact that serum factors were usually evaluated at only one point in time. This failed to take into account the dynamic state of some surface antigens and their corresponding antibodies, which in turn most likely reflects the kinetics of the immune response. It was not until 1975 that the sequence of serological events occurring during the subcutaneous growth of a particular tumor was determined by means of immuno-fluorescence (46). Following subcutaneous inoculation of a transplantable aminoazo-dye-induced rat hepatoma, serum levels of antigen, antibody, and immune complexes were correlated with in vitro blocking and inhibition of immune cytotoxic lymph node cells for cultured tumor cells. Seven to 14 days after tumor implantation, sera from rats bearing small subcutaneous hepatomas contained tumor specific antigen. Sera from rats bearing intermediate sized tumors had high levels of both blocking (against target tumors) and inhibitory factors (against effector cells) when neither free antibody nor antigen could be detected (presumably in the presence of antigen-antibody complexes). Sera taken 24 to 28 days after implantation had tumor-specific immune complexes in antibody excess (46). Consideration of the kinetics of the response may help reconcile the different results obtained in different laboratories both with regard to the presence and identity of factors in the sera of tumor bearers following subcutaneous tumor implantation.

In addition, the site of tumor implantation may also affect the types of serum factors detected. The intravenous injection of the same aminoazo dye-induced hepatoma described above resulted in grossly visible nodules in the lungs and a different pattern of factors in the serum (45). Complexed antigen appeared at day 10, but free tumor-specific antigen was not detected until day 14. Both rose to high levels, which persisted thereafter; antibody was not detected at any stage (45). If, however, tumor cells were admixed with BCG prior to inoculation, visible lung nodules did not develop, free tumor antigen was detected from as early as 3 to 10 days after inoculation, and free tumor-specific antibody was found from day 10 onward at the time antigen-antibody complexes were also detected (45).

Sequential studies using the isotopic antiglobulin technique for evaluating the humoral response to several virally induced tumors in syngeneic murine hosts showed that the kinetics of the antibody response also varied between different tumors (257). In general, antitumor antibodies could be detected at an early stage of tumor growth and were generally higher in progressors. In the SV 40 system, rechallenge with the same tumor after surgical amputation of the tumor transplant produced a secondary humoral antibody response which eventually declined. In contrast, antibody titers constantly rose in the progressors in parallel to the size of the tumor (257).

It has been established that some human and animal tumor cells are coated in vivo with Ig (272). In the case of ascites mouse tumors, such Ig is in dynamic equilibrium with the Ig in ascitic fluid (216). Sequential studies of syngeneic, in vivo propagated polyoma-virus-induced tumor cells showed they became progressively coated with IgG during the second week (48). This correlated directly with an increase in the coating of cells with potentially cytotoxic antitumor antibodies, which could be demonstrated by the addition of exogenous complement (48). Cell populations propagated in vivo for longer than 3 weeks became less sensitive to exogenous complement although their IgG coating remained high suggesting that antibodies coating young tumor cell populations have the capacity to activate complement, whereas those coating older cell populations cannot. Antibody-coated tumor cells incubated in vitro at 37°C but not at 4°C lost some of the molecules coating the cell surface (48).

Antigenic Modulation

Conceivably, antigenic modulation mediated by the reaction of antibody with cell surface TSTA (201) which is then shed could account for in vivo tumor escape. A comparison of the immunoferritin technique with the cytotoxicity test for murine mammary-tumor virus (MuMTV) antigens, Thy 1.2, and H-2.8, indicated that preincubation of GR mouse ascites leukemia (GRSL) cells with anti-MuMTV serum at 37°C but not at 0°C resulted in shedding from the cell surface of only the MuMTV antigen-antibody complexes (54). Evidence for antigenic modulation causing in vivo escape derives from the finding of MuMTV antigen-antibody complexes in GRSL ascitic fluid (265).

In another in vitro system, isoantiserum to the murine mastocytoma, P 815, resulted in antigenic modulation at 37°C such that 20% of specifically bound ^{125}I labeled antibodies were released following incubation for 30 min and 40% after 5 hours (81). The rate was apparently controlled by active metabolism of the mastocytoma, for less than 10% of bound antibody was released during incubation at 4°C (81).

The concept of antibody induced antigenic modulation (201) has not been taken into account in evaluating the in vitro tests used to detect blocking of target cells or inhibition of lymph node cell cytotoxicity by tumor bearer serum. All those assays which include incubation at 37°C for several days (e.g., 126) would provide ample opportunity for antigenic modulation to occur. Thus, in addition to the interactions of antibody, antigen, or antigen-antibody complexes with lymphoid or tumor cell surface antigens, the possibility that these reactants perform their functions after release from these surfaces should be considered. The subject of antigenic modulation is covered in detail elsewhere in this work (240).

Immunological Enhancement

A consideration of the role of serum in escape mechanisms must take into account immunological enhancement. This was originally defined as the enhanced growth of tumor allografts following active or passive immunization procedures intended to accelerate their rejection (147). Functionally, immunologic enhancement is manifested by reduced cellular immunity such that the growth of the enhanced tumor exceeds that of the tumor in the untreated allografted host wherein it is rejected. This phenomenon has conclusively been shown to be passively transferred by immunoglobulins with H-2 specificity (84, 147) primarily of the 7 S class (IgG_1 and IgG_2) if used in precisely defined doses (219), although IgM can also be effective (56, 219). Recent evidence showed that the $F(ab')_2$ fraction but not Fc fraction of passively administered IgG alloantibody was responsible for suppressing cellular immunity (148). In this situation, suppression of the cell-mediated response by antibody is considered to be a consequence of complexes being formed between the antibody and the stimulating antigen (231, 245). This may operate by antigen masking (peripheral blocking) (245), or by direct action on the immunopotent cell (central blocking) (232).

In a guinea pig model using a syngeneic methylcholanthrene-induced sarcoma, concomitant immunity and in vitro T cell cytotoxicity were shown to exist, yet tumor cells were not rejected in vivo (31). The isotopic antiglobulin assay showed that antibodies were present on the tumor cells in vivo suggesting that antibody mediated efferent enhancement was the mechanism of tumor escape either due to masking of tumor antigens or shedding of soluble antigen-antibody complexes (31).

In contrast to the hypotheses depending on antibody-mediated interference with the immune response to the tumor, other observations suggest that immunological enhancement is the result of a direct effect of antibody on neoplastic cells (10, 108, 109, 225–227). Direct stimulation of mitotic activity in allogeneic tumors by small amounts of specific antibody was first observed by Gorer (108, 109). This was later ascribed to a direct effect of antibody on tumor cells resulting in cell injury accompanied by uncoupling of oxidative phosphorylations, with a subsequent secondary rebound and resultant increased tumor growth (10). Short-term experiments in vitro have shown that antibodies exert a dual action on tumor cell growth: cytotoxic effects at high antibody concentrations but stimulation of cell growth at low antibody concentrations. Limiting amounts of anti-L-cell antibody were found to stimulate nucleoside incorporation, DNA synthesis, and cell growth in mouse L cells (225–227). Complement also enhanced the stimulatory as well as the inhibitory effects of antibody. Complement activated through the third component reduced the quantity of antibody needed to stimulate cell growth by as much as 1000-fold (224). Antibody stimulation of tumor growth has also been observed in vivo in T-cell-depleted mice using allogeneic (91) or syngeneic (32) antisera, suggesting that the antibody effect was one of direct stimulation rather than interference with cellular immunity.

Facilitation, Blocking in Vivo

The preceding evidence for a role for serum (either antigen, antigen-antibody complexes, or antibody) in blocking the cell-mediated response to TSTA has been based largely on in vitro studies. What is the evidence that factors in the sera of tumor bearers can block immunity in vivo? A frequently cited example of in vivo blocking (23) employed either sera from rats carrying progressively growing polyoma tumors which had blocking activity in vitro or low pH tumor eluates. These were inoculated either simultaneously with, or at intervals up to 8 days after, sc inoculation of syngeneic tumors. The resulting tumor growth was significantly faster than that in controls. Such accelerated rates of growth have been termed "facilitation." These are an example of inhibition of an immune response in the sense that tumor growth in a normal syngeneic host elicits an immune response without which the tumor might grow faster. Presumably the administration of sera inhibited the efferent arc of the immune response for tumor growth in treated rats did not differ from controls until after 8 days of growth in vivo, at a time when immunity was most likely fully developed. This is further substantiated by the fact that evaluation of sera from these treated rats in vitro revealed blocking activity for 3 days after inoculation, yet lymph node cell cytotoxicity was not abrogated, findings consistent with an efferent blockade (23).

Another frequently cited example of in vivo blocking used sera from mice treated with 400 rads of whole body X-irradiation followed by twice daily intraperitoneal and subcutaneous administration of irradiated cells for 6 consecutive days (263). The systemic administration of this serum into immune mice somewhat depressed their tumor immunity as measured by host resistance to challenge (263). The problem with this experiment is that the method of eliciting the "blocking sera" was not physiologic. It assumed that irradiated animals would not respond immunologically to the irradiated cells and that the serum contained soluble tumor antigens. One cannot conclude that this occurs in vivo.

Still another example of facilitated tumor growth in vivo implicated serum factors only indirectly (262). Mice who had been immunized by tumor growth and excision were injected at the time of challenge with a 4 day course of irradiated tumor cells. Resistance was significantly impaired if the challenge and irradiated cells were injected 16–22 days after the initiation of the immune response. It is noteworthy that the same quantity of irradiated tumor cells that could depress resistance at this susceptible stage assisted the development of resistance if injected at the time of its initiation and boosted resistance at the time of its decline (262).

Another in vivo study used IgG_2-containing eluates dissociated from chemically induced sarcomas by low pH glycine buffer (217). They had no cytotoxic effect on tumor cells but were thought to be blocking antibodies. These eluates were incubated with trypsinized tumor cell suspensions for 30–60 mins and then injected intramuscularly in syngeneic mice (217). The results were variable. Less than half of the experiments indicated an increased incidence of tumor takes for those cells incubated with autologous eluates. Isologous eluates had a still smaller effect. These experiments can be critized on several technical grounds as well as on the fact that the eluate would be rapidly diluted as the tumor grew so that its effect would rapidly wane. These results are far from conclusive evidence of in vivo enhancement of tumor growth by IgG_2.

In the interval there have been no new reports of in vivo blocking of antitumor immunity by factors in the serum of tumor bearing hosts.

We have developed a murine model of BCG potentiated antitumor immunity for the purpose of determining whether BCG potentiated immunity is subject to the same regulatory mechanisms which enable tumor escape in the "normal" tumor bearing animal. The model employs the injection of isologous irradiated cells into subcutaneous sites prepared by a prior injection of BCG; a challenge located remotely in the footpad is then monitored for evidence of delayed type hypersensitivity (DTH) and specific antitumor resistance (120). Using the poorly immunogenic, methylcholanthrene induced, murine ascites mastocytoma, P 815 (MA), in this prevention model, information has been obtained regarding optimal conditions, time course (123), dimensions (119), and the cells involved (120) in BCG-potentiated antitumor immunity. Attempts at immunotherapy using these optimal conditions failed to produce detectable tumor resistance in situ (Fig. 1) when started as soon as 1 or 7 days after tumor implantation. Yet lymphoid cells from such mice were able to transfer local antitumor immunity against admixed MA which was almost as effective on a cell:cell comparison as that transferred from normal

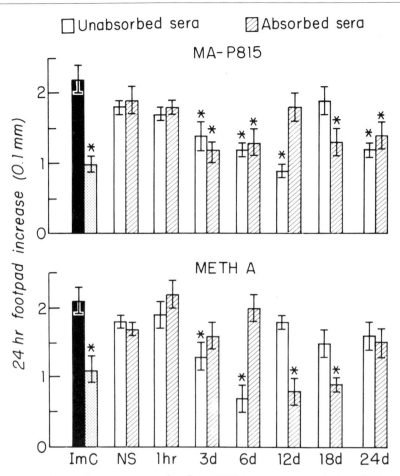

Fig. 1. Comparison of tumor growth after BCG immunopotentiation (Px) was begun 7 (A) or 1 (B) day(s) after, or 5 (C) or 17 (D) days prior to tumor implantation. For each panel, groups of control (●---●) and immunized (●——●) mice were inoculated in the right hind footpad with mastocytoma cells (MA) at day 0. The immunized groups were injected with BCG and irradiated MA at sc sites at times indicated along the abscissa except in (D), where BCG and irradiated MA were injected 17 and 7 days respectively before challenge. The expected onset of immunity 7 days after the injection of irradiated MA was only evident in the pretreated groups in (C) and (D). In (D) the immune group (I) had a significant DTH reaction (*inset*), p < 0.005 compared to controls.

immunized mice and considerably more potent than that transferred from unimmunized tumor bearing mice who possessed concomitant immunity. Despite the fact that immunized tumor bearers had 3 to 4 times as many lymph node lymphocytes as the unimmunized tumor-bearing mice, this increased number of cells failed to overcome factors inhibiting the expression of antitumor immunity in the tumor bearing host (121). The ease with which antitumor immunity was adoptively transferred from the immunized tumor bearing hosts was consonant with the possibility that serum and other factors were blocking BCG-potentiated antitumor immunity. Injection of sera from mice with progressively growing MA into recipients immunized with BCG and irradiated MA inhibited the efferent arc of the immune response (both DTH and antitumor immunity) in vivo, while the afferent arc was largely unaffected. Absorption of the progressor sera with viable syngeneic tumor cells at room temperature for the purpose of removing antibody increased such blocking, three absorptions being more effective than one (122). Because the results with the poorly immunogenic MA were not dramatic parallel experiments were performed with the more antigenic methylcholanthrene-induced sarcoma, Meth A. Unlike the MA, whose irradiated cells alone failed to immunize without prior priming with BCG, irradiated Meth A alone could immunize but prior priming with BCG increased this response. Thus studies with Meth A enabled a comparison of the effects of serum blocking factors on the response in the BCG-potentiated groups and those immunized with irradiated Meth A alone. Appropriately absorbed progressor sera from Meth A tumor bearers inhibited both the induction and expression of DTH and antitumor immunity elicited by sc irradiated Meth A regardless of prior priming with BCG. The expression of the BCG-potentiated response could be inhibited by absorbed progressor sera as early as 15 min after the injection of irradiated Meth A into sites previously primed with BCG (122).

The preceding experiments used sera from mice bearing 18-day growths originating from 10^6 viable tumors injected into the hind footpad. If mice with either progressing MA or Meth A were bled at intervals after tumor inoculation and these sera were subsequently injected into the respective syngeneic BCG-potentiated host at the peak of the expression of the immune response, 10 days after the injection of irradiated tumor cells into the BCG-primed sites, similar patterns of sequential change in the nature of serum factors which could block the expression of both DTH (Fig. 2) and antitumor immunity became apparent. For each time point, the effect of progressor sera was compared with that of sera absorbed with syngeneic tumor cells to determine what role, if any, antibody played.

In general, during the very early phase of tumor growth, blocking activity was not affected by absorption with syngeneic tumor cells and

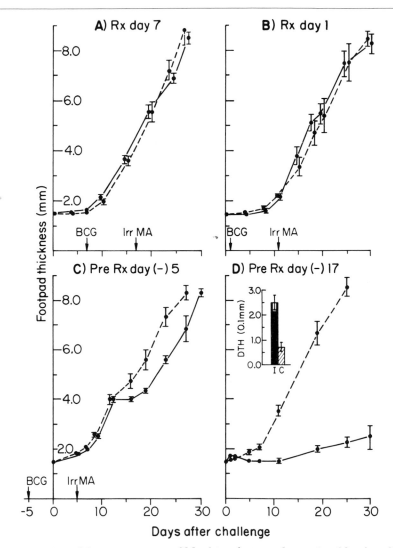

Fig. 2. Kinetics of the appearance of blocking factors, determined by the effect of sera from mice bearing MA (*above*) or Meth A (*below*), to suppress the expression of BCG potentiated DTH to their respective tumors. Unabsorbed (white columns) or absorbed (hatched columns) progressor sera from mice exsanguinated at time points indicated along the abscissa were injected i.v. in 0.5 ml aliquots into immunized mice at the peak of the immune response. These results are compared to DTH in BCG-potentiated mice (Imo) and controls (C) who were challenged with 10^6 tumor cells. Normal sera (NS) had no effect in either tumor system. *P at least < 0.05 compared to immune groups. Means of 6 ± SEM for MA and 5 ± SEM for Meth A.

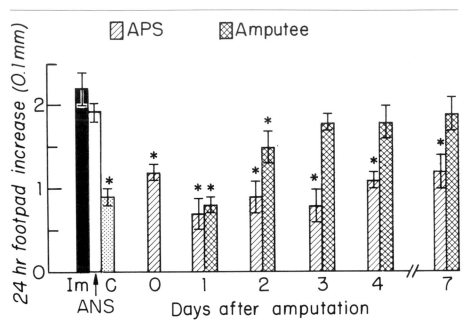

Fig. 3. Disappearance of blocking of BCG-potentiated DTH to Meth A by absorbed progressor sera (APS) following tumor amputation. DTH of immune mice injected iv 1 hour prior to footpad challenge with either APS from 12-day tumor bearers obtained before (day 0) or at intervals after amputation of either the footpad tumor (double-hatched columns) or contralateral normal limb (single-hatched columns) was compared with that of immune mice who were (ANS) or were not (Im) inoculated with absorbed normal mouse sera. Controls, C, were injected with 10^6 Meth A only. *P at least < 0.05 vs. immune control. Means of 5 ± SEM.

therefore presumed to be mediated by tumor antigens. Subsequently blocking was accomplished by serum factors which could be absorbed by specific tumor (antibody?), whereas later sera had increased activity after absorption, presumably due to antigen-antibody complexes left after antibody removal. Amputation of late-phase tumors resulted in the disappearance of blocking factors within 2 to 3 days (Fig. 3).

These results help explain why BCG potentiated immunotherapy of large tumors has generally met with poor success (28). Factors in the sera of mice bearing either poorly or highly immunogenic tumors can block the efferent arc of BCG-potentiated DTH and antitumor resistance *in vivo*. Sera from mice bearing a more antigenic tumor can also block the afferent limb of the immune response. If the tumor is small or of short duration, BCG-potentiated immunization can increase the number of immune lymphoid cells in the tumor-bearing host (121), although they may not produce detectable resistance in situ. However, if the tumor is amputated, the blocking factors rapidly disappear and the BCG-potentiated lymphoid cells should then be effective in mediating antitumor resistance (122).

ROLE OF LYMPHOID CELLS IN TUMOR ESCAPE

Immunologic Eclipse

That animals bearing a progressively growing tumor in one anatomic location can reject a subsequent challenge with the same tumor in another location was originally termed "concomitant immunity" in 1908 (25). Renewed interest in this area (69, 101, 261) has centered not so much on the immunity engendered but on the observation that at large tumor volumes (69) or in the presence of residual or reinjected killed tumor cells (162), specific immunity in vivo was depressed yet the host could still respond to other tumors. The concept of immunologic eclipse derived from studies of the growth of a chemically induced syngeneic sarcoma, in which it was found that host peritoneal cells initially inhibited tumor growth in vitro but later these responses were specifically suppressed or "eclipsed" (30, 275). This in vitro sequence paralleled in vivo responses to autologous tumor challenge (30). If the tumor were surgically amputated both in vitro cytotoxicity and in vivo antitumor immunity reappeared (30). Subsequently, it was shown that sera from tumor bearers inhibited the effector peritoneal cells but not the target cells (275).

A similar pattern of stimulation followed by specific suppression of the immune response was found in studies measuring DTH to transplanted SV 40 and methylcholanthrene induced fibrosarcomas (205). In this case splenic lymphocytes from the anergic tumor bearing mice were able to adoptively transfer a DTH reaction when mixed with tumor cells and inoculated into the footpad of normal mice (205). (This reaction, which depends on the interaction of lymphocytes with macrophages, is considered hereafter.) The question in this section is whether such patterns of reactivity followed by suppression indicate that the ability of lymphoid cells to mediate specific cytotoxicity in vitro or adoptively transfer antitumor immunity or DTH to the autochthonous tumor in vivo varies with the stage of disease.

Some investigavors have found in vitro lymphocyte reactivity limited to situations in which tumors were small (29, 132, 171, 203, 256), whereas others did not (15, 135). For example, in a sequential clinical study of 10 patients with malignant melanoma it was shown that the degree of tumor immunity mediated by their peripheral blood lymphocytes in vitro against cultivated melanoma cells was higher in those with little or no residual tumor than in those with large tumor loads, although the latter were also reactive (132). Sera from those patients with clinically detectable melanoma were shown to block lymphocyte cytotoxicity but this effect disappeared as the clinical situation improved (132).

Adult mice develop tumors at the site of inoculations with the murine Moloney sarcoma virus (MSV) which have a high incidence of spontaneous regression (83). Regressors have lymphocytes which are cytotoxic in vitro, whereas tumor bearers have lymphocytes that are significantly less active both specifically (157, 170–172) and nonspecifically (157). This model has been used extensively to show the effects of blocking serum (see previous section) but the question of intrinsic lymphocyte hyporeactivity has not been resolved.

A comparison of the effects of in vitro cocultivation of lymphoid cells from either immune or tumor-bearing mice with autologous tumor cells from a methylcholanthrene induced sarcoma indicated that after 6 days the cells from the tumor bearers were inactive whereas those from the mice immunized in vivo by tumor transplantation followed by excision were specifically cytotoxic to the appropriate target cells (149, 150). The lymph node cells from tumor bearers were shown to exert a suppressor function, but it was not demonstrated whether this was due to cellular contact or a cellular product (128).

The strength of the specific spleen cell mediated in vitro microcytotoxicity of multiparous BALB/cfC3H female mice bearing large progressively growing MTV-induced mammary tumors, was similar to that effected by similar tumor free multiparous females (35) but there was a qualitative change in the response of the former, namely the loss of detectable antibody dependent cell-mediated cytotoxicity (173). Although some cells capable of secreting specific antibody in culture were detected in the spleens of tumor-bearing females, their relative numbers were low. The apparent lack of a non-T cell immune reactivity in the spleens of these females was attributed to a diminution both in the number of antibody-secreting cells and the number of effector cells (36). Further studies showed that cells from tumor bearers were least active in assays testing the effectiveness of specific recruiting antibodies in the sera of tumor-bearing mice that mediate spleen cell cytotoxicity toward the autologous tumor (37). This was presumed to indicate a decrease in the number of recruitable cells (37).

It has been shown that hyporeactivity of tumor bearer lymphocytes, detected as decreased in vitro cytotoxicity, is at least in part a result of their interaction with either circulating soluble tumor-specific antigens or antigen-antibody complexes (see previous sections). The in vivo counterpart of the first of these interactions, paralysis of stimulated lymphocytes by antigen in the lymph nodes draining the tumor has already been discussed. Clinical data which support this concept come from studies in which cells from lymph nodes draining large tumors could not be stimulated by autologous, freshly biopsied, tumor cells which had been treated with mitomycin C, whereas peripheral blood lymphocytes from the same patients gave positive reactions (243). Such paralysis was considered to be due to excess antigen because lymph node cells from the draining lymph node could stimulate the autologous peripheral lymphocytes (243).

Other possible causes of lymphocyte hyporeactivity in tumor bearers include deficiency of lymphocytes (for which there are no experimental data), anatomic barriers that prevent the interaction of lymphocytes with appropriate targets, alterations of lymphocyte traffic such as lymph node trapping, interaction with regulatory lymphocytes such as suppressor cells, and interactions with factors (which may or may not be the same as those described in previous sections) that affect the function of lymphocytes, such as their proliferative ability. The latter two situations will be considered below.

Suppressor Cells in Vitro

The concept of feedback inhibition as a mechanism for regulation of antibody production by specific antibody has been generally accepted (88, 260). More recently, immunoregulatory T cells (100, 151), which function as either helpers, amplifiers, or suppressors, have been demonstrated not only in antibody production (85, 88) but also in cell-mediated reactions, such as DTH reactions (142, 264, 276) and chronic allotype suppression (137).

Suppressor effects have been elicited by T cells activated by soluble or cell-bound antigens (85, 144, 200, 250, 251), and by mitogens (72, 209). The suppressor T cells have been either specific to the inducing antigen (85, 200, 276) or non-specific, that is, able to suppress responses to other antigens as well (55, 72, 137, 144, 209, 250). Some forms of suppression have been mediated by cell-free supernatants (72, 85, 209, 250, 276). The target for T cell suppression can be either a T (55, 165, 276) or a B cell (52, 86).

The role of suppressor cells in tumor escape has only recently begun to be explored. Several studies have attempted to characterize the suppressor cell in tumor systems (75, 106, 161), but not all have indicated whether it is the suppressor cell or its product which mediates suppressor function. One of the earliest studies of suppressor cells in tumor systems showed that spleen cells from mice with progressing MSV-induced tumors failed to express immunity in migration inhibition assays against soluble 3*M* KCl extracts of the tumor (106). Separation of the cells by velocity sedimentation revealed that large and small cells could express immunity, but they were suppressed by the addition of intermediate sized (4.8–6.0 mm/hr) cells which had surface immunoglobulins and were therefore presumably B cells (106). The effects of these suppressors were non-specific, since induction of protein synthesis in T cells in response to the mitogen, phytohemagglutinin, was also suppressed (106, 158).

In other studies, MSV-induced tumors reached maximum size 12 to 16 days after virus inoculation, and regressed by 21 days (161). This paralleled specific spleen cell-mediated cytotoxicity measured as the percentage ^{51}Cr released from syngeneic lymphoma cells and was inversely related to the phytohemagglutinin (PHA)-induced proliferative response, which was maximally depressed at 15 days (161). The inhibition of PHA responsiveness was attributed to a suppressor cell since admixture of spleen cells from tumor bearers, 12–16 days after MSV, inhibited the activity of syngeneic normal spleen cells when added before PHA (161). Subsequent studies showed that these cells could suppress the proliferative response of normal spleen cells if added up to 24 hours after the addition of PHA, but after that time the normal spleen cells were no longer susceptible to the action of the suppressor cells (162). The suppressor cell was characterized as belonging to the monocyte/macrophage series (161).

In contrast to the depression of PHA-induced DNA synthesis in MSV spleen cell cultures, their PHA-induced cytotoxicity was elevated compared with that of normal spleen cells (162). This dissociation implied that proliferation dependent lymphocyte effector functions were the target of suppressor cell action (162). It was reasoned that if cytotoxic T cells were generated before suppressor cells, the activity of the latter could not be detected. To test this idea, spleens from 14-day MSV-infected tumor bearing mice (which were at the peak of both the cytotoxic antitumor response and PHA suppressor activity) were depleted of T cells thereby eliminating the cytotoxic cell population while retaining suppressor functions (104). Such spleen cell populations markedly inhibited the *in vitro* secondary cytotoxic antitumor response of immune spleen cells taken from regressors infected with M-MuSV 30 days earlier (104). Thus, it was proposed that suppressor cells account at least in part for the inability of tumor bearing hosts to reject their tumor despite their ability to mount a specific immune response against TSTAs. This conclusion may not be accurate, for the MSV system is characterized by the fact that the majority of the tumors do regress despite the presence of these suppressor cells, and MSV-induced tumors are susceptible to inhibition by antibody both *in vitro* and *in vivo* (208).

In other *in vitro* studies, spleen cells from mice bearing methylcholanthrene induced tumors could non-specifically suppress the ability of lymphocytes from normal mice to be immunized *in vitro* against transplant alloantigens. The suppressor cells were non-θ bearing and nylon adherent. They did not mediate their effects via soluble factors (75).

A series of *in vitro* studies which clearly indicate that suppressor effects were mediated by soluble factors has been performed (191–193). *In vitro* production of blocking factors by spleen cells from tumor bearing mice was shown to be dependent on T cell function (191). These blocking factors which were absorbed on anti-mouse immunoglobulin columns could inhibit specific lymphocyte destruction of cultivated tumor cells and mediate antibody dependent cytotoxicity (ADCC) with control lymphoid cells (191, 192). However, spleen cells passed through Sephadex G-10 which removed plasma cells and macrophages did not continue to synthesize factors with ADCC activity although the synthesis of blocking factors continued (192). Lysis of Thy-1 positive lymphocytes with antiserum and complement abolished the synthesis of blocking factors (192). Supernatants of cultured spleen cells which had been treated with cycloheximide or puromycin, both inhibitors of protein synthesis, failed to block or promote ADCC activity indicating that both these activities of culture supernatants were dependent on active protein synthesis *in vitro* (193). It was not indicated whether some tumor cells were present in the spleens at the initiation of the cultures which could provide a source of antigen for there was no need for antigen priming in this system. These results support the concept that lymphoid cells act as suppressors of specific antitumor responses by producing blocking substances such as complexes between tumor antigens and IgG antibodies which are capable of preventing sensitized T lymphocytes from killing their targets (128).

Factors Which Suppress Lymphocyte Proliferation

In addition to suppressor cells which can inhibit the proliferative response of lymphoid cells (162), sera from mice with various types of tumors have been shown to contain a factor(s) inhibiting the proliferative response of normal spleen and lymph node cells to mitogens, allogeneic cells, and specific antigens (176, 269, 270). Comparable inhibition of the proliferative response of normal human peripheral blood lymphocytes has also been observed when sera from patients with various tumors were added to cultures (50, 114, 247). The inhibitory factor in sera from tumor-bearing mice increased in titer with progressive tumor growth (269) and disappeared rapidly after surgical resection (271). It suppressed allogeneic and xenogeneic lymphoid cells as effectively as it inhibited syngeneic cells (270). It inhibited lymphocyte proliferation even of those cells fully activated to DNA synthesis (271). As little as one hour exposure to sera from mice with a transplantable 3-methylcholanthrene-induced tumor reduced the ability of normal mouse spleen cells to respond to subsequent mitogen stimulation, an effect which was not reversed by washing. This irreversible inhibition was shown to be produced by a monomeric immunoglobulin, ~150,000 molecular weight, which was not dissociable into lower molecular weight moieties (271). It remains to be seen whether this serum inhibitor bears a relation to the suppressor cells in mice with MSV-induced tumors which inhibited PHA-induced lymphocyte proliferation (106, 161). However, in contrast with the action of the serum factor (271), those suppressor cells did not inhibit the PHA response when added after DNA synthesis was underway.

Suppressor Cells in Vivo

Evidence for an in vivo role for suppressor cells as a cause of the apparent ineffectiveness of the immune response in tumor-bearing mice has been presented in studies of mice bearing an antigenic, syngeneic, methylcholanthrene-induced sarcoma (96). Mice were immunized by surgical excision of the growing tumor. They were then infused with either sera or 4×10^7 thymus or spleen cells from donor mice bearing 7 day old syngeneic tumors. The transferred cells partially and temporarily reduced the immune rejection of 10^6 subcutaneous syngeneic tumor cells administered simultaneously, or the ongoing immune rejection of challenges administered 5 days earlier. The tumor bearer sera failed to affect the immunity. Microscopically the tumors in recipients of suppressor cells had diminished mononuclear cell infiltrates.

These immunosuppressor cells were generated in tumor-bearing mice within 24 hours after subcutaneous tumor inoculation and persisted through at least 16 days of tumor growth (97). They were detected in the thymuses, spleens, draining lymph nodes, and bone marrow of tumor bearers but not in the peripheral blood (97). Their effect was abolished by anti-θ sera treatment and complement but not by cortisone (97).

Immunostimulation by Lymphoid Cells

The immunostimulation hypothesis proposed that, in the initial stages of the immune response to TSTA, the low level of immune reactivity stimulated rather than inhibited tumor growth (213). Later, as the immune response matured, it became inhibitory, but by that time the tumor had proliferated beyond the capacity of an inhibitory immune response to contain its further extension and progressive tumor growth ensued (213). Support for this concept was divided into three categories, those studies relating to (1) pregnancy which showed that the existence of stable histocompatibility polymorphism in mice and men was at least partly dependent on immunologic reinforcement of fetal survival; (2) lymphoid and/or immune stimulation of normal tissues; and (3) lymphoid and/or immune stimulation of tumors, such as occurs in immunological enhancement. The reader is referred to the exposition for more details (213).

Since this concept was proposed in 1971 (213), few new pieces of experimental evidence have supported it. These derive mainly from *in vitro* cytotoxicity assays employing lymph node or peripheral blood lymphocytes from tumor bearers, which when taken early in the course of tumor development (145), stimulated tumor growth if used in small effector:target cell ratios [i.e., 100:1] (90, 145, 185). This effect was potentiated by the addition of autologous serum (90, 145, 185), whereas high effector:target cell ratios (i.e. 1000:1) (90) or cells taken at later time points (145) inhibited growth. These studies are hampered by the failure to include stringent specificity controls, for the well-known "feeder effect" employed in tissue culture systems can be mediated by nonlymphoid cells (244) and/or the "conditioned media" in which they have grown (218).

Another set of *in vitro* studies which may support the immunostimulation concept employed the sensitization of lymphoid cells to tumor antigens by co-cultivation (149). After 3 days' co-incubation, specifically increased numbers of tumor cells were detected by the microcytotoxicity assay (149). By 5 days, however, specific cytotoxic effects were predominant (149).

ROLE OF THE MACROPHAGE

Activated Macrophages

The concept that immunologically committed lymphocytes mediate most of their effects through "activated" macrophages has been well documented for the cell-mediated responses to facultative intracellular organisms such as *Mycobacteria, Listeria monocytogenes,* and *Brucella* (179, 180, 195). A similar mechanism has been demonstrated in the case of antitumor resistance (6, 78–80). *In vitro* studies have shown that immune T cells, after culture with specific antigen, release humoral substances which adhere to the surface of normal macrophages (6, 79). Such "armed" macrophages on coming into contact with the sensitizing tumor antigen become specifically activated and can subsequently kill in a nonspecific manner (6, 79). Nonspecifically activated macrophages induced by proteoses (153, 155), adjuvants (99, 139), or Toxoplasma infection (138) can also inhibit the growth of neoplastic cells *in vitro* in a nonspecific manner. Some investigators have found that such macrophages do not affect normal cells (26, 66, 187), while there is other evidence that all rapidly replicating cells, whether derived from normal or transformed tissues, are affected although the degree of cytostasis and cytotoxicity differs markedly from one cell line to another (156). A distinction has been made between cytostasis and cytotoxicity which often depends on the *in vitro* tests used to evaluate macrophage function. In general, the *in vitro* studies of macrophage-mediated cytostasis used short interactions lasting in the vicinity of 24 hours (102, 169, 202). If the incubations were extended to 48 or 72 hours, tumor target cells subsequently renewed DNA synthesis, indicating that the activated macrophages did not irreversibly damage or kill them (168). However, activated macrophages cultured for long periods prior to addition to target cells have been shown to lose some of their cytostatic capabilities (169, 202). *In vivo*, however, they would be subject to the continuing presence of sensitized lymphocytes or the substances which activated them initially. Therefore, it is not clear whether these *in vitro* models would have relevance to tumor escape *in vivo*.

Another report which raises the question of whether such *in vitro* studies are relevant to the *in vivo* situation showed that peritoneal macrophages from conventionally housed nude mice were highly tumoricidal and very responsive to chemotactic stimuli *in vitro*, presumably due to environmental stimuli, since macrophages from germ-free nude mice were not tumoricidal (186). Yet it is generally accepted that transplanted tumors are not rejected in conventionally housed nude mice *in vivo* (274).

Anergy in Tumor Bearers

Patients with solid tumors and lymphomas often fail to express cutaneous delayed-type hypersensitivity (DTH) to antigens with which they have been previously sensitized (136, 211, 239). Initially this was viewed as a manifestation of immunological anergy, although humoral responses to the same antigen which failed to elicit DTH might be normal (e.g., 12). A similar pattern of responsiveness followed by specific suppression was found in murine models of DTH to transplanted SV 40 and methylcholanthrene-induced fibrosarcomas (205). For the first week after subcutaneous tumor implantation, specific DTH correlated with tumor size, but, as it continued to increase in size, DTH declined to undetectable levels. If the tumor were amputated, DTH returned to high levels. The splenic lymphocytes from the anergic tumor-bearing mice did, however, support a vigorous DTH reaction when admixed with tumor cells and inoculated into the footpads of normal mice (205). Similarly, mice given large intravenous doses of facultative intracellular organisms, such as 10^8 viable BCG, failed to react to PPD at an appropriate interval (60). Their spleen cells, however, were capable of adoptively transferring DTH to normal recipients (60). Since cells from the bone marrow are required for the expression of DTH (178) and it has been demonstrated that normal peritoneal but not lymph node cells admixed with antigen and administered intradermally in irradiated sensitized guinea pigs, restored their ability to express a cutaneous DTH reaction to PPD (267), it seemed likely that the failure to elicit cutaneous DTH in tumor-bearing hosts was due to a deficiency of cells of the monocyte-macrophage series.

The old observation that certain tumors are infiltrated with histiocytes (110) has been updated by studies which showed by trypsinization and mincing procedures that primary and transplanted fibrosarcomas grown intramuscularly or subcutaneously in rats and mice had a macrophage content ranging from 4 to 55% of the total cell population (77). Tumor cells freed of macrophages and transplanted into syngeneic recipients regained the macrophage content typical of that tumor, demonstrating that they originated from the host (77). Since blood monocytes are precursors of macrophages in DTH reactions (266), studies were made to determine if those reactions were in competition with tumors for available blood monocytes (74). Tumor-bearing animals sensitized to either sheep red blood cells or PPD were found to have both depressed DTH reactions and decreased numbers of macrophages in induced peritoneal exudates (74, 238). These phenomena correlated directly with the increase in the size of tumors having the greater macrophage content (74). Yet such anergic tumor-bearing rats that had been sensitized to BCG could adoptively transfer reactivity to PPD to normal rats (74). DTH to PPD could also be restored in the tumor bearing host by admixing antigen with glycogen-induced peritoneal exudate cells obtained from normal rats (74). These studies clearly made the point that the magnitude of DTH suppression was related to the total number of macrophages in the tumor rather than the tumor size alone. Additional studies detected an inverse correlation between the capacity for metastasis and macrophage content in both experimental and human (5, 73) tumor systems.

More recently, studies of the Moloney sarcoma showed that the percentage of macrophages in regressing tumors was greater than in the progressing tumors although the absolute numbers in both groups were similar (220). This suggests that perhaps there is a limit to the number of macrophages the host can produce. Histological examination revealed that the regressing tumors had widely distributed mononuclear cells, whereas they were confined to the periphery of the progressing tumors. Significantly, regressors had a lower tumor mitotic index, since wherever mononuclear cells were found in either progressing or regressing tumors the tumor cell mitotic activity was negligible (220). If these observations apply in general, then the role of intratumoral macrophages calls for elucidation.

Function of Macrophages from Tumor Bearing Host

Some time ago it was demonstrated that tumor antigens from chemically induced tumors could specifically inhibit the migration of peritoneal exudate cells from sensitized guinea pigs in the macrophage migration inhibition assay (42), an in vitro correlate of DTH (68), which could account for the in vivo DTH reaction. Macrophages isolated from two rat sarcomas by unit gravity sedimentation at 12 and 35 days after implantation were capable of inhibiting tumor growth in vitro as assayed by both colony inhibition and the microcytotoxicity assay (117). On a cell:cell comparison the macrophages extracted from the tumor not only inhibited colony growth better than spleen cells, but the macrophage colony inhibition was nonspecific whereas the lymphoid spleen cells inhibition was specific (117). Yet despite the presence of large numbers of macrophages in tumors, they continue to grow (e.g., 5, 73).

Numerous studies have shown that tumor bearing hosts have a deficiency in macrophage chemotaxis towards non-specific inflammatory stimuli both in vivo (238, 241) and in vitro (43, 118, 194, 237). The in vivo results may merely indicate a deficiency of circulating monocytes but the possibility that these monocytes are dysfunctional cannot be ruled out. The in vitro studies are not hampered by considerations of inadequate numbers of cells and clearly indicate malfunction towards inflammatory and other stimuli such as phytohemagglutinin (238). That they may be specifically "armed" and unable to respond to other antigens has not been evaluated.

The important question with regard to tumor escape is how the macrophages react to their autochthonous tumor antigens, not only at the primary site but also at metastatic sites. Surprisingly, the chemotactic response of monocytes from tumor bearers to their own tumor antigens has not been evaluated. Are the monocytes subject to the other factors in the sera of tumor bearers such as tumor antigens, antigen-antibody complexes, or cytophilic antibodies, whose role has been considered mainly in relation to their effects on immune lymphoid or target tumor cells which are employed in in vitro cytotoxicity tests?

Studies specifically addressing this question have been undertaken, using Nippostrongylus brasiliensis-infected rats in whom the growth of the Walker carcinosarcoma can be either suppressed or enhanced, depending on the timing of the inoculation of tumor cells in relation to the parasitic infection. Tumor elimination is attributed to activated macrophages not specifically immune to the tumor (154). Serum from rats immune to *Nippostrongylus brasiliensis* enhanced tumor growth *in vivo* and nonspecifically inactivated rat as well as mouse macrophages *in vitro* although such sera injected intraperitoneally did not affect peptone induced intraperitoneal migration. Such exudates, however, adhered less well to culture dishes (154). The *in vitro* results implied that the blocking factor disturbed metabolic functions of macrophages without actually killing them (154).

In the tube leukocyte adherence inhibition assay (LAI) peripheral blood monocytes from patients with early or localized tumors react with specific antigens in tumor extracts and fail to adhere to glass (112). The specific tumor antigen is bound to cytophilic IgG antitumor antibody bound to the Fc receptor on the surface of the monocyte (183). Normal peripheral blood monocytes can be "armed" or made specifically reactive to the tumor extract following incubation with sera from patients with limited cancer containing free cytophilic IgG antitumor antibody, whereas sera of patients with metastatic tumors whose leukocytes did not react in the tube LAI contained no free cytophilic antitumor antibody capable of arming normal leukocytes (183). Nonreactive monocytes from patients with metastatic cancer failed to bind free cytophilic antitumor antibody because their monocytes were coated with antigen (113). Serum from nonreactive cancer patients inhibited LAI of reactive leukocytes in an immunologically specific manner. It contained tumor antigen that specifically bound free cytophilic antitumor IgG and removed the arming capacity of serum from reactive cancer patients (113). These results suggest that it is antigen that exerts a blocking effect by coating the monocyte surface because only sera from bearers of the same type tumor blocked. If immune complexes were blocking then sera from any advanced cancer patient would be expected to block for they bind nonspecifically to monocytes via Fc (113). These results are consistent with the concept that primary tumors which initially stimulate an antitumor response eventually escape immunologic destruction by the release of tumor antigens in the microenvironment which coat and neutralize monocytes and other host effector cells entering the tumor (252). As the tumor increases in mass, tumor antigen is shed systemically and such antigen competes with the tumor for the effector processes of the immune response (254, 255).

Molecules Suppressing Macrophage Function in Vivo and in Vitro

Supernatants of four sonicated murine neoplasms injected subcutaneously into normal mice suppressed the intraperitoneal macrophage accumulation in response to phytohemagglutinin (210). Nonneoplastic tissues, including inflammatory exudate cells and lymphocytes, did not contain detectable inhibitory activity (210). Characterization of the supernatant from one of these tumors, the hepatoma 129, indicated that a molecule weighing 6–10,000 Daltons inhibited not only macrophage accumulation in vivo but also chemotaxis toward endotoxin-activated mouse serum in vitro (210). However, the critical question whether such a molecule affected the intraperitoneal macrophage accumulation in response to the tumor from which it was extracted was not evaluated.

Another small molecule, weighing between 10^3 and 10^4 daltons, has been found to be produced by mouse teratocarcinomas (82). In vitro, it prevents macrophages from interacting with these antigenic tumors and, in vivo, impairs inflammatory responses in the vicinity of the tumor (82).

Still another small molecule of less than 12,000 molecular weight which apparently affects macrophage function has been found in serum within 8 hours of subcutaneous injection of syngeneic murine tumors (196). Quantities as small as 0.015 ml of such sera suppressed the capacity of normal syngeneic recipients to resist infection with Listeria monocytogenes (196). Since macrophages are the cells which destroy this micro-organism albeit the reaction is mediated by T lymphocytes, it would appear that the serum factor either directly or indirectly interferes with the antibacterial function of mononuclear phagocytic cells (196). The rapid appearance of the small molecule is reminiscent of the soluble antigen found in sera after subcutaneous tumor injection which has been ascribed to autolysis of tumor cells (254). This similarity is consistent with the finding that the suppressor factor was short-lived and that following the state of decreased anti-bacterial resistance, increased antibacterial resistance appeared in parallel to increased antitumor resistance. These last two findings may indicate that both mechanisms have a final common pathway via the macrophage (197).

CONCLUSION

It is readily apparent that mechanisms by which tumors avoid destruction by the immune system are to a great extent linked to immunoregulatory mechanisms involving interactions between the tumor, serum factors, lymphocytes and macrophages. The presence of soluble tumor-specific antigens in the sera of tumor bearers is obviously useful in making diagnoses or prognoses. It is not clear under which circumstances they represent the results of an immune response, spontaneous shedding or autolysis following experimental implantation (62, 254). The detection of antibodies or antigen-antibody complexes in the sera of tumor bearers may very well depend on the kinetics of the immunoregulatory feedback response to a particular tumor. The apparent hyporeactivity of lymphoid cells from tumor bearers seems to be in part at least due to interactions with soluble tumor antigens or antigen-antibody complexes (61, 232). The former presumably interact with specific receptors on the lymphocyte surface. The latter may function via a specific or non-specific mechanism (107). The specific mechanism involves antigen reacting with the specific receptor on the surface of the T lymphocyte. Nonspecific inhibition depends on binding of the antigen-antibody complex to the lymphocyte surface via an Fc receptor. Only a small fraction of T lymphocytes would be expected to be blocked by antigen via the specific mechanism, but a large fraction would have to be blocked via the nonspecific mechanism in order to exercise significant control over the immune response. Or the immune complex or antibody alone might produce efferent blockade by means of the interaction with tumor specific antigens on target tumor cells. The in vitro data (Section III) show that both blocking of target cells by antibody or antigen-antibody complexes and inhibition of lymph node cells by either antigen or antigen-antibody complexes can occur. More studies are needed to demonstrate the in vivo counterparts of the in vitro reactions.

The role of suppressor cells and/or their products also needs to be clarified. Are there several different suppressor mechanisms? For example, they may be mediated by: B cells which inhibit T cells, most likely by production of antibody that reacts with antigen from the tumor and nonspecifically binds to the surface of T lymphocytes producing nonspecific inhibition (107); T-T collaboration, mediated not by cell contact but by production of complexes of antigen with receptor (87); or macrophages which can inhibit secondary cytotoxic T cell responses by an as yet unknown mechanism (104).

The role of macrophages and monocytes in antitumor immunity is still not well elucidated. Their role in tumor escape is even more obscure. What role do intratumoral macrophages play? Are macrophages also blocked by tumor antigens or antigen-antibody complexes (113)? Do these factors interfere with their migration into nonspecific inflammatory foci? Is there any evidence that their migration is impaired at sites of tumor implantation? Is there an upper limit to the production of macrophages by the host?

The intriguing possibility that a physical complex of H-2 and viral antigens would form a hybrid antigen (70, 223) and that both antiviral (167) and anti-H-2 sera (166) can block lysis of virally infected cells is consistent with the view that T cell receptors bind to a physical complex of viral and H-2 antigens. Thus either antiviral antibody or anti-H-2 sera could provide effective means of tumor escape.

The mechanisms by which tumors avoid destruction by the immune response are only beginning to be understood. This is a multidisciplinary problem involving not only the field of immunology but also the fields of virology, endocrinology, and embryology, to name a few. It is the hope and expectation that knowledge of these mechanisms will provide insight into ways to reverse such escape, the ultimate goal of immunotherapy. Whether or not this will prove true does not detract from the challenge to understand these fascinating means of escape.

ACKNOWLEDGMENTS

The author thanks Dr. Osias Stutman for his helpful comments on this manuscript.

The experimental work in this paper was supported by Grant Nos. CA-18351, CA-15988, and CA-17818, awarded by the National Cancer Institute, DHEW, and Faculty Research Award FRA-150 from the American Cancer Society.

REFERENCES

1. Abelev, G. I. 1963. Study of the antigenic structure of tumors. *Acta Un. Int. Cancer.* 19: 80–82.

2. Alexander, P. 1972. Foetal "antigens" in cancer. *Nature* 235: 137–140, 181.

3. Alexander, P. 1974. Escape from immune destruction by the host through shedding of surface antigens: is this a characteristic shared by malignant and embryonic cells? *Cancer Res.* 34: 2077–2082.

4. Alexander, P. 1975. Mechanisms of escape of antigenic tumours from host control. In E. J. Ambrose and F. J. C. Roe (eds.), *Biology of Cancer, 1975*, pp. 252–278. Ellis Horwood, Ltd., Chichester.

5. Alexander, P., Eccles, S. A., and Gauci, C. L. L. 1976. The significance of macrophages in human and experimental tumors. *Ann. N.Y. Acad. Sci.* 276: 124–133.

6. Alexander, P., Evans, R., and Grant, C. K. 1972. The interplay of lymphoid cells and macrophages in tumor immunity. *Ann. Inst. Pasteur* 122: 645–658.

7. Alexander, P., and Hall, J. G. 1970. The role of immunoblasts in host resistance and immunotherapy of primary sarcomata. *Adv. Cancer Res.* 13: 1–37.

8. Algire, G. H., and Chalkley, H. W. 1945. Vascular reactions of normal and malignant tissues *in vivo*; vascular reactions of mice to wounds and to normal and neoplastic transplants. *J. Natl. Cancer Inst.* 6: 73–85.

9. Ambrose, E. J. 1975. The surface properties of tumour cells. In E. J. Ambrose and F. J. C. Roe (eds), *Biology of Cancer*, 2nd ed., pp. 27–57. Ellis Horwood, Ltd., Chichester.

10. Amos, D. B., Prioleau, W. H., and Hutchin, P. 1968. Biochemical changes during growth of C3H ascites tumor BP8 in C57B1 mice. *J. Surg. Res.* 8: 122–127.

11. Aoki, T., and Takahashi, T. 1972. Viral and cellular surface antigens of

murine leukemias and myelomas. *J. Exp. Med.* 135: 443–457.

12. Ashikawa, K., Motoya, K., Sekiguchi, M., and Ishibashi, Y. 1967. Immune response in tumor-bearing patients and animals. II. Incidence of tuberculin anergy in cancer patients. *Gann* 58: 565–573.

13. Baldwin, R. W., Bowen, J. G., and Price, M. R. 1973. Detection of circulating hepatoma D23 antigen and immune complexes in tumour bearer serum. *Brit. J. Cancer* 28: 16–24.

14. Baldwin, R. W., and Embleton, M. J. 1974. Neoantigens on spontaneous and carcinogen-induced rat tumors defined by in vitro lymphocytotoxicity assays. *Int. J. Cancer* 13: 433–443.

15. Baldwin, R. W., Embleton, M. J., Jones, J. S. P., and Langman, M. J. S. 1973. Cell-mediated and humoral immune reactions to human tumors. *Int. J. Cancer* 12: 73–83.

16. Baldwin, R. W., Embleton, M. J., and Price, M. R. 1973. Inhibition of lymphocyte cytotoxicity for human colon carcinoma by treatment with solubilized tumour membrane fractions. *Int. J. Cancer* 12: 84–92.

17. Baldwin, R. W., Embleton, M. J., and Robins, R. A. 1973. Cellular and humoral immunity to rat hepatoma-specific antigens correlated with tumour status. *Int. J. Cancer* 11: 1–10.

18. Baldwin, R. W., and Glaves, D. 1972. Solubilization of tumour-specific antigen from plasma membrane of an aminoazo-dye-induced rat hepatoma. *Clin. Exp. Immunol.* 11: 51–56.

19. Baldwin, R. W., and Pimm, M. V. 1971. Influence of BCG infection on growth of 3-methylcholanthrene-induced rat sarcomas. *Rev. Eur. Etudes Clin. Biol.* 16: 875–881.

20. Baldwin, R. W., Price, M. R., and Robins, R. A. 1972. Blocking of lymphocyte-mediated cytotoxicity for rat hepatoma cells by tumour-specific antigen-antibody complexes. *Nature New Biol.* 238: 185–187.

21. Baldwin, R. W., Price, M. R., and Robins, R. A. 1973. Inhibition of hepatoma-immune lymph-node cell cytotoxicity by tumour-bearer serum, and solubilized hepatoma antigen. *Int. J. Cancer* 11: 527–535.

22. Baldwin, R. W., and Robins, R. A. 1975. Humoral factors abrogating cell-mediated immunity in the tumor-bearing host. *Curr. Top. Microbiol. Immunol.* 72: 21–53.

23. Bansal, S. C., Hargreaves, R., and Sjögren, H. O. 1972. Facilitation of polyoma tumor growth in rats by blocking sera and tumor eluate. *Int. J. Cancer* 9: 97–108.

24. Bartlett, G. L., and Zbar, B. 1972. Tumor-specific vaccine containing Mycobacteria bovis and tumor cells: safety and efficacy. *J. Natl. Cancer Inst.* 48: 1709–1726.

25. Bashford, E. F. 1908. Third Scientific Report of the Imperial Cancer Research Fund. Taylor and Francis, Ltd., pp. 262–292, London, England.

26. Bašíc, I., Milas, L., Grdina, D. J., and Withers, H. R. 1975. In vitro destruction of tumor cells by macrophages from mice treated with Corynebacterium granulosum. *J. Natl. Cancer Inst.* 55: 589–596.

27. Basombrio, M. A., and Prehn, R. T. 1972. Antigenic diversity of tumors chemically induced within the progeny of a single cell. *Int. J. Cancer* 10: 1–8.

28. Bast, R. C., Zbar, B., Borsos, T., and Rapp, H. J. 1974. BCG and cancer. *New Engl. J. Med.* 290: 1413–1420, 1458–1469.

29. Bean, M. A., Pees, H., Fogh, J. E., Grabstald, H., and Oettgen, H. F. 1974. Cytotoxicity of lymphocytes from patients with cancer of the urinary bladder: detection by a ^{3}H-proline microcytotoxicity test. *Int. J. Cancer* 14: 186–197.

30. Belehradek, J., Jr., Barski, G., and Thonier, M. 1972. Evolution of cell-mediated antitumor immunity in mice bearing a syngeneic chemically induced tumor. Influence of tumor growth, surgical removal and treatment with irradiated tumor cells. *Int. J. Cancer* 9: 461–469.

31. Berczi, I., Tsay, H.-M., and Sehon, A. H. 1976. Efferent enhancement of a methylcholanthrene-induced sarcoma transplantable in strain 13 guinea pigs. *Eur. J. Immunol.* 6: 453–455.

32. Biddle, C. 1976. Stimulation of transplanted 3-methylcholanthrene-induced sarcomas in mice by specific immune and by normal serum. *Int. J. Cancer* 17: 755–764.

33. Birbeck, M. S. C., and Hall, J. G. 1967. Transformation *in vivo* of basophilic lymph cells into plasma cells. *Nature* 214: 183–185.

34. Blair, P. B., and Lane, M. A. 1974. Serum factors in mammary neoplasia: enhancement and antagonism of spleen cell activity *in vitro* detected by different methods of serum factor assay. *J. Immunol.* 112: 439–453.

35. Blair, P. B., and Lane, M. A. 1975. *In vitro* detection of immune responses to MTV-induced mammary tumors: Qualitative differences in response detected by time studies. *J. Immunol.* 114: 17–23.

36. Blair, P. B., and Lane, M.-A. 1975. Non-T cell killing of mammary tumor cells by spleen cells: secretion of antibody and recruitment of cells. *J. Immunol.* 115: 184–189.

37. Blair, P. B., Lane, M.-A., and Mar, P. 1976. Antibody in the sera of tumor-bearing mice that mediates spleen cell cytotoxicity toward the autologous tumor. *J. Immunol.* 116: 606–609.

38. Blair, P. B., Lane, M.-A., and Mar, P. 1976. Complexity of factors in sera of different mice that affect MTV-induced mammary tumor cells. *J. Immunol.* 116: 610–614.

39. Blair, P. B., Lane, M. A., and Yagi, M. J. 1974. *In vitro* detection of immune responses to MTV-induced mammary tumors: activity of spleen cell preparations from both MTV-free and MTV-infected mice. *J. Immunol.* 112: 693–705.

40. Blanden, R. V. 1974. Mechanisms of cell-mediated immunity in viral infection. In L. Brent and J. Holborow (eds), *Progress in Immunology* II, Vol. 4 1974, pp. 117–125. North-Holland Publishing Co., Amsterdam.

41. Blank, K. J., Freedman, H. A., and Lilly, F. 1976. T-lymphocyte response to Friend virus-induced tumour cell lines in mice of strains congenic at H-2. *Nature* 260: 250–252.

42. Bloom, B. R., Bennett, B., Oettgen, H. F., McLean, E. P., and Old, L. J. 1969. Demonstration of delayed hypersensitivity to soluble antigens of chemically induced tumors by inhibition of macrophage migration. *Proc. Natl. Acad. Sci. USA* 64: 1176–1180.

43. Boetcher, D. A., and Leonard, E. J. 1974. Abnormal monocyte chemotactic response in cancer patients. *J. Natl. Cancer Inst.* 52: 1091–1099.

44. Bonavida, B. 1974. Studies on the induction and expression of T cell-mediated immunity. I. Blocking of cell-mediated cytolysis by membrane antigens. *J. Immunol.* 112: 926–934.

45. Bowen, J. G., and Baldwin, R. W. 1976. Serum factor levels during the growth of rat hepatoma nodules in the lungs. *Int. J. Cancer* 17: 254–260.

46. Bowen, J. G., Robins, R. A., and Baldwin, R. W. 1975. Serum factors modifying cell-mediated immunity to rat hepatoma D23 correlated with tumour growth. *Int. J. Cancer* 15: 640–650.

47. Boyse, E. A., Old, L. J., and Chouroulinkov, I. 1964. Cytotoxic test for demonstration of mouse antibody. *Methods Med. Res.* 10: 39–47.

48. Braslawsky, G., Ran, M., and Witz, I. P. 1976. Tumor bound immuno-globulins: the relationship between the *in vivo* coating of tumor cells by potentially cytotoxic anti-tumor antibodies, and the expression of immune complex receptors. *Int. J. Cancer* 18: 116–121.

49. Brawn, R. J. 1970. Possible association of embryonal antigen(s) with several primary 3-methylcholanthrene-induced murine sarcomas. *Int. J. Cancer* 6: 245–249.

50. Brooks, W. H., Netsky, M. G., Normansell, D. E., and Horowitz, D. A. 1972. Depressed cell-mediated immunity in patients with primary intracranial tumors. Characterization of a humoral immunosuppressive factor. *J. Exp. Med.* 136: 1631–1646.

51. Burk, K. H., and Drewinko, B. 1976. Cell cycle dependency of tumor antigens. *Cancer Res.* 36: 3535–3538.

52. Burns, F. D., Marrack, P. C., Kappler, J. W., and Janeway, C. A., Jr. 1975. Functional heterogeneity among the T-derived lymphocytes of the mouse. IV. Nature of spontaneously induced suppressor cells. *J. Immunol.* 114: 1345–1347.

53. Cahill, R. N. P., Frost, H., and Trnka, Z. 1976. The effects of antigen on the migration of recirculating lymphocytes through single lymph nodes. *J. Exp. Med.* 143: 870–888.

54. Calafat, J., Hilgers, J., Van Blitterswijk, W. J., Verbeet, M., and Hageman, P.C. 1976. Antibody-induced modulation and shedding of mammary tumor virus antigens on the surfaces of GR ascites leukemia cells as compared with normal antigens. *J. Natl. Cancer Inst.* 56: 1019–1029.

55. Cantor, H., and Simpson, E. 1975. Regulation of the immune response by subclasses of T lymphocytes. I. Interactions between pre-killer T cells and regulatory T cells obtained from peripheral lymphoid tissues of mice. *Eur. J. Immunol.* 5: 330–336.

56. Cantrell, J. L., and Kaliss, N. 1975. Modification by passive IgM of the immune response of mice to a tumor allograft. *J. Natl. Cancer Inst.* 52: 1619–1625.

57. Chatterjee, S. K., Kim, U., and Bielat, K. 1976. Plasma membrane associated enzymes of mammary tumours as the biochemical indicators of metastasizing capacity. Analyses of enriched plasma membrane preparations. *Brit. J. Cancer* 33: 15–26.

58. Coggin, J. H., Jr., Ambrose, K. R., and Anderson, N. G. 1970. Fetal antigen capable of inducing transplantation immunity against SV 40 hamster tumor cells. *J. Immunol.* 105: 524–526.

59. Coggin, J. H., Jr., and Anderson, N. G. 1974. Cancer, differentiation and

embryonic antigens: some central problems. *Adv. Cancer Res.* 19: 105–165.

60. Collins, F. M., and Mackaness, G. B. 1970. The relationship of delayed hypersensitivity to acquired antituberculous immunity. I. Tuberculin sensitivity and resistance to reinfection in BCG-vaccinated mice. *Cell. Immunol.* 1: 253–265.

61. Currie, G. 1973. The role of circulating antigen as an inhibitor of tumour immunity in man. *Brit. J. Cancer* 28: Suppl. I: 153–161.

62. Currie, G. A., and Alexander, P. 1974. Spontaneous shedding of TSTA by viable sarcoma cells: its possible role in facilitating metastatic spread. *Brit. J. Cancer* 29: 72–75.

63. Currie, G. A., and Bagshawe, K. D. 1968. The role of sialic acid in antigenic expression: further studies of the Landschütz ascites tumor. *Brit. J. Cancer* 22: 843–853.

64. Currie, G. A., and Bagshawe, K. D. 1969. Tumour specific immunogenicity of methylcholanthrene-induced sarcoma cells after incubation in neuraminidase. *Brit. J. Cancer* 23: 141–149.

65. Currie, G. A., and Basham, C. 1972. Serum-mediated inhibition of the immunological reactions of the patient to his own tumour: a possible role for circulating antigen. *Brit. J. Cancer* 26: 427–438.

66. Currie, G. A., and Basham, C. 1975. Activated macrophages release a factor which lyses malignant cells but not normal cells. *J. Exp. Med.* 142: 1600–1605.

67. Currie, G. A., Lejeune, F., and Fairley, G. H. 1971. Immunization with irradiated tumour cells and specific lymphocyte cytotoxicity in malignant melanoma. *Brit. Med. J.* II: 305–310.

68. David, J. R. 1973. Lymphocyte mediators and cellular hypersensitivity. *N. Engl. J. Med.* 288: 143–149.

69. Deckers, P. J., Pardridge, D. H., Wang, B. S., and Mannick, J. A. 1976. The specificity of concomitant tumor immunity at large tumor volumes. *Cancer Res.* 36: 3690–3694.

70. Doherty, P. C., and Zinkernagel, R. M. 1975. H-2 compatibility is required for T-cell-mediated lysis of target cells infected with lymphocytic choriomeningitis virus. *J. Exp. Med.* 141: 502–508.

71. Doherty, P. C., and Zinkernagel, R. M. 1975. Capacity of sensitized thymus-derived lymphocytes to induce fatal lymphocytic choriomeningitis is restricted by the H-2 gene complex. *J. Immunol.* 114: 30–33.

72. Dutton, R. W. 1972. Inhibitory and stimulatory effects of concanavalin A on the response of mouse spleen cell suspensions to antigen. I. Characterization of the inhibitory cell activity. *J. Exp. Med.* 136: 1445–1460.

73. Eccles, S. A., and Alexander, P. 1974. Macrophage content of tumours in relation to metastatic spread and host immune reaction. *Nature (Lond.)* 250: 667–669.

74. Eccles, S. A., and Alexander, P. 1974. Sequestration of macrophages in growing tumours and its effect on the immunological capacity of the host. *Brit. J. Cancer* 30: 42–49.

75. Eggers, A. E., and Wunderlich, J. R. 1975. Suppressor cells in tumor-bearing mice capable of nonspecific blocking of *in vitro* immunization against transplant antigens. *J. Immunol.* 114: 1554–1556.

76. Ehrlich, P. 1909. Über den jetzigen Stand der Karzinom-forschung. In F. Himmelweit (ed.), The Collected Papers of Paul Ehrlich. Vol. II. Immunology and Cancer Research 1957, pp. 550–562. Pergamon Press.

77. Evans, R. 1972. Macrophages in syngeneic animal tumours. Transplantation 14: 468–473.

78. Evans, R., and Alexander, P. 1970. Cooperation of immune lymphoid cells with macrophages in tumour immunity. Nature 228: 620–622.

79. Evans, R., and Alexander, P. 1972. Mechanism of immunologically specific killing of tumour cells by macrophages. Nature (Lond.) 236: 168–170.

80. Evans, R., and Alexander, P. 1972. Role of macrophages in tumour immunity. I. Cooperation between macrophages and lymphoid cells in syngeneic tumour immunity. Immunology 23: 615–626.

81. Faanes, R. B., and Choi, Y. S. 1974. Interaction of isoantibody and cytotoxic lymphocytes with allogeneic tumor cells. J. Immunol. 113: 279–288.

82. Fauve, R. M., Hevin, B., Jacob, H., Gaillard, J. A., and Jacob, F. 1974. Antiinflammatory effects of murine malignant cells. Proc. Natl. Acad. Sci. USA 71: 4052–4056.

83. Fefer, A., McCoy, J. L., Kalman, P., and Glynn, J. P. 1968. Immunologic, virologic, and pathologic studies of regression of autochthonous Moloney sarcoma virus-induced tumors in mice. Cancer Res. 28: 1577–1585.

84. Feldman, J. D. 1972. Immunological enhancement: A study of blocking antibodies. Adv. Immunol. 15: 167–214.

85. Feldmann, M. 1974. T cell suppression in vitro. I. Role in regulation of antibody responses. Eur. J. Immunol. 4: 660–666.

86. Feldmann, M. 1974. T-cell suppression in vitro. II. Nature of specific suppressor factor. Eur. J. Immunol. 4: 667–674.

87. Feldmann, M., and Kontiainen, S. 1976. Suppressor cell induction in vitro. II. Cellular requirements of suppressor cell induction. Eur. J. Immunol. 6: 302–305.

88. Feldmann, M., and Nossal, G. J. V. 1972. Tolerance, enhancement and the regulation of interactions between T cells, B cells and macrophages. Transplant. Rev. 13: 3–34.

89. Fenyö, E. M., Klein, E., Klein, G., and Swiech, K. 1968. Selection of an immunoresistant Moloney lymphoma subline with decreased concentration of tumor-specific surface antigens. J. Natl. Cancer Inst. 40: 69–89.

90. Fidler, I. J., Brodey, R. S., and Bech-Nielsen, S. 1974. In vitro immune stimulation-inhibition to spontaneous canine tumors of various histologic types. J. Immunol. 112: 1051–1060.

91. Fink, M. P., Parker, C. W., and Shearer, W. T. 1975. Antibody stimulation of tumour growth in T-cell depleted mice. Nature 255: 404–405.

92. Foley, E. J. 1953. Antigenic properties of methylcholanthrene-induced tumors in mice of the strain of origin. Cancer Res. 13: 835–837.

93. Folkman, J. 1974. Tumour angiogenesis. Adv. Cancer Res. 19: 331–358.

94. Folkman, J., Merler, E., Abernathy, C., and Williams, G. 1970. Isolation of a tumor factor responsible for neovascularization. J. Clin. Invest. 49: 30a.

95. Freund, J. 1956. The mode of action of immunologic adjuvants. Adv. Tuberc. Res. 7: 130–148.

96. Fujimoto, S., Greene, M. I., and Sehon, A. H. 1976. Regulation of the immune response to tumor antigens. I. Immunosuppressor cells in tumor-bearing hosts. *J. Immunol.* 116: 791–799.

97. Fujimoto, S., Greene, M. I., and Sehon, A. H. 1976. Regulation of the immune response to tumor antigens. II. The nature of immunosuppressor cells in tumor-bearing hosts. *J. Immunol.* 116: 800–806.

98. Gardner, I., Bowern, N. A., and Blanden, R. V. 1975. Cell-mediated cytotoxicity against ectromelia virus-infected target cells. III. Role of the H-2 gene complex. *Eur. J. Immunol.* 5: 122–127.

99. Germain, R. N., Williams, R. M., and Benacerraf, B. 1973. Specific and nonspecific antitumor immunity. II. Macrophage-mediated nonspecific effector activity induced by BCG and similar agents. *J. Natl. Cancer Inst.* 54: 709–718.

100. Gershon, R. K. 1975. T cell control of antibody production. *Contemp. Top. Immunobiol.* 3: 1–40.

101. Gershon, R. K., Carter, R. L., and Kondo, K. 1967. On concomitant immunity in tumor-bearing hamsters. *Nature* 213: 674–676.

102. Ghaffar, A., Cullen, R. T., Dunbar, N., and Woodruff, F. A. 1974. Antitumour effect *in vitro* of lymphocytes and macrophages from mice treated with Corynebacterium parvum. *Brit. J. Cancer* 29: 199–205.

103. Gillette, R. W., and Boone, C. W. 1976. Augmented immunogenicity of tumor cell membranes produced by surface budding viruses: parameters of optimal immunization. *Int. J. Cancer* 18: 216–222.

104. Glaser, M., Kirchner, H., Holden, H. T., and Herberman, R. B. 1976. Brief communication: Inhibition of cell-mediated cytotoxicity against tumor-associated antigens by suppressor cells from tumor-bearing mice. *J. Natl. Cancer Inst.* 56: 865–867.

105. Gold, P., and Freedman, S. O. 1965. Specific carcinoembryonic antigens of the human digestive system. *J. Exp. Med.* 122: 467–481.

106. Gorczynski, R. M. 1974. Immunity to murine sarcoma virus-induced tumors. II. Suppression of T-cell-mediated immunity by cells from progressor animals. *J. Immunol.* 112: 1826–1838.

107. Gorczynski, R., Kontiainen, S., Mitchison, N. A., and Tigelaar, R. E. 1974. Antigen-antibody complexes as blocking factors on the T lymphocyte surface. In G. M. Edelman (ed.), *Cellular Selection and Regulation in the Immune Response 1974*, pp. 143–154. Raven Press, New York.

108. Gorer, P. A. 1958. Some reactions of H-2 antibodies *in vitro* and *in vivo*. *Ann. N.Y. Acad. Sci.* 73: 707–721.

109. Gorer, P. A. 1960. Interactions between sessile and humoral antibodies. In G. E. W. Wolstenholme and M. O'Connor (eds.), *Ciba Foundation Symposium on Cellular Aspects of Immunity 1960*, pp. 330–346. Little, Brown, Boston.

110. Gorer, P. A. 1961. The antigenic structure of tumors. *Adv. Immunol.* 1: 345–393.

111. Greenblatt, M., and Shubik, P. 1968. Tumor angiogenesis: Transfilter diffusion studies in the hamster by the transparent chamber technique. *J. Natl. Cancer Inst.* 41: 111–124.

112. Grosser, N., Marti, J. H., Proctor, J. W., and Thomson, D. M. P. 1976. Tube leukocyte adherence inhibition assay for the detection of anti-tumour im-

munity. I. Monocyte is the reactive cell. *Int. J. Cancer* 18: 39–47.

113. Grosser, N., and Thomson, D. M. P. 1976. Tube leukocyte (monocyte) adherence inhibition assay for the detection of antitumor immunity. III. "Blockade" of monocyte reactivity by excess free antigen and immune complexes in advanced cancer patients. *Int. J. Cancer* 18: 58–66.

114. Gutterman, J. U., Hersh, E. M., McCredie, K. B., Bodey, G. P., Rodriguez, V., and Freireich, E. J. 1972. Lymphocyte blastogenesis to human leukemia cells and their relationship to serum factors, immunocompetence, and prognosis. *Cancer Res.* 32: 2524–2529.

115. Habel, K. 1969. Antigens of virus-induced tumors. *Adv. Immunol.* 10: 229–250.

116. Hall, J. G., and Morris, B. 1965. The immediate effect of antigens on the cell output of a lymph node. *Brit. J. Expt. Pathol.* 46: 450–454.

117. Haskill, J. S., Proctor, J. W., and Yamamura, Y. 1975. Host responses within solid tumors. I. Monocytic effector cells within rat sarcomas. *J. Natl. Cancer Inst.* 54: 387–393.

118. Hausman, M. S., Brosman, S., Snyderman, R., Mickey, M. R., and Fahey, J. L. 1973. Defective monocyte function in patients with genitourinary carcinoma. *Clin. Res.* 21: 646.

119. Hawrylko, E. 1975. Immunopotentiation with BCG: dimensions of a specific antitumor response. *J. Natl. Cancer Inst.* 54: 1189–1197.

120. Hawrylko, E. 1975. BCG immunopotentiation of an antitumor response: Evidence for a cell-mediated mechanism. *J. Natl. Cancer Inst.* 55: 413–423.

121. Hawrylko, E. 1977. Influence of BCG-potentiated immunotherapy in tumor-bearing mice. *J. Natl. Cancer Inst.* 59: 359–365.

122. Hawrylko, E. 1977. Serum-mediated escape from BCG-potentiated antitumor immunity *in vivo. J. Natl. Cancer Inst.* 59: 367–375.

123. Hawrylko, E., and Mackaness, G. B. 1973. Immunopotentiation with BCG. IV. Factors affecting the magnitude of an antitumor response. *J. Natl. Cancer Inst.* 51: 1683–1688.

124. Hellström, I., Evans, C. A., and Hellström, K. E. 1969. Cellular immunity and its serum-mediated inhibition in Shope-virus-induced rabbit papillomas. *Int. J. Cancer* 4: 601–607.

125. Hellström, I., and Hellström, K. E. 1969. Studies on cellular immunity and its serum mediated inhibition in Moloney-virus-induced mouse sarcomas. *Int. J. Cancer* 4: 587–600.

126. Hellström, I., and Hellström, K. E. Colony inhibition and cytotoxicity assays. In B. R. Bloom and P. R. Glade (eds.), *In vitro Methods in Cell-mediated Immunity 1971*, pp. 409–414. Academic Press, New York and London.

127. Hellström, I., and Hellström, K. E. 1975. Cytotoxic effect of lymphocytes from pregnant mice on cultivated tumor cells. I. Specificity, nature of effector cells and blocking by serum. *Int. J. Cancer* 15: 1–16.

128. Hellström, I., Hellström, K. E., Kall, M. A., Nelson, K., and Pollack, S. 1976. Suppression of cell-mediated cytotoxicity by lymphocytes from tumor-bearing animals. *Trans. Proc.* 8: 255–264.

129. Hellström, I., Hellström, K. E., and Sjögren, H. O. 1970. Serum mediated inhibition of cellular immunity to methylcholanthrene-induced murine sarcomas.

Cell. Immunol. 1: 18–30.

130. Hellström, I., Hellström, K. E., Sjögren, H. O., and Warner, G. A. 1971. Demonstration of cell-mediated immunity to human neoplasms of various histological types. *Int. J. Cancer* 7: 1–16.

131. Hellström, I., Sjögren, H. O., Warner, G., and Hellström, K. E. 1971. Blocking of cell-mediated tumor immunity by sera from patients with growing neoplasms. *Int. J. Cancer* 7: 226–237.

132. Hellström, I., Warner, G. A., Hellström, K. E., and Sjögren, H. O. 1973. Sequential studies on cell-mediated tumor immunity and blocking serum activity in ten patients with malignant melanoma. *Int. J. Cancer* 11: 280–292.

133. Hellström, K. E., and Hellström, I. 1974. Lymphocyte-mediated cytotoxicity and blocking serum activity to tumor antigens. *Adv. Immunol.* 18: 209–277.

134. Heppner, G. H., and Pierce, G. E. 1969. *In vitro* demonstration of tumor-specific antigens in spontaneous mammary tumors of mice. *Int. J. Cancer* 4: 212–218.

135. Heppner, G. H., Stolbach, L., Byrne, M., Cummings, F. J., McDonough, E., and Calabresi, P. 1973. Cell-mediated and serum blocking reactivity to tumor antigens in patients with malignant melanoma. *Int. J. Cancer* 11: 245–260.

136. Hersh, E. M., Gutterman, J. U., Mavligit, G. M., Mountain, C. W., McBride, C. M., Burgess, M. A., Lurie, P. M., Zelen, M., Takita, H., and Vincent, R. G. 1976. Immunocompetence, immunodeficiency and prognosis in cancer. *Ann. N.Y. Acad. Sci.* 276: 386–406.

137. Herzenberg, L. A., Okumura, K., and Metzler, C. M. 1975. Regulation of immunoglobulin and antibody production by allotype suppressor T cells in mice. *Transplant. Rev.* 27: 57–83.

138. Hibbs, J. B., Jr., Lambert, L. H., and Remington, J. S. 1972. Possible role of macrophage-mediated nonspecific cytotoxicity in tumour resistance. *Nature New Biol.* 235: 48–50.

139. Hibbs, J. B., Jr., Lambert, L. H., and Remington, J. S. 1972. *In vitro* nonimmunologic destruction of cells with abnormal growth characteristics by adjuvant-activated macrophages. *Proc. Soc. Exp. Biol. Med.* 139: 1049–1052.

140. Holland, J. F. 1975. The acute leukemias. *In* P. B. Beeson and W. McDermott (eds.), *Textbook of Medicine 1975*, pp. 1485–1492. W. B. Saunders Co., Philadelphia.

141. Holland, J. F., and Bekesi, J. G. 1976. Immunotherapy of human leukemia with neuraminidase-modified cells. *Med. Clin. North Amer.* 60:539–549.

142. Huber, B., Devinsky, O., Gershon, R. K., and Cantor, H. 1976. Cell-mediated immunity: delayed-type hypersensitivity and cytotoxic responses are mediated by different T-cell subclasses. *J. Exp. Med.* 143: 1534–1539.

143. Hunsmann, G., Moennig, V., and Schäfer, W. 1975. Properties of mouse leukemia viruses. IX. Active and passive immunization of mice against Friend leukemia with isolated viral "gp 71 Glycoprotein" and its corresponding antiserum. *Virology* 66: 327–329.

144. Janeway, C. A., Jr., Sharrow, S. O., and Simpson, E. 1975. T-cell populations with different functions. *Nature* 253: 544–546.

145. Jeejeebhoy, H. F. 1974. Stimulation of tumor growth by the immune response. *Int. J. Cancer* 13: 665–678.

146. Jose, D. G., and Skvaril, F. 1974. Serum inhibitors of cellular immunity in human neuroblastoma. IgG subclass of blocking activity. *Int. J. Cancer* 13: 173–178.

147. Kaliss, N. 1972. Immunological enhancement. *In* J. S. Najarian and R. L. Simmons (eds.), *Transplantation, 1972,* pp. 195–206. Lea & Febiger, New York.

148. Kaliss, N., Sinclair, N. R. St. C., and Cantrell, J. L. 1976. Immunological enhancement of a murine tumor allograft by passive alloantibody IgG and F(ab')$_2$. *Eur. J. Immunol.* 6: 38–42.

149. Kall, M. A., and Hellström, I. 1975. Specific stimulatory and cytotoxic effects of lymphocytes sensitized *in vitro* to either alloantigens or tumor antigens. *J. Immunol.* 114: 1083–1088.

150. Kall, M. A., Hellström, I., and Hellström, K. E. 1975. Different responses of lymphoid cells from tumor-bearing as compared to tumor-immunized mice when sensitized to tumor-specific antigens *in vitro. Proc. Natl. Acad. Sci. USA* 72: 5086–5089.

151. Katz, D. H., and Benacerraf, B. 1972. The regulatory influence of activated T cells on B cell responses to antigen. *Adv. Immunol.* 15: 1–94.

152. Katz, D. H., Hamaoka, T., and Benacerraf, B. 1973. Cell interactions between histoincompatible T and B lymphocytes. II. Failure of physiologic cooperative interactions between T and B lymphocytes from allogeneic donor strains in humoral response to hapten-protein conjugates. *J. Exp. Med.* 137: 1405–1418.

153. Keller, R. 1973. Cytostatic elimination of syngeneic rat tumor cells *in vitro* by nonspecifically activated macrophages. *J. Exp. Med.* 138: 625–644.

154. Keller, R. 1973. Evidence for compromise of tumour immunity in rats by a non-specific blocking serum factor that inactivates macrophages. *Brit. J. Exp. Path.* 54: 298–305.

155. Keller, R. 1974. Mechanisms by which activated normal macrophages destroy syngeneic rat tumour cells *in vitro.* Cytokinetics, non-involvement of T lymphocytes, and effect of metabolic inhibitors. *Immunol.* 27: 285–298.

156. Keller, R. 1976. Susceptibility of normal and transformed cell lines to cytostatic and cytocidal effects exerted by macrophages. *J. Natl. Cancer Inst.* 56: 369–374.

157. Kiessling, R., Bataillon, G., Lamon, E. W., and Klein, E. 1974. The lymphocyte response to primary Moloney sarcoma virus tumors: Definition of a nonspecific component of the *in vitro* cellular hyporeactivity of tumor bearing hosts. *Int. J. Cancer* 14: 642–648.

158. Kilburn, D. G. Smith, J. B., and Gorczynski, R. M. 1974. Non-specific suppression of T lymphocyte responses in mice carrying progressively growing tumors. *Eur. J. Immunol.* 4: 784–788.

159. Kim, U., Baumler, A., Carruthers, C., and Bielat, K. 1975. Immunological escape mechanism in spontaneously metastasizing mammary tumors. *Proc. Natl. Acad. Sci. USA* 72: 1012–1016.

160. Kindred, B., and Shreffler, D. C. 1972. H-2 dependence of cooperation between T and B cells *in vivo. J. Immunol.* 109: 940–943.

161. Kirchner, H., Chused, T. M., Herberman, R. B., Holden, H. T., and Lavrin, D. H. 1974. Evidence of suppressor cell activity in spleens of mice bearing primary tumors induced by Moloney sarcoma virus. *J. Exp. Med.* 139: 1473–1487.

162. Kirchner, H., Muchmore, A. V., Chused, T. M., Holden, H. T., and Herberman, R. B. 1975. Inhibition of proliferation of lymphoma cells and T lymphocytes by suppressor cells from spleens of tumor-bearing mice. *Immunol.* 114: 206–210.

163. Klein, G., and Klein, E. 1962. Antigenic properties of other experimental tumors. *Cold Spring Harbor Symp. Quant. Biol.* 27: 463–470.

164. Knight, R. A., Mitchison, N. A., and Shellam, G. R. 1975. Studies on a Gross-virus-induced lymphoma in the rat. II. The role of cell-membrane-associated and serum p30 antigen in the antibody and cell-mediated response. *Int. J. Cancer* 15: 417–428.

165. Kontiainen, S., and Feldmann, M. 1976. Suppressor cell induction *in vitro*. I. Kinetics of induction of antigen-specific suppressor cells. *Eur. J. Immunol.* 6: 296–301.

166. Koszinowski, U., and Ertl, H. 1975. Lysis mediated by T cells and restricted by *H-2* antigen of target cells infected with vaccinia virus. *Nature* 255: 552–554.

167. Koszinowski, U., and Thomssen, R. 1975. Target cell-dependent T-cell-mediated lysis of vaccinia-virus-infected cells. *Eur. J. Immunol.* 5: 245–251.

168. Krahenbuhl, J. L., Lambert, L. H., Jr., and Remington, J. S. 1976. The effects of activated macrophages on tumor target cells: escape from cytostasis. *Cellular Immunol.* 25: 279–293.

169. Krahenbuhl, J. L., and Remington, J. S. 1974. The role of activated macrophages in specific and nonspecific cytostasis of tumor cells. *J. Immunol.* 113: 507–516.

170. Lamon, E. W., Hale, P., and Whitten, H. D. 1976. Antibody-dependent, cell-mediated cytotoxicity with autochthonous lymphocytes and sera after infection with Moloney sarcoma virus. *J. Natl. Cancer Inst.* 56: 349–355.

171. Lamon, E. W., Skurzak, H. M., and Klein, E. 1972. The lymphocyte response to a primary viral neoplasm (MSV) through its entire course in BALB/c mice. *Int. J. Cancer* 10: 581–588.

172. Lamon, E. W., Wigzell, H., Klein, E., Andersson, B., and Skurzak, H. M. 1973. The lymphocyte response to primary Moloney sarcoma virus tumors in BALB/c mice: Definition of the active subpopulations at different times after infection. *J. Exp. Med.* 137: 1472–1493.

173. Lane, M. A., Roubinian, J., Slomich, M., Trefts, P., and Blair, P. B. 1975. Characterization of cytotoxic effector cells in the mouse mammary tumor system. *J. Immunol.* 114: 24–29.

174. Law, L. W. 1970. Studies of tumor antigens and tumor-specific immune mechanisms in experimental systems. *Transplant. Proc.* 2: 117–132.

175. Lerner, R. A., Oldstone, M. B. A., and Cooper, N. R. 1971. Cell cycle-dependent immune lysis of Moloney virus-transformed lymphocytes: presence of viral antigen, accessibility to antibody, and complement activation. *Proc. Natl. Acad. Sci. USA* 68: 2584–2588.

176. Levy, J. G., Smith, A. G., Whitney, P. B., McMaster, R., and Kilburn, D. G.

1976. Characterization of a T lymphocyte inhibitor in the serum of tumour-bearing mice. *Immunol.* 30: 565–573.

177. Lubaroff, D. M., and Waksman, B. H. 1968. Bone marrow as source of cells in reactions of cellular hypersensitivity. I. Passive transfer of tuberculin sensitivity in syngeneic systems. *J. Exp. Med.* 128: 1425–1433.

178. Lubaroff, D. M., and Waksman, B. H. 1968. Bone marrow as source of cells in reactions of cellular hypersensitivity. II. Identification of allogeneic or hybrid cells by immunofluorescence in passively transferred tuberculin reactions. *J. Exp. Med.* 128: 1437–1447.

179. Mackaness, G. B. 1969. The influence of immunologically committed lymphoid cells on macrophage activity *in vivo*. *J. Exp. Med.* 129: 973–992.

180. Mackaness, G. B., and Blanden, R. V. 1967. Cellular immunity. *Prog. Allergy* 11: 89–140.

181. MacLennan, I. C. M. 1973. Cytotoxic cells. In A. J. S. Davies and R. L. Carter (eds.), *Contemporary Topics in Immunobiology*, Vol. II. *Thymus Dependency*, pp. 175–187. Plenum Press, New York.

182. MacLeod, C. M. 1972. The Pneumococci. In R. J. Dubos and J. G. Hirsch (eds.), *Bacterial and Mycotic Infections in Man*, 4th ed., pp. 391–411. J. B. Lippincott Co., Philadelphia.

183. Marti, J. H., Grosser, N., and Thomson, D. M. P. 1976. Tube leukocyte adherence inhibition assay for the detection of anti-tumour immunity. II. Monocyte reacts with tumour antigen via cytophilic anti-tumor antibody. *Int. J. Cancer* 18: 48–57.

184. Medawar, P. B., and Hunt, R. 1976. The significance of embryonic reexpression in cancer. *Cancer Res.* 36: 3453–3454.

185. Medina, D., and Heppner, G. 1973. Cell-mediated immunostimulation induced by mammary tumour virus-free BALB/c mammary tumours. *Nature* 242: 329–330.

186. Meltzer, M. S. 1976. Tumoricidal responses *in vitro* of peritoneal macrophages from conventionally housed and germ-free nude mice. *Cell. Immunol.* 22: 176–181.

187. Meltzer, M. S., Tucker, R. W., Sanford, K. K., and Leonard, E. J. 1975. Interaction of BCG-activated macrophages with neoplastic and nonneoplastic cell lines *in vitro*: quantitation of the cytotoxic reaction by release of tritiated thymidine from prelabeled target cells. *J. Natl. Cancer Inst.* 54: 1177–1184.

188. Möller, E., and Möller, G. 1962. Quantitative studies of the sensitivity of normal and neoplastic cells to the cytotoxic action of isoantibodies. *J. Exp. Med.* 115: 527–553.

189. Murgita, R. A., and Tomasi, T. B., Jr. 1975. Suppression of the immune response by α-fetoprotein on the primary and secondary antibody response. *J. Exp. Med.* 141: 269–286.

190. Murgita, R. A., and Tomasi, T. B., Jr. 1975. Suppression of the immune response by α-fetoprotein. II. The effect of mouse α-fetoprotein on mixed lymphocyte reactivity and mitogen induced lymphocyte transformation. *J. Exp. Med.* 141: 440–452.

191. Nelson, K., Pollack, S. B., and Hellström, K. E. 1975. Specific anti-tumor responses by cultured immune spleen cells. I. *In vitro* culture method and initial

characterization of factors which block immune cell-mediated cytotoxicity *in vitro. Int. J. Cancer* 15: 806–814.

192. Nelson, K., Pollack, S. B., and Hellström, K. E. 1975. Specific anti-tumor responses of cultured immune spleen cells. III. Further characterization of cells which synthesize factors with blocking and antiserum-dependent cellular cytotoxicity (ADC) activities. *Int. J. Cancer* 16: 539–549.

193. Nelson, K., Pollack, S. B., and Hellström, K. E. 1975. *In vitro* synthesis of tumor-specific factors with blocking and antibody-dependent cellular cytotoxicity (ADC) activities. *Int. J. Cancer* 16: 932–941.

194. Normann, S. J., and Sorkin, E. 1976. Cell-specific defect in monocyte function during tumor growth. *J. Natl. Cancer Inst.* 57: 135–140.

195. North, R. J. 1974. Cell-mediated immunity and the response to infection. *In* R. T. McCluskey and S. Cohen (eds.), *Mechanisms of Cell-Mediated Immunity,* 1974, pp. 185–219. John Wiley & Sons, New York and London.

196. North, R. J., Kirstein, D. P., and Tuttle, R. L. 1976. Subversion of host defense mechanisms by murine tumors. I. A circulating factor that suppresses macrophage mediated resistance to infection. *J. Exp. Med.* 143: 559–573.

197. North, R. J., Kirstein, D. P., and Tuttle, R. L. 1976. Subversion of host defense mechanisms by murine tumors. II. Counterinfluence of concomitant antitumor immunity. *J. Exp. Med.* 143: 574–584.

198. Obata, Y., Ikeda, H., Stockert, E., and Boyse, E. A. 1975. Relation of G_{IX} antigen of thymocytes to envelope glycoprotein of murine leukemia virus. *J. Exp. Med.* 141: 188–197.

199. Ohanian, S. H., Borsos, T., and Rapp, H. J. 1973. Lysis of tumor cells by antibody and complement. I. Lack of correlation between antigen content and lytic susceptibility. *J. Natl. Cancer Inst.* 50: 1313–1320.

200. Okumura, K., and Tada, T. 1973. Suppression of hapten-specific antibody response by carrier-specific T cells. *Nature New Biol.* 245: 180–182.

201. Old, L. J., Stockert, E., Boyse, E. A., and Kim, J. H. 1968. Antigenic modulation. Loss of TL antigen from cells exposed to TL antibody. Study of the phenomenon *in vitro. J. Exp. Med.* 127: 523–539.

202. Olivotto, M., and Bomford, R. 1974. *In vitro* inhibition of tumour cell growth and DNA synthesis by peritoneal and lung macrophages from mice injected with *Corynebacterium parvum. Int. J. Cancer* 13: 478–488.

203. O'Toole, C., Perlmann, P., Unsgaard, B., Moberger, G., and Edsmyr, F. 1972. Cellular immunity to human urinary bladder carcinoma. I. Correlation to clinical stage and radiotherapy. *Int. J. Cancer* 10: 77–91.

204. Panem, S., and Schauf, V. 1974. Cell-cycle-dependent appearance of murine leukemia sarcoma virus antigens. *J. Virol.* 13: 1169–1175.

205. Paranjpe, M. S., and Boone, C. W. 1974. Kinetics of the antitumor delayed hypersensitivity response in mice with progressively growing tumors: stimulation followed by specific suppression. *Int. J. Cancer* 13: 179–186.

206. Parmely, M. J., and Hsu, H. F. 1973. Rat alpha-fetoprotein: inhibitory activity on lymphocyte cultures. *Fed. Proc.* 32: 979.

207. Parmely, M. J., and Thompson, J. S. 1974. Inhibition of rat lymphocyte cultures by serum fractions rich in alpha-fetoprotein. *Fed. Proc.* 33: 812.

208. Pearson, G. R., Redmon, L. W., and Bass, L. R. 1973. Protective effect of

immune sera against transplantable Moloney virus-induced sarcoma and lymphoma. *Cancer Res.* 33: 171–178.

209. Peavy, D. L., and Pierce, C. W. 1974. Cell-mediated immune responses *in vitro*. I. Suppression of the generation of cytotoxic lymphocytes by concanavalin A and concanavalin A-activated spleen cells. *J. Exp. Med.* 140: 356–369.

210. Pike, M. C., and Snyderman, R. 1976. Depression of macrophage function by a factor produced by neoplasms: a mechanism for abrogation of immune surveillance. *J. Immunol.* 117: 1243–1266.

211. Pinsky, C. M., Wanebo, H., Mike, V., and Oettgen, H. 1976. Delayed cutaneous hypersensitivity reactions and prognosis in patients with cancer. *Ann. N.Y. Acad. Sci.* 276: 407–410.

212. Prehn, R. T. 1967. The significance of tumor-distinctive histocompatibility antigens. In J. J. Trentin (ed.), *Cross-reacting Antigens and Neoantigens, 1967*, pp. 105–117. Williams and Wilkins Co., Baltimore.

213. Prehn, R. T., and Lappé, M. A. 1971. An immunostimulation theory of tumor development. *Transplant. Rev.* 7: 26–54.

214. Prehn, R. T., and Main, J. M. 1957. Immunity to methylcholanthrene-induced sarcomas. *J. Natl. Cancer Inst.* 18: 769–778.

215. Price, M. R., and Baldwin, R. W. 1974. Immunogenic properties of rat hepatoma subcellular fractions. *Brit. J. Cancer* 30: 394–400.

216. Ran, M., Fish, F., Witz, I. P., and Klein, G. 1974. Tumour-bound immunoglobulins. The *in vitro* disappearance of immunoglobulin from the surface of coated tumour cells, and some properties of released components. *Clin. Exp. Immunol.* 16:355–365.

217. Ran, M., and Witz, I. P. 1972. Tumour-associated immunoglobulins: enhancement of syngeneic tumours by IgG2-containing tumour eluates. *Int. J. Cancer* 9: 242–247.

218. Rubin, H. 1966. A substance in conditioned medium which enhances the growth of small numbers of chick embryo cells. *Exp. Cell Res.* 41: 138–148.

219. Rubinstein, P., Decary, F., and Streun, E. W. 1974. Quantitative studies on tumor enhancement in mice. I. Enhancement of sarcoma I induced by IgM, IgG1 and IgG2. *J. Exp. Med.* 140: 591–596.

220. Russell, S. W., Doe, W. F., and Cochrane, C. G. 1976. Number of macrophages and distribution of mitotic activity in regressing and progressing Moloney sarcomas. *J. Immunol.* 116: 164–166.

221. Sambrook, J., Westphal, H., Srinivasan, P. R., and Dulbecco, R. 1968. The integrated state of viral DNA in SV 40-transformed cells. *Proc. Natl Acad. Sci. USA* 60: 1288–1295.

222. Sanford, B. H., 1967. An alteration in tumor histocompatibility induced by neuraminidase. *Transplant.* 5: 1273–1279.

223. Schrader, J. W., Cunningham, B. A., and Edelman, G. M. 1975. Functional interactions of viral and histocompatibility antigens at tumor cell surfaces. *Proc. Natl. Acad. Sci. USA* 72: 5066–5070.

224. Shearer, W. T., Atkinson, J. P., Frank, M. M., and Parker, C. W. 1975. Humoral immunostimulation. IV. Role of complement. *J. Exp. Med.* 141: 736–752.

225. Shearer, W. T., Philpott, G. W., and Parker, C. W. 1973. Stimulation of cells by antibody. *Science* 182: 1357–1359.

226. Shearer, W. T., Philpott, G. W., and Parker, C. W. 1974. Humoral immunostimulation. I. Increased [^{125}I]iododeoxyuridine and [^{3}H]thymidine into TNP-cells treated with anti-TNP antibody. *J. Exp. Med.* 139: 367–379.

227. Shearer, W. T., Philpott, G. W., and Parker, C. W. 1975. Humoral immunostimulation. II. Increased nucleoside incorporation, DNA synthesis, and cell growth in L cells treated with anti-L cell antibody. *Cell. Immunol.* 17: 447–462.

228. Shearer, G. M., Rehn, T. G., and Garbarino, C. A. 1975. Cell-mediated lympholysis of trinitrophenyl-modified autologous lymphocytes. Effector cell specificity to modified cell surface components controlled by the H-2K and H-2D serological regions of the murine major histocompatibility complex. *J. Exp. Med.* 141: 1348–1363.

229. Shipley, W. U. 1971. Immune cytolysis in relation to the growth cycle of Chinese hamster cells. *Cancer Res.* 31: 925–929.

230. Simmons, R. L., and Rios, A. 1975. Comparative immunotherapeutic effect of concanavalin A and neuraminidase-treated cancer cells. *Transplant. Proc.* 7: 247–251.

231. Sinclair, N. R. St. C., Lees, R. K., Fagan, G., and Birnbaum, A. 1975. Regulation of the immune response. VIII. Characteristics of antibody-mediated suppression of an *in vitro* cell-mediated immune response. *Cell. Immunol.* 16: 330–347.

232. Sjögren, H. O., Hellström, I., Bansal, S. C., and Hellström, K. E. 1971. Suggestive evidence that the "blocking antibodies" of tumor-bearing individuals may be antigen-antibody complexes. *Proc. Natl. Acad. Sci. USA* 68: 1372–1375.

233. Sjögren, H. O., Helström, I., Bansal, S. C., Warner, G. A., and Hellström, K. E. 1972. Elution of "blocking factors" from human tumors, capable of abrogating tumor-cell destruction by specifically immune lymphocytes. *Int. J. Cancer* 9: 274–283.

234. Sjögren, H. O., Hellström, I., and Klein, G. 1961. Resistance of polyoma virus immunized mice to transplantation of established polyoma tumors. *Exp. Cell Res.* 23: 204–208.

235. Skipper, H. E. 1969. Improvement of the model systems. *Cancer Res.* 29: 2329–2333.

236. Skurzak, H. M., Klein, E., Yoshida, T. O., and Lamon, E. W. 1972. Synergistic or antagonistic effect of different antibody concentrations on *in vitro* lymphocyte cytotoxicity in the Moloney sarcoma virus system. *J. Exp. Med.* 135: 997–1002.

237. Snyderman, R., Dickson, J., Meadows, L., and Pike, M. C. 1974. Deficient monocyte chemotactic responsiveness in humans with cancer. *Clin. Res.* 22: 430a.

238. Snyderman, R., Pike, M. C., Blaylock, B. L., and Weinstein, P. 1976. Effects of neoplasms on inflammation: depression of macrophage accumulation after tumor implantation. *J. Immunol.* 116: 585–589.

239. Southam, C. M. 1968. The immunologic states of patients with nonlymphomatous cancer. *Cancer Res.* 28: 1433–1440.

240. Stackpole, C. 1978. Antigenic modulation. In H. Waters (ed.), *The Handbook of Cancer Immunology, Vol. 2: Cellular Escape from Immune Destruction*, pp. 55–159. Garland STPM Press, New York and London.

241. Stevenson, M. M., and Meltzer, M. S. 1975. Defective macrophage

chemotaxis in tumor-bearing mice. *Fed. Proc.* 34: 991.

242. Stillman, A., and Zamcheck, N. 1970. Recent advances in immunologic diagnosis of digestive tract cancer. *Digestive Dis.* 15: 1003–1018.

243. Stjernswärd, J., and Vánky, F. 1972. Stimulation of lymphocytes by autochthonous cancer. *J. Natl. Cancer Inst. Monogr.* 35: 237–242.

244. Stoker, M., and Sussman, M. 1965. Studies on the action of feeder layers in cell culture. *Exp. Cell Res.* 38: 645–653.

245. Stuart, F. P., McKearn, T. J., and Fitch, F. W. 1974. Immunological enhancement of renal allografts. *Transplant. Proc.* 6: 53–58.

246. Stutman, O. 1975. Immunodepression and malignancy. *In Adv. Cancer Res.* 22: 261–422.

247. Suciu-Foca, N., Buda, J., McManus, J., Thiem, T., and Reemtsma, K. 1973. Impaired responsiveness of lymphocytes and serum-inhibitory factors in patients with cancer. *Cancer Res.* 33: 2373–2377.

248. Symposium: Cancer and Chemistry. *In* J. H. Coggin, Jr., and N. G. Anderson (eds.), *Fourth Conference on Embryonic and Fetal Antigens in Cancer,* 1976. *Cancer Res.* 36: 3382–3544.

249. Tatarinov, I. U. S. 1964. Obnaruzhenie embriospetsificheskogo alpha-globulina v. syvorotke krovi bol'nogo pervichnym rakom pecheni. *Vop. Med. Khim.* 10: 90–91.

250. Taussig, M. J. 1974. Demonstration of suppressor T cells in a population of "educated" T cells. *Nature* 248: 236–238.

251. Thomas, D. W., Roberts, W. K., and Talmage, D. W. 1975. Regulation of the immune response: Production of a soluble suppressor by immune spleen cells *in vitro. J. Immunol.* 114: 1616–1622.

252. Thomson, D. M. P. 1975. Soluble tumour-specific antigen and its relationship to tumour growth. *Int. J. Cancer* 15: 1016–1029.

253. Thomson, D. M. P., Eccles, S., and Alexander, P. 1973. Antibodies and soluble tumor-specific antigens in blood and lymph of rats with chemically induced sarcomata. *Brit. J. Cancer* 28: 6–15.

254. Thomson, D. M. P., Sellens, V., Eccles, S., and Alexander, P. 1973. Radioimmunoassay of tumour specific transplantation antigen of a chemically induced rat sarcoma: circulating soluble tumour antigen in tumour bearers. *Brit. J. Cancer* 28: 377–388.

255. Thomson, D. M. P., Steele, K., and Alexander, P. 1973. The presence of tumour-specific membrane antigen in the serum of rats with chemically induced sarcomata. *Brit. J. Cancer* 27: 27–34.

256. Ting, A., and Terasaki, P. I. 1974. Depressed lymphocyte-mediated killing of sensitized targets in cancer patients. *Cancer Res.* 34: 2694–2698.

257. Ting, C.-C. 1976. Detection of anti-tumor antibody in virally induced tumors and its relationship to tumor growth. *Int. J. Cancer* 18: 205–215.

258. Ting, C.-C., Lavrin, D. H., Shiu, G., and Herberman, R. B. 1971. Tumor-specific cell surface antigens in papova-virus-induced tumors and their relationship to fetal antigens. *In* N. G. Anderson and J. H. Coggin, Jr. (eds.), *Proceedings of the First Conference and Workshop on Embryonic and Fetal Antigens in Cancer,* Oak Ridge Natl. Lab., pp. 223–237.

259. Todd, R. F., III, Stulting, R. D., and Amos, D. B. 1975. Lymphocyte-

mediated cytolysis of allogeneic tumor cells in vitro. I. Search for target antigens in subcellular fractions. Cell. Immunol. 18: 304–323.

260. Uhr, J. W., and Möller, G. 1968. Regulatory effect of antibody on the immune response. Adv. Immunol. 8: 81–127.

261. Vaage, J. 1971. Concomitant immunity and specific depression of immunity by residual or reinjected syngeneic tumor tissue. Cancer Res. 31: 1655–1662.

262. Vaage, J. 1973. Influence of tumor antigen on maintenance versus depression of tumor specific immunity. Cancer Res. 33: 493–503.

263. Vaage, J. 1974. Circulating tumour antigens versus immune serum factors in depressed concomitant immunity. Cancer Res. 34: 2979–2983.

264. Vadas, M. A., Miller, J. F. A. P., McKenzie, I. F. C., Chism, S. E., Shen, F.-W., Boyse, E. A., Gamble, J. R., and Whitelaw, A. M. 1976. Ly and Ia antigen phenotypes of T cells involved in delayed-type hypersensitivity and in suppression. J. Exp. Med. 144: 10–19.

265. Van Blitterswijk, W. J., Emmelot, P., Hilgers, J., Kamlag, D., Nusse, R., and Feltkamp, C. A. 1975. Quantitation of virus-induced (MLr) and normal (Thy.1.2) cell surface antigens in isolated plasma membranes and the extracellular ascites fluid of mouse leukemia cells. Cancer Res. 35: 2743–2751.

266. Volkman, A., and Collins, F. M. 1968. Recovery of delayed-type hypersensitivity in mice following suppressive doses of X-radiation. J. Immunol. 101: 846–859.

267. Volkman, A., and Collins, F. M. 1971. The restorative effect of peritoneal macrophages on delayed hypersensitivity following ionizing radiation. Cell. Immunol. 2: 552–566.

268. Warren, B. A., and Shubik, P. 1966. The growth of the blood supply to melanoma transplants in the hamster cheek pouch. Lab. Invest. 15: 464–478.

269. Whitney, R. B., and Levy, J. G. 1974. Suppression of mitogen responses by serum from tumour-bearing mice. Eur. J. Cancer 10: 739–745.

270. Whitney, R. B., and Levy, J. G. 1975. Effects of sera from tumor-bearing mice on mitogen and allogeneic cell stimulation of normal lymhpoid cells. J. Natl. Cancer Inst. 54: 733–741.

271. Whitney, R. B., and Levy, J. G. 1975. Mode of action of immunosuppressive substances in sera of tumor-bearing mice. J. Natl. Cancer Inst. 55: 1447–1452.

272. Witz, I. P. 1973. The biological significance of tumor-bound immunoglobulins. Curr. Top. Microbiol. Immunol. 61: 151–171.

273. Wolf, A., Steele, K. A., and Alexander, P. 1976. Estimation in sera by radioimmunoassay of a specific membrane antigen associated with a murine lymphoma. Brit. J. Cancer 33: 144–153.

274. Wortis, H. H. 1974. Immunological studies of nude mice. In M. D. Cooper and N. L. Warner (eds.), Contemporary Topics in Immunobiology, Vol. 3, 1974, pp. 243–263. Plenum Press, New York.

275. Youn, J. K., LeFrançois, D., and Barski, G. 1973. In vitro studies on mechanism of the "eclipse" of cell-mediated immunity in mice bearing advanced tumors. J. Natl. Cancer Inst. 50: 921–926.

276. Zembala, M., and Asherson, G. L. 1974. T cell suppression of contact sensitivity in the mouse. II. The role of soluble suppressor factor and its interac-

tion with macrophages. *Eur. J. Immunol.* 4: 799–804.

277. Zinkernagel, R. M., and Doherty, P. C. 1974. Restriction of *in vitro* T-cell-mediated cytotoxicity in lymphocytic choriomeningitis within a syngeneic or semiallogeneic system. *Nature* 248: 701–702.

278. Zinkernagel, R. M. 1974. Restriction by H-2 gene complex of transfer of cell-mediated immunity to *Listeria monocytogenes. Nature (Lond.)* 251: 230–233.

CHAPTER 2

ANTIGENIC MODULATION

Christopher W. Stackpole and
Janet B. Jacobson

Memorial Sloan-Kettering
Cancer Center
Rye, New York   10580

Antibody-induced desensitization of cells to lysis by complement is considered as a mechanism for tumor cell escape from immune destruction. In vitro, modulation may occur by: (1) retention of modulated antigen-antibody complexes on the cell surface, effectively masked from immune intervention by localized aggregation and intercalation of complement component C3 (TL and H-2 antigens); (2) loss of modulated complexes from the cell surface by capping and internalization (surface Ig); or (3) loss of modulated complexes from the cell surface by capping and shedding (measles virus-related antigens). TL modulation occurs in vivo in the same manner as TL modulation in vitro, but how modulation affords protection against immune destruction in this case remains unclear. Certain virus-related and tumor-specific antigens on mouse and human tumor cells may also modulate, but the significance of this phenomenon as a general means for tumor escape remains to be established.

I. INTRODUCTION

The development and growth of malignancies in higher animals must involve complex and subtle interactions between tumor cell and host, since the very aberrancies that distinguish these cells from their normal counterparts should render them susceptible to host defense mechanisms. The highly developed immune system should be especially effective in preventing tumor progression since tumor cells generally express novel cell surface antigenicities. And yet, for a variety of reasons not yet fully appreciated, tumors too often "escape" immunological destruction, and effective therapy of cancer no doubt will require that these escape routes be blocked.

On certain malignant as well as normal cells, a specific, rapid, and reversible loss of sensitivity to lysis by surface antigen-directed antibody and complement may result from prior exposure to that antibody alone. The purpose of this review is to appraise this phenomenon of antigenic modulation[1] (25) as a means by which tumor cells may escape immune destruction.

A. Immunological Surveillance of Tumors and Tumor Immunity

According to the concept of immunological surveillance proposed formally by Burnet (36), the immune systems of higher vertebrates can utilize the capacity of distinguishing self from non-self to eradicate aberrant cells arising in the host as a result of somatic mutation or neoplastic transformation. This proposal is based on the assumption that all such cells possess antigenicities capable of eliciting an immune response—at least under certain conditions—and is patterned after (and potentially explains) thymus-dependent (T) cell-mediated homograft rejection phenomena. In fact, the presence of tumor-specific transplantation antigens (TSTA) on the surfaces of cells comprising experimental tumors in general is well established, as is host responsiveness to these antigens, although the response may be complex and variable (88, 107, 146, 192). In man, the evidence for existence of TSTA is inconclusive, but there are indications of host immune responses elicited towards specific determinants on human tumor cells (88, 107, 144). However, the demonstration of an immune response to tumor-specific antigens of established tumors is insufficient evidence for the existence of a surveillance system designed to destroy newly arising tumor cells, and, therefore, these responses may more accurately be categorized as examples of tumor immunity (49, 212).

Establishing the existence or generality of an immune system with a surveillance function has proven extremely difficult, largely because certain predictions regarding consequences of alterations in that system that ought to be fulfilled often are not. Among these predictions are the following: (1) the development and growth of tumors should be facilitated in hosts with immunological dysfunction or in which immune responsiveness has been depressed, as well as within immunologically privileged sites; (2) hosts bearing well-developed malignancies would be expected to possess defective immune systems, particularly with regard to cell-mediated immunity; and (3) oncogenic agents should depress immune functions. Experimental evidence bearing on these predictions has been reviewed extensively elsewhere (49, 107, 212) and need not be discussed here.

In general, then, even if an immune surveillance mechanism is operative against neoplastic cells, it is obviously quite ineffective since the incidence of tumors developing in immunologically normal and abnormal animals is so nearly comparable. At best, current evidence tends to support the existence of effective surveillance only in certain restricted cases, such as exceptionally antigenic chemically-induced tumors and tumors involving strong virus-related antigen systems that are regularly encountered by most individuals within a species (107, 161).

Prehn (161) has emphasized that while most neoplasms are probably not subjected to surveillance controls, there is a late-acting and relatively inefficient immune defense mechanism directed against established tumors. Tumor immunity seems to involve complex humoral and cell-mediated effector mechanisms, the precise nature of which may be somewhat characteristic of a particular system. For example, Currie and Sime (50) have demonstrated that cytophilic immunoglobulin in serum from syngeneic mice immunized against a spontaneous lymphoma attaches to the surfaces of these cells and also inhibits the motility of cells from this tumor established in culture. Similar tumor cell-specific motility-inhibiting activity has been demonstrated in remission sera from leukemia patients (49). Cytostatic or cytolytic effects may also be exerted on tumor cells by membrane-reactive TSTA antibodies in cooperation with unsensitized killer (K) lymphocytes (129, 159) or together with complement (102). Lysis of tumor cells in vitro may occur when the cells are exposed to specifically immunized (TSTA antibody-sensitized) or nonspecifically activated T lymphocytes or lymphoid cell precursors to antibody-producing (B) cells, without the requirement for intervention of complement (39, 88, 91, 158); intimate contact between target cell and lymphoid effector cell seems to be essential for lysis to occur.

There is also increasing evidence implicating macrophages in mediation of tumor immunity. These cells may have several roles, including: (1) processing of tumor antigens and presentation to immunocompetent cells; (2) effecting cytolysis of neoplastic cells following nonspecific activation by a variety of stimuli or specific activation by immune lymphocytes or cytophilic antibody; (3) inhibition of tumor cell migration or growth following nonspecific or specific activation; or (4) production of complement components (39, 44, 49, 68, 123).

B. Escape of Tumor Cells from Immune Destruction

Despite the capacity for the immune system to marshal such a multifaceted response against tumor cells, the end result of such onslaught is invariably continued tumor progression, even though comparable attacks on invading pathogens are generally devastatingly successful. The difference must be attributable to unique characteristics of proliferating tumor cells that render them relatively insensitive to potentially lethal attacks. Active tumor cells seem to escape immune destruction in a variety of ways (many of which are undoubtedly interrelated) involving, almost paradoxically, direct interactions between the tumor cells and the host immune system.

1. IMMUNOLOGICAL TOLERANCE OR PARALYSIS. The failure of an immunologically competent host to elicit a detectable immune response against a tumor may result from induction of immunological tolerance or paralysis during prior contact with the same tumor-specific antigen, or perhaps an oncogenic virus-related antigen. Acquisition of tolerance seems to involve the rendering of normally antigen-sensitive T and B cells insensitive to appropriate activation signals, either by altering the cells' reactivity to antigen, by saturating antigen receptors on the cell surface with nonimmunogenic antigen and thus preventing stimulation of the cell by immunogenic antigen, or by eliminating specific cell clones through direct antigen contact (141). The structural nature of the antigen, and especially the number of determinants on an individual molecule, may be a critical parameter determining the exact manner of tolerance induction. Polymeric, multivalent, and highly immunogenic antigens may tolerize B cells directly when present in high doses, possibly by reducing antibody secretion rate through direct attachment to the cell surface. On the other hand, soluble, oligovalent, and poorly immunogenic antigens may suppress B cell function indirectly by activating suppressor T cells, or they may be directly tolerogenic to T cells. Antigen-antibody complexes seem capable of tolerizing both T and B cells. With regard to tumor immunity, the important considerations in effecting tolerance induction ap-

pear to be the age of the host at the time of initial encounter with the antigen, the dose of antigen, and the molecular nature of the antigen (141).

It is important to point out, however, that concepts of immunological tolerance are based on the lack of a *detectable* host immune response to tumor antigens, which should not necessarily be equated with a complete lack of response. The AKR strain of mouse, for example, which has a high incidence of spontaneous leukemia, was long considered immunologically tolerant to antigens associated with the causative agent, Gross murine leukemia virus (Gross MuLV), since no antibody to these antigens could be detected in the serum of leukemic mice (146). Subsequently, antibody to Gross MuLV structural components and to virus-related cell surface antigens was demonstrated in kidney eluates from these animals, and antigen-antibody complexes were visualized in kidney glomeruli by immunofluorescence (8, 152). These results indicate that the AKR mouse does in fact elicit an immune response, albeit extremely weak, to Gross MuLV-associated antigens. Perhaps because of a tremendous excess of antigen, much of it shed from the cell surface with virus, antibody is demonstrable only in the form of antigen-antibody complexes trapped and concentrated within the kidney. Actually, rapid destruction of advanced leukemias in these animals can be achieved by infusion of the C5 component of complement, which is genetically absent from the AKR mouse strain (102). At least in this case, then, a specific immune deficiency rather than tolerance may be responsible for tumor escape from destruction.

2. IMMUNOLOGICAL ENHANCEMENT.

Kaliss (100) was the first to discover that the growth of certain allografted tumors, which normally would be rejected, could actually be facilitated by injection of tumor-specific alloantibody into tumor-bearing animals. This paradoxical phenomenon, designated immunological enhancement, has never been demonstrated in a syngeneic tumor system (49) and only occurs with certain tumors, most notably sarcomas and carcinomas. Enhancement by antibody is effective following either passive or active immunization, or introduction of antibody-coated tumor cells into unimmunized hosts, and also occurs with univalent (Fab) antibody fragments (48). Enhanced growth of the mouse leukemia EL4 has only been observed when the number of leukemic cells inoculated was quite high relative to the amount of antibody present in the host (21).

There seem to be two possible mechanisms responsible for immunological enhancement that are most supported by current evidence: (1) attachment of antibody to cell surface TSTA hinders metabolic release of these antigens into the environment, thus diminishing TSTA-induced stimulation of the immune system; and (2) antibody attachment to TSTA may interfere with the establishment of direct contact between host im-munocompetent lymphoid cells and tumor cells, thus preventing lytic interaction (48). Alternately, antibody, after attaching to cell surface anti-gens, might be shed as antigen-antibody complexes that could activate suppressor T cells which in turn would inhibit B cell function (105).

3. BLOCKING FACTORS. Hellström and Hellström (88) have demonstrated that sera from animals and humans bearing progressively growing tumors can "block" the cytolytic interaction of specifically TSTA-sensitized lymphocytes with the tumor cells *in vitro*. This effect, since demonstrated in a number of different systems, was initially attrib-uted to "blocking" antibody and suggested that humoral responses in the animal might antagonize cell-mediated immune responses. It now seems unlikely that antibody alone is responsible for this blocking effect, since such effects are not demonstrable with sera from animals bearing regress-ing tumors, and these sera may even counteract the protective influence of blocking sera (87). Present indications are that blocking is caused by tumor antigens and/or antigen-antibody complexes shed into the circula-tion (13, 89, 190), and that "unblocking" regressor sera represent a shift-ing of the imbalance from antigen excess to antibody excess as a conse-quence of tumor decline (89).

4. IMMUNORESISTANCE. Because of the generally incom-plete destruction of tumor cells resulting from immune attack even under the best of circumstances, it is often possible for variant cell clones to arise with altered antigenicity such that they are rendered unsusceptible to immune destruction. For example, Fenyö et al. (70) showed that the de-velopment of immunoresistance by a Moloney MuLV-induced murine lymphoma to virus-specific antiserum was accompanied by a significant decrease in the amount of virus-determined cell surface antigenicity as measured by quantitative absorption and membrane immunofluores-cence. When virus isolated from variant cells was used to infect sensitive indicator cells growing in culture, the virus multiplied normally within the cells but virus-related cell surface antigenicity was reduced from the normal amount (71). In this case, selective outgrowth of a cell occurred because a virus variant arose that failed to induce production of normal amounts of antigen. Undoubtedly, a variety of other mechanisms could similarly result in development of immunoresistant cell clones based on the acquisition of an antigen-negative phenotype.

5. "SNEAKING THROUGH." While studying the effects of cell dosage on the growth of the highly antigenic chemically induced BALB/c sarcoma Meth A in syngeneic hosts, Old et al. (147) obtained a most unexpected result. Moderate cell doses (1, 250–62,500 cells) were rejected in typical fashion, while both larger (> 62,500 cells) and very small (40–200 cells) doses grew unimpeded. While growth of the large cell dose is readily explainable as an overpowering of a relatively weak immune response, growth of the very small dose is not likely to be explained in the same way. Similar results have subsequently been obtained with a variety of viral and chemically induced tumors (107), so the phenomenon seems to be real. Relevant to these findings, several investigators have shown that development of polyoma- or SV40-induced tumors in neonatally infected animals could be prevented by administering a second virus dose, or heavily irradiated tumor cells induced by the same virus, toward the end of the oncogenic latency period (62, 78). It is conceivable that when a tumor is extremely small an insufficient amount of shed TSTA reaches the immune system to effect stimulation, and that by the time the immune system is triggered, a threshold level of growth has been achieved which is then insensitive to a full onslaught by the immune system. If antigen is administered prior to that threshold level being reached, then the tumor can presumably be suppressed (107). Thus, the host is not tolerant of the tumor antigen, but the immune system is simply not efficient enough to detect and/or respond to extremely small antigen doses.

6. ANTIGEN MASKING. In a number of studies, transplantation of cultured tumor or transformed cells into syngeneic hosts has resulted in alterations in the quantitative expression of cell surface antigens, generally in the direction of decreased expression (42, 56, 57, 95). Ohno et al. (145) examined the alterations in expression of H-2 and other surface antigens on IgA-synthesizing 58-8 plasmacytoma cells induced in BALB/c mice occurring during continued transplantation into syngeneic hosts. They obtained indications that decreased antigenicity resulted from "masking" of antigen determinants. Antigen expression decreased progressively during the first 13 transplant generations, but was restored by treating the cells with the proteolytic enzyme pronase. Pronase-treated cells also lost their antigenicity upon retransplantation or culturing in vitro, but this loss was prevented by actinomycin D or puromycin. A protein-like material synthesized by the cells was, therefore, suspected of masking the antigens (steric hindrance?) so that antibody attachment was reduced.

Tumor cells growing in vivo are often coated with immunoglobulins (Ig) that are of uncertain biological significance, but may at least partly represent adsorbed tumor-specific antibody (61, 234, 235). Dorval et al. (61) have found that an Ig "coat" on Moloney MuLV-induced lymphoma cells masks some tumor-associated antigens without affecting the expression of other cell surface antigens; virus antibody-dependent complement-mediated cytolysis is effectively blocked by this coat of Ig molecules. An active role of the host in contributing some tumor-bound Ig was indicated by the decreased amounts of such molecules on cells inoculated into irradiated hosts, and by the increased binding observed with progressively longer periods of growth in normal unimmunized animals (235).

Why does tumor-bound Ig have no apparent detrimental effect on the progressive growth of tumor cells in vivo? It may be that many of the bound molecules represent irrelevant Ig that effectively masks the cells from immune attack dependent upon cell attachment of tumor-specific antibody (234). The relatively small numbers of specific antibody molecules capable of attaching may be prevented from promoting complement- or cell-mediated cytodestruction, perhaps by steric hindrance.

7. ANTIGENIC MODULATION, SHEDDING, AND INTERNALIZATION.

In 1963, Old and his associates (148) described a cell surface antigen that was detectable only on certain mouse leukemias and on normal thymocytes from some, but not all, mouse strains. The antigen, designated thymus-leukemia (TL) because of this restricted occurrence, was defined with antisera raised in C57BL/6 mice by hyperimmunization with viable cell suspensions from allogeneic and histoincompatible spontaneous or radiation-induced A, (C57BL/6 × A)F$_1$, or C58 strain leukemias. Eight of nine such antisera reacted positively with the C57BL/6 radiation-induced leukemia ERLD when tested by complement-mediated in vitro cytotoxicity (24, 79); guinea pig serum was used as a source of lytic complement since mouse complement is virtually nonlytic for mouse cells in vitro (233).

A particularly potent antiserum raised against the A-strain spontaneous leukemia ASL1 (C57BL/6 anti-ASL1) reacted positively with the cells from 14 of 18 radiation-induced syngeneic C57BL/6 leukemias tested, as well as one urethan-induced C57BL/6 leukemia (148). No cytotoxic effect of this antiserum was observed on normal C57BL/6 thymus, spleen, lymph node, or bone marrow cells, however, indicating that TL is a leukemia-specific antigen in that mouse strain. By absorption of specific cytotoxic activity against ERLD from this antiserum, thymocytes from A, (C57BL/6 × A)F$_1$, and C58 mice were also shown to possess TL antigen, but all other normal cells tested (spleen, lymph node, erythrocytes, and liver) failed to absorb TL antibody activity from the antiserum. Subsequently, bone marrow, kidney, brain and lung tissue from these strains were also found to be TL− (25).

Due to the presence of TL antigen on A-strain thymocytes, these mice failed to produce antibodies against TL+ C57BL/6 leukemias that would react with TL+ A-strain leukemias (148). At the same time, however,

C57BL/6 anti-ASL1 serum, which contained H-2 histocompatibility (H-2^b and H-2^a) antibodies in addition to TL antibody, could be made specific for TL by in vivo absorption in A-strain mice; the TL antibody titer was unaffected by absorption, presumably because TL antigen on A thymocytes is not accessible to circulating antibody (23). TL antiserum could be raised by immunization of TL− mice with TL+ thymocytes, but could only be distinguished when host and donor histocompatibilities were chosen so as to avoid production of antibodies to H-2 antigens as well (25).

Because of the anomalous appearance of TL antigen on certain leukemias induced in otherwise TL− C57BL/6 mice, hyperimmunization of these mice with TL+ leukemias would be expected to engender these animals with a strong immunity to transplanted syngeneic TL+ leukemias. When these experiments were performed (e.g., ERLD was passaged into C57BL/6 mice hyperimmunized with the TL+ leukemia ASL1), rather unexpectedly there was no indication of active immunity to the tumor transplants, all of which grew progressively and killed the hosts within the normal length of time (13–17 days when tumor cells were inoculated intraperitoneally, 21–28 days when inoculated subcutaneously), despite the continued presence of high levels of cytotoxic TL antibody in the serum (22). The addition of rat serum as a source of supplemental complement had no effect, indicating that complement deficiency was probably not responsible for the animals' failure to reject their tumors. Surprisingly, when tumor cells transplanted to immunized mice were removed following outgrowth (12–28 days), they had become completely insensitive to the cytotoxic effects of TL antiserum and guinea pig complement. This acquired TL− phenotype was maintained for as long as the leukemia cells were passaged in immunized mice, but the original TL+ phenotype was totally restored by a single transplant passage (12–14 days) into normal unimmunized C57BL/6 mice. Suppression of TL antigenicity was not accompanied by detectable modulation of H-2 antigenicity. This specific and reversible loss of the TL+ phenotype from leukemias was designated antigenic modulation by Boyse et al. (25).

The possibility that antigenic modulation might represent the emergence of a resistant cell population as a result of immunoselection was dismissed by Boyse et al. (22) for the following reasons: (1) under optimum conditions, virtually all cells of a TL+ leukemia such as ERLD were sensitive to TL antiserum and complement, so that inherently resistant cells would have to represent an exceedingly small proportion of the total population of leukemia cells; (2) outgrowth of TL+ leukemias in actively immunized animals occurred at essentially the same rate as in unimmunized animals, indicating participation of most inoculated cells; and (3) totally resistant populations of leukemia cells from immunized hosts reverted to totally sensitive populations during a single passage in unimmunized mice, much more rapidly than would be expected for a variant cell population (106). Most likely, then, antigenic modulation is an adaptive phenotypic change that affects the entire cell population.

Immunological enhancement was also ruled out as a probable explanation for modulation (22), since enhancement of mouse leukemias had only been observed when the ratio of inoculated cells to reactive antibody present in the host was high (21). The conditions leading to modulation were just the opposite, that is, a low cell-to-antibody ratio.

Modulation of TL antigenicity was subsequently demonstrated with both TL+ leukemias and thymocytes in TL+ mouse strains by passive immunization of the hosts with TL antiserum (26); modulation occurred on ASL1 leukemia cells within 1 day, and on A-strain thymocytes within 3 days after passive immunization was initiated. TL+ thymocytes of suckling mice have also been modulated by transfer of maternal antibody, with the TL+ phenotype returning to normal within several weeks after weaning (26). Thus, TL antigens on leukemia cells and thymocytes from TL+ mouse strains were as susceptible to modulation as TL antigens appearing anomalously on leukemia cells from TL− strains. When three additional TL antigens were defined (TL.2, TL.3 and TL.4; the original antigen was designated TL.1), they were also found to undergo modulation (26, 29). A fifth TL antigen specificity has been identified recently, and it apparently also modulates (76).

Similar modulation of TL antigens was also found to occur in vitro within minutes to several hours in a temperature- and energy-dependent process apparently requiring cellular metabolic activity (26, 150). Modulation of leukemia cells in vitro was completely reversible within 1–2 days after removal of unbound TL antibody from the medium and further incubation of the cells at 37°C in fresh medium. Modulation in vivo was also completely reversible in vitro, but 5–6 days were required for the normal TL+ phenotypic expression to return in this case (150). Transfer of in vivo-modulated leukemia cells into unimmunized mice has, however, resulted in complete restoration of TL antigenicity within 24 hours (97).

Modulation in vitro was also achieved by use of univalent (Fab) fragments of TL antibody prepared by papain digestion (114). While these fragments lacked the Fc, or complement-binding, portion of the antibody molecule and were thus unable to fix or activate complement, TL antigens were nevertheless modulated by the criterion of loss of sensitivity of treated cells to fresh TL antiserum (containing intact antibody) and guinea pig complement. Modulation by Fab fragments also appeared to require cellular metabolic activity.

Because of the energy requirements for in vitro modulation, an active cellular process rather than a passive blocking or masking of TL antigens (perhaps by antibody lacking the capacity to fix or activate complement) was favored as an explanation for antigenic modulation (30). An actual loss of TL antigens from the cell surface was supported by several observations. In the first place, modulated cells were incapable of absorbing TL antibody from antiserum. Secondly, modulation of TL antigenicity both in vivo and in vitro was accompanied by a compensatory increase in the amount of H-2 antigen (specifically those antigens determined by the D end of the H-2 complex) detectable on the cell surface by quantitative absorption (26, 150); other studies had shown that expression of TL antigens on thymocytes results in a decreased expression of H-2D antigens on the same cells (26, 27). And, finally, modulating TL antibody was not detected on the cell surface by indirect membrane immunoflourescence (26, 150).

Thus, the prevalent views until recently have been that modulated TL antigens were either shed from the cell surface as a consequence of antibody attachment, perhaps in concert with normal cellular processes of membrane turnover, or internalized by the cell in a temperature- and energy-dependent pinocytotic process (18, 150, 240).

Modulation-like phenomena have been reported for a variety of other cell surface receptors (see Section III), and in many instances a loss of antigens from the cell surface by shedding or internalization was also considered the most likely explanation.

Shedding of antigens from the cell surface may occur to a significant extent in certain tumors and may, in the presence of antibody, form circulating "blocking" factors important in preventing immune destruction of tumor cells in certain cases (see Section I, B, 3). However, antigen shedding is not necessarily dependent upon exposure of the cells to specific antibody (60, 104). Davey et al. (51), for example, have found that metastasizing and nonmetastasizing mouse lymphoma cells spontaneously shed H-2 antigens that are readily detectable in soluble form in sera of tumor-bearing mice and in supernatant fluids from cultures. Shedding of antigens from metastasizing cells occurred at a greater rate than from nonmetastasizing cells.

Antigens shed from the cell surface may set up a "smoke-screen" effect in masking the tumor proper from an antibody barrage, since the shed antigen could presumably engage antibody and, therefore, compete with the cell surface for unbound antibody (2). Boyse et al. (26) and Old et al. (150) had previously noted that the rate of TL antigenic modulation both in vivo and in vitro seemed to be related to the metabolic activity and growth characteristics of the particular cell type. Thus, modulation in vitro occurred in a shorter length of time with rapidly growing leukemias than with the slow-growing leukemia cells and normal thymocytes (67,

150, 203, 240). Similarly, H-2 antibody-sensitized metastasizing mouse lymphoma cells lose sensitivity to lytic complement more rapidly than nonmetastasizing cells, consistent with the tendency for the respective cells to spontaneously shed their H-2 antigens (51). However, shedding of antigens was not demonstrated under modulating conditions, and even if it did occur might simply be a consequence of high metabolic activity and short generation time, reflecting rapid cell surface membrane and antigen turnover (60); shedding may, therefore, not necessarily entail a net loss of cell surface antigenicity even though it might be highly significant as a mechanism by which tumor cells may escape immune destruction. On the other hand, surface antigens, especially those specified by enveloped viruses, may in certain instances be virtually completely lost from the cell surface by shedding, following interaction with antibody (see Section III, C, 1).

Internalization of cell surface receptors by pinocytosis following attachment of ligands seems to be a general cellular process that is dependent on temperature and metabolic activity (181, 198), as is modulation. For this reason, it is quite logical to assume that pinocytosis could account for a complete loss of TL antigens during the course of modulation, particularly in light of the rapid and virtually complete internalization of surface Ig molecules that occurs on lymphocytes following antibody attachment and topographical redistribution of the labeled complexes into "caps" (54, 181, 216, 221). In fact, internalization of antibody-bound surface antigens is undoubtedly a significant mechanism available to tumor cells for the purpose of escape from immune destruction (117, 120).

While modulation of TL antigens is now known to be accompanied by capping and some internalization of antigen-antibody complexes (67, 203, 240), this mechanism does not account for a complete loss of modulated antigens from the cell surface either in vivo or in vitro (97, 203). Instead, modulation appears to result primarily from TL antibody-induced lateral displacement of antigen within the cell surface membrane into "microaggregates" resistant to a subsequent exposure to TL antibody and cytolytic guinea pig complement. TL antigens remain detectable on the surfaces of modulated cells when rabbit complement is substituted for guinea pig complement, and TL antigen-antibody complexes are demonstrable by direct or indirect membrane immunofluorescence. Retention of much of the original quantity of cell surface TL antigens on in vitro modulated cells has since been verified by use of an indirect radioimmunoassay (66, 67).

In the remainder of this chapter, modulation of TL antigens and other antigens will be discussed in greater detail, with the purpose of ascertaining the underlying mechanism(s) and the potential significance of this phenomenon as a general means for tumors to avoid the consequences of immune attack.

II. MODULATION OF TL ANTIGENS

Antigens of the TL system in the mouse exhibit a number of unique characteristics that might help to explain the unusual tendency for these molecules to undergo antigenic modulation. At the same time, in certain ways, TL antigens show a remarkable resemblance to other cell surface molecules, molecules bearing antigens that display considerably less tendency to modulate. In order to arrive at a clearer understanding of the nature of modulation, available information regarding the genetics, biology, and biochemistry of TL antigens will first be considered.

A. Genetics of TL Antigens

At present, five distinct antigens are recognizable on the surfaces of mouse thymocytes and/or leukemia cells (Table 1) as TL antigens on the basis of several criteria (29, 76). In addition to being restricted to thymocytes and leukemia cells and undergoing antigenic modulation, all of these antigens are specified by genes linked to a common *Tla* (thymus-leukemia-antigen) locus. The cell surface expression of TL antigens is also characteristically related in reciprocal fashion to the expression of antigens specified by the *H-2D* locus (27). Another feature of TL antigens (with the exception of TL.3) is their anomalous appearance on leukemias of mice that do not normally express TL antigenicity on their thymocytes. And yet, while basically similar, each specificity also has unique characteristics in terms of phenotypic expression on normal and leukemic cells (Table 2). The TL.1 specificity is universally expressed on leukemias; so is TL.2, but it is the only specificity that may be expressed alone. TL.3 appears only on leukemias in mice in which that specificity is also expressed on thymocytes, and it is always accompanied by TL.1 and TL.2, while TL.4 seems to be leukemia-specific, not having been detected on thymocytes (29). The recently identified specificity TL.5 accompanies TL.1,2,3 expression on thymocytes from certain strains but may be lacking from other TL.1,2,3+ thymocytes (76). Further analysis of the phenotypic expression of TL antigens provides considerable insight into mechanisms operative in the genetic control of TL antigen expression.

1. ACTIVATION OF TL ANTIGEN DETERMINANTS IN LEUKEMIA CELLS.

In the mouse, leukemias generally tend to develop within the thymus and, therefore, presumably consist of transformed thymocytes (103, 131, 186). The anomalous appearance of TL.1, TL.2, TL.4 and TL.5 antigens on the surfaces of leukemia cells arising in mice that do not normally express those specificities on their thymocytes suggests that all mice carry repressed structural *Tla* genes that may be derepressed (or otherwise activated) as a specific consequence of

Table 1. Mouse alloantisera defining the five TL antigen specificities[a]

Antiserum	Antigens Recognized	Cytotoxicity for Thymocytes of Strains				Cytotoxicity for TL+ Leukemias of Strains			
		A	C57BL/6	BALB/c	DBA/2	A	C57BL/6	BALB/c	DBA/2
C57BL/6 [TL−; H-2^b] anti-A strain spontaneous leukemia ASL1 [TL.1,2,3,5; H-2^a], absorbed in vivo in A mice to remove H-2^a histo-compatibility antibodies	TL.1,2,3,−,5	+	−	±	±	+	+	+	+
(C57BL/6 × A/TL−)F$_1$ [TL−] anti-ASL1, unabsorbed,[b] or A/TL− anti-ASL1, unabsorbed									
(C57BL/6 × A/TL−)F$_1$ anti-A thymocytes [TL.1,2,3,5], unabsorbed									
(BALB/c × C3H)F$_1$ [TL.2]anti-ASL1, unabsorbed	TL.1,−,3,−,5	+	−	−	−	+	+	+	+
(C57BL/6 × A/TL−)F$_1$ anti-ASL1, absorbed in vitro with BALB/c thymocytes [TL.2][b]									

Antiserum	TL designation							
(BALB/c × C3H)F$_1$ anti-ASL1, absorbed in vivo in (C57BL/6 × A)F$_1$ male mice bearing advanced transplants of the C57BL/6 leukemia ERLD [TL.1,2,4]	TL.−,−,3,−,5[c]	+	−	−	−	+	−	−
(C57BL/6 × A/TL−)F$_1$ anti-ASL1, absorbed in vitro with ERLD[b]		−	−	−	−	−	−	−
C57BL/6 anti-129 thymocytes [TL.2], unabsorbed[b]	TL.−,2,−,−,−	±	−	±	±	±	±	±
(C57BL/6 × A/TL−)F$_1$ anti-ASL1, absorbed in vitro with the DBA/2 leukemia SL2	TL.−,−,3,−,−[d]	+	−	−	−	+	−	−
C57BL/6/TL+ [TL.1,2,3,5] anti-ERLD, unabsorbed[b]	TL.−,−,−,4,−	−	−	−	−	+	+	+ or −
(B10.A(2R) × A.CA)F$_1$ anti-B10 lymphoid cells, absorbed in vitro with BALB/c and/or C57BL/6 lymph node cells	TL.−,−,−,−,5	+	−	+	−	+	−	+

a. Modified from Klein (108) and based on Boyse et al. (25, 26, 27), Old et al. (150), Stackpole et al. (203), Flaherty et al. (76), and unpublished results. TL.1-specific antiserum has not been obtained.
b. Antisera used in co-capping experiments described in Table 3.
c. Positive on A.CM thymocytes.
d. Negative on A.CM thymocytes.

Table 2. Phenotypic expression of TL antigens on normal mouse thymocytes and leukemia cells[a]

Tla Haplotype	Thymocyte Phenotype	Leukemia Cell Phenotype[b]	Representative Strains
a	1,2,3,–, 5	1,2,3,–, 5	A, C57BL/6/TL+, C58
b	–,–,–,–, –	1,2,–,4,–,	C57BL/6, A/TL–, AKR, C3H
c	–,2,–,–, –	1,2,–,–, –	
			BALB/c, DBA/2
	–,2,–,–, –	1,2,–,4,5,	
d	1,2,3,–, –	?	A.CM, B10.M

a. Adapted from Boyse et al. (29), Boyse and Old (19), and Flaherty et al. (76).
b. Leukemias arising in TL+ or TL– mouse strains may also be phenotypically TL–.

leukemic transformation of thymocytes; transformation of other cell types is not accompanied by *Tla* gene derepression (19, 29).

In certain mouse strains, TL.1 and TL.2 represent normal thymocyte "differentiation" antigens, being characteristic of that particular cell type (19), but the structural genes for both specificities (*Tla.1* and *Tla.2*) are present in all strains and may be derepressed in leukemia cells. Expression of TL.4 antigen is strictly dependent upon leukemogenic derepression of *Tla.4*, since that antigen is not present on thymocytes. There is no evidence, however, that mice normally expressing TL.1,2,3,5 antigens or certain mice expressing TL.2 antigen possess the *Tla.4* structural gene. By the same reasoning, *Tla.3* is either not derepressed in leukemias of TL.3– mouse strains or is lacking altogether, but in either event there is no known example of *Tla.3* derepression. There is a possibility that *Tla.3* and *Tla.4* could be alleles at the same locus, since the two determinants never occur together in a *Tla* homozygote, but their different characteristics tend to argue against this possibility (29).

A close association between the *Tla* and the *H-2* loci is indicated by the results of Boyse et al. (32) regarding an H-2-loss variant line of leukemia cells obtained by immunoselection of a (C57BL/6 × A)F$_1$ (*H-2^b/H-2^a*) transplanted leukemia. This variant line lacked H-2^a haplotype cell surface antigens, the specific consequence of immunoselection. However, there were also changes in quantitative expression of TL.1,2,3,5 antigens[2] on these cells that indicated deletion of the *Tla* locus along with the *H-2^a* determinants of the chromosome contributed by the A-strain parent. Functional deletion of *Tla* did not occur by specific immunoselection, since TL.1,2,4 antigens, contributed by the derepressed structural genes of the chromosome contributed by the C57BL/6 parent, were expressed.

The precise relationship between leukemogenesis and derepression of *Tla* structural genes is somewhat unclear, although Boyse *et al.* (25) have noted several interesting aspects of the incidence of TL+ leukemias. While TL+ leukemias may arise in TL+ as well as TL− mouse strains, TL− leukemias also develop in TL+ animals. Leukemias developing spontaneously in TL+ or TL− mouse strains that generally have a low incidence of such neoplasms (e.g., C57BL/6, TL−; A, TL+) are often TL+, whereas leukemias arising in TL+ or TL− high incidence strains (e.g., AKR, TL−; C58, TL+) are usually TL−. A large number of leukemias induced by natural or experimental infection with leukemia viruses are TL−, while most radiation-induced leukemias and tumors arising in mice of strains that are not overtly infected with leukemia viruses (e.g., C57BL/6) are TL+, irrespective of the TL status of the host. Thus, TL phenotypic derepression in leukemia cells may depend upon the manner of transformation, with radiation more likely to induce a TL+ phenotype than viruses. Possible relevance of the *Tla* locus to leukemogenesis has been discussed more extensively by Boyse and Old (19) and Boyse *et al.* (32, 33).

2. CONTROL OF TL PHENOTYPE IN THYMOCYTES.

The occurence of TL antigenic modulation might suggest that lack of TL antigen expression by thymocytes of TL− mouse strains may result from continuous "modulation" of nascent TL antigens by circulating TL antibodies. There is not the slightest evidence to support such a possibility, however (194; see Section II, B, 2).

It should be evident from the discussion in the previous section that in addition to *structural* genes encoding for TL.1, TL.2, TL.3, TL.4 and TL.5 antigens, the phenotypic appearance of these antigens on the cell surface requires activation of the appropriate *regulatory* alleles controlling expression versus nonexpression of the structural genes. (The environment provided by the thymus is also essential for expression of TL antigens by normal cells—see Section II, B, 1.) Four *Tla* haplotypes are currently recognized on the basis of normal thymocyte phenotypes, and each haplotype behaves as a separate allele (Table 2): Tla^a (TL.1,2,3,5), Tla^b (TL−), Tla^c (TL.2), and Tla^d (TL.1,2,3) (76, 185). These alleles control expression of the *Tla.1–5* structural genes.

Genetic studies by Boyse *et al.* (23) indicated that the *Tla* locus behaves like an autosomal gene with mendelian inheritance characteristics: progeny of a cross between A (Tla^a) and C57BL/6 (Tla^b) mice had half as much TL antigen on their thymocytes as cells from the parental A strain, as measured by quantitative absorption; upon backcrossing these F_1 hybrids to C57BL/6 mice, 50% of the progeny were TL+, indicating segregation of a single dominant gene. In these and subsequent studies, linkage of the Tla locus to the H-2 complex on linkage group IX (chromosome 17) and specifically with the D end of that complex (1.5 map units distance), was established on the basis of incidence of cross-overs between Tla, H-$2D$, and H-$2K$ (23, 25, 27).

According to Schlesinger (174), Tla structural genes need not necessarily reside in the same locus or even on the same chromosome as their regulatory alleles. Since $Tla.1$ and $Tla.2$ are present and identical in all mouse strains, then in the experiments of Boyse et al. (23), segregation in the backcross (A × C57BL/6)F_1 × C57BL/6 (Tla^a/Tla^b × Tla^b/Tla^b) would affect the regulatory rather than the structural genes. In this case, it is the regulatory alleles that are linked to H-$2D$, and the structural genes could be anywhere within the genome. Boyse and Old (20) have presented a rather compelling argument, however, in favor of the structural genes also being located within the Tla locus.

There are also indications that the Tla locus contains weak histocompatibility loci. Two reciprocal pairs of Tla congenic mouse lines were developed by Boyse et al. (25) that resulted from transfer of the Tla^b (TL−) chromosome from strain C57BL/6 onto an A-strain background and transfer of the Tla^a (TL.1,2,3,5) chromosome from A to C57BL/6. The A/Tla^b (A/TL−) congenic line was produced by 26 backcrossing generations, and the C57BL/6/Tla^a (C57BL/6/TL+) line by 15 generations, so both lines should be histocompatible with their inbred partners (108). However, skin grafts and leukemia transplants exchanged between A and A/Tla^b or between C57BL/6 and C57BL/6/Tla^a congenic lines were rejected (34).

After so many backcrossing generations, it is unlikely that these congenic lines differ chromosomally except for the Tla region and, therefore, the observed histoincompatibility is most likely associated with that region. Similar skin graft rejections ascribable to the Tla region have been obtained by other investigators (59, 72, 73, 195). Rejections most frequently occurred only with first grafts and were more pronounced between females than between males.

These histocompatibility effects have been assigned to an $H(Tla)$ locus linked to, yet separable from, the Tla locus (74, 231). The Tla locus itself is known not to be histoincompatible since, for example, C57BL/6 mice do not reject the syngeneic TL+ leukemia ERLD. Also, $H(Tla)$-specified antigens are recognizable on skin, fibroblast, melanoma and leukemia cells, a tissue distribution not in common with TL antigens. Two distinct $H(Tla)$ loci are now distinguishable on the basis of recombination. The $H(Tla$-$1)$, or H-31, locus has not been separated from Tla, but its expression does not depend upon the Tla genotype, while the $H(Tla$-$2)$, or H-32, locus is separable from both Tla and $H(Tla$-$1)$ (75).

Quantitative absorption has been used by Boyse *et al.* (27) to analyze interactions occurring between *Tla* alleles contributed by different chromosomes that might affect cell surface representation of TL antigens. No interaction between alleles on separate chromosomes was apparent in a *Tla^a* (TL.1,2,3,5)/*Tla^b* (TL−) cross, the amount of both TL.1 and TL.3 antigens being reduced by 50% compared with the *Tla^a* homozygote (TL.2 antigen was not measured). This would be the predicted result if each active allele were producing one "dose" of antigen and no chromosomal interactions were occurring, since there were two active *Tla.1* and *Tla.3* genes in the homozygote, but only one each in the heterozygote. If the "silent" *Tla.1* gene from the TL− parent (also the *Tla.3* gene, if present) were being repressed by some sort of a diffusible inactivator, then the *Tla^a*/*Tla^b* heterozygote should be totally devoid of TL.1 antigen. Alternately, if the repressed *Tla.1* gene from the TL− parent were somehow derepressed by the presence of a chromosome with an activated *Tla.1* gene, a 100% representation of TL.1 antigen on heterozygous thymocytes would be expected.

Interestingly, in these experiments of Boyse *et al.* (27), there was some indication of chromosomal interaction affecting quantitative representation of TL.1 and TL.2 antigens on thymocytes of a *Tla^a* (TL.1,2,3,5)/*Tla^c* (TL.2) heterozygote. As expected from a dosage effect, only half of the amount of TL.3 expressed on *Tla^a* homozygotes was expressed on these *Tla^a*/*Tla^c* heterozygotes, while surprisingly, the full complement of TL.1 antigen was expressed. Possibly, a repressed *Tla.1* gene on the *Tla^c* chromosome was activated by the presence of an active *Tla.1* gene on the *Tla^a* chromosome, although this possibility could not be tested. If such an explanation were to prove correct, it might indicate that the *Tla^c* chromosome lacks the *Tla.3* structural gene.

Only about 80% of the homozygous (*Tla^a*) amount of TL.2 antigen was present on *Tla^a*/*Tla^c* thymocytes, despite contributions by both chromosomes. However, homozygous *Tla^c*/*Tla^c* thymocytes express only 60% as much TL.2 antigens as *Tla^a* thymocytes, while heterozygous *Tla^b*/*Tla^c* mice express only 30% as much of this antigen as *Tla^a* mice. If each *Tla^c* chromosome produces only 60% as much TL.2 antigen as each *Tla^a* chromosome, for whatever reason, then the observed results might be explained on a simple "dosage" basis.

Unfortunately, the situation is almost certainly not that simple. Similar quantitative studies by Boyse *et al.* (27) on cell surface representation of H-2 antigens on thymocytes expressing TL antigens to varying degrees indicate that a dosage effect does not adequately account for reduced representation of TL antigens on heterozygous thymocytes. Rather, results obtained relative to *Tla* allelic interactions were probably influenced by interactions between the *Tla* locus and the adjoining *H-2* complex.

3. INTERACTIONS BETWEEN TL AND H-2 ANTIGEN DE-TERMINANTS.

By examining the quantitative effects of TL phenotype on expression of H-2 antigens on the surfaces of thymocytes, Boyse et al. (26, 27) noted that while antigens specified by the K region of the H-2 complex were not quantitatively affected by TL phenotype, H-$2D$-specified antigens were profoundly influenced. Thymocytes of Tla^a (TL.1,2,3,5) and Tla^c (TL.2) homozygotes also homozygous for H-2 express significantly smaller quantities (about one-third to one-half less) of H-2D antigens (regardless of H-2 haplotype: H-2^a, H-2^b, or H-2^k) than do Tla^b (TL−) H-2 homozygous thymocytes. The reduction in H-2D antigens is approximately the same whether thymocytes express the Tla^a or Tla^c haplotype. Moreover, H-2D antigen reduction in Tla^a homozygotes heterozygous for H-2 (H-2^a/H-2^b) is nearly twice that occurring in Tla^a homozygotes also homozygous for H-2^a or H-2^b. In this case, H-$2D$-specified antigens of both haplotypes are reduced to the same extent. Antigen reduction occurs irrespective of whether Tla and H-$2D$ loci are inherited in a cis or trans configuration, indicating that extrachromosomal interaction between the cell surface products of these loci is most likely occurring.

Other investigators have noted a similar reduction in reactivity of H-2 antigens concomitant with the acquisition of tumor-specific antigens (86, 218), suggesting that the TL-H-2D interaction is not necessarily unique.

A similar relationship observed between cell surface expression of TL and H-2D antigens relative to TL modulation (26, 150) supports a phenotypic rather than a genotypic basis to this interaction. The exact nature of this TL-H-2D interrelationship has not been explained adequately, but it might reflect the existence of steric hindrance between the respective antigens at the cell surface (27). Apparently, TL and H-2D antigens are sufficiently close together on the cell surface that attachment of antibody to either antigen will interfere with, or block, subsequent binding of antibody to the other antigen (28). This subject will be considered further in Section II, C, 9.

B. Biology of TL Antigens

Cell surface antigens or other distinctive molecules that are confined to one particular cell type are often implicated as "recognition units" vital to the processes of differentiation (cf. 15). By distinguishing presumptive tissue types, such molecules could mediate cell-cell interactions to create order out of chaos during embryonic morphogenesis. At the other end of the scale, they may simply reflect the differentiated state of a cell, the product of a select genomic program.

1. TL ANTIGENS AND THYMOCYTE DIFFERENTIATION.

Since TL antigens do not appear on thymocytes of all mouse strains, it would seem that these cell surface antigens are certainly not essential for thymocyte differentiation (30). Since these molecules are only discernible as antigens, however, it is conceivable that functionally related molecules determined by currently unrecognized alleles within the *Tla* locus populate the surfaces of thymocytes not expressing known TL antigens. Thymocytes, of course, are not fully differentiated cells since they eventually become T lymphocytes. Therefore, residence within the thymus is only a transient, albeit essential, step in that pathway of differentiation. Acquisition of TL antigens accompanies only that one step, thymocyte progenitor cells from bone marrow, spleen, or lymph nodes, as well as newly emergent T cells being TL− (115, 180). Therefore, TL antigens probably do not represent distinctive cell surface molecules essential for morphogenetic differentiation.

Establishment of a functional role for TL antigens and possible homologous nonantigenic molecules is an extraordinarily difficult proposition, so information relative to that aspect of TL antigens is not likely to be forthcoming in the near future.

Since TL antigens are expressed only on cells within the thymus, that tissue must provide the environment necessary to effect their phenotypic expression. Schlesinger et al. (180) established this thymus requirement experimentally. When these investigators repopulated lethally irradiated A (TL+ or *Tla^a*) or C57BL/6 (TL− or *Tla^b*) mice with TL− bone marrow cells from either strain, they found that the thymuses of the resulting chimeras became repopulated with thymocytes expressing the *Tla* genotype of the donor, not the host. The repopulating cells were in fact derived from donor cells, as indicated by expression of H-2 antigenicity characteristic of the donor strain. There was a remote possibility that an undetectably small number of bone marrow cells from TL+ mice were actually TL+ and that these cells proliferated selectively and populated the TL− thymus. This conclusion is unlikely to have merit, however, since similar results were obtained when bone marrow cells from TL+ donors were exposed to TL antiserum and guinea pig complement *in vitro* (a procedure which should lyse any TL+ cells) prior to introduction into irradiated hosts. Thus, the thymus affects expression of the normal cellular *Tla* genotype, and this influence is provided by the thymuses of TL− as well as TL+ mice. The TL phenotype expressed is strictly determined by the *Tla* genotype of the cell.

Relative to these observations, Komura et al. (111) demonstrated that TL antibodies could be made by TL− (*Tla^b*) mice inoculated with bone marrow, spleen or lymph node cells from TL+ (*Tla^a*) mice. While once again it is possible that the inoculated cells contained some TL+ cells, it is more likely that the TL− inoculum populated the thymus, was induced to express TL antigens, and thus effectively elicited an antibody response from the host. Furthermore, no antibody was produced when the same experiment was performed with thymectomized hosts.

Within the thymuses of TL+ mouse strains, approximately 80–90% of the thymocytes express detectable quantities of TL antigens. These TL+ thymocytes are relatively small dense cells that also express considerable amounts of Thy-1, G_{IX}, and Ly antigens, but relatively few H-2 antigens (112, 113). The remaining TL− population consisted of larger, less dense cells expressing much greater amounts of H-2 antigens but relatively small quantities of Thy-1 and Ly antigens, and no G_{IX} antigen. This minor population seems to represent mature T lymphocytes just prior to peripheralization (112, 116, 164, 175), since they are resistant to cortisone treatment and whole-body irradiation (113, 178). The results of such studies should be interpreted with caution, however, due to possible contamination of thymocyte preparations with peripheral T lymphocytes from thymus-associated lymph nodes (116).

It seems likely that T lymphocytes are derived from the TL+ population of thymocytes, but this has not been absolutely established (112, 175). If that is the case, then the transient acquisition of TL antigens by cells only while in residence within the thymus is unique among known T lymphocyte surface antigens (with the possible exception of the MuLV-related thymocyte antigen G_{IX}—see Section III, C, 1). Other thymocyte antigens (e.g., Thy-1, H-2, Ly) undergo quantitative changes, but do not disappear from the cell surface when the cells leave the thymus.

Recently, it has been possible to duplicate the influence of the thymus on precursor thymocytes in vitro by treating bone marrow or spleen cells with thymus extracts (110). The active substance in these extracts has been identified as a polypeptide designated thymin or thymopoietin (14). Similar induction of thymocyte differentiation from precursor cells has been achieved with agents such as cyclic AMP, poly A:U and bacterial endotoxin, suggesting that thymopoietin provides nonspecific differentiation "signals" (173).

2. INTRACELLULAR REPRESENTATION OF TL ANTIGENS.

Is the phenotypic expression of TL antigens restricted to the cell surface or are these antigens also demonstrable intracellularly? Given that cell surface expression of TL antigens requires thymopoietin and that TL antigenicity may be modulated from the cell surface by antibody, is it possible that phenotypically TL− cells synthesize TL antigens but appearance on the cell surface is blocked by antibody or lack of thymopoietin?

Smith *et al.* (194) addressed these questions by examining subcellular fractions of various TL+ and TL− cell types for the presence of TL antigens demonstrable by inhibiting the cytotoxic effect of TL antisera on TL+ test cells. By this criterion, TL.1,2,3,5 antigens were present on microsomal and mitochondrial fractions of cells expressing these antigens on the cell surface, but were absent from nuclear and cytosol fractions. TL antigens were not demonstrable in any fractions from TL− cells. Therefore, phenotypic expression of TL antigens appears to involve genomic controls rather than selective controls operative at the cell surface.

3. ONTOGENY OF TL ANTIGENS.

Analysis of TL antigen expression in TL+ mouse strains during embryogenesis has indicated that TL+ thymocytes are first recognizable by 15–16 days of development, the same time that small lymphocytes can be detected, H-2 antigens appear, and other characteristics of thymocytes become apparent (175, 179). By 18 days, the full adult complement of TL antigens is present on thymocytes. No expression of TL antigens on thymocytes of TL− mouse strains has been detected at any period of embryonic development.

In order to determine whether TL− cells residing in the thymus primordium can directly give rise to TL+ cells, or whether TL+ cells are contributed by cells migrating into the thymus subsequently, Owen and Raff (156) cultured TL− 14-day A-strain thymic rudiments in diffusion chambers on chick chorioallantoic membranes. Normal numbers of TL+ cells were present in these rudiments within 4 days, evidence that TL+ cells developed from TL− cells present in the undifferentiated thymus.

4. BIOCHEMISTRY OF TL ANTIGENS.

As indicated in Sections I, B, 7 and II, A, 3, a peculiar relationship exists in quantitative representation of TL and H-2D antigens on the surfaces of mouse thymocytes and leukemia cells. As a result, phenotypic expression of TL antigens entails a significant reduction in the number of H-2D antigens detectable on thymocytes by quantitative absorption (27), while modulation of TL antigenicity results in a compensatory increase in H-2D antigens (26, 150).

This TL-H-2D phenotypic interaction suggested that antigens of both systems might reside on a common cell surface molecule and stimulated early attempts to solubilize and characterize TL antigens. These initial studies (52, 53) demonstrated that TL and H-2D antigens resided on separable molecules.

In the studies of Davies *et al.* (52), H-2 and TL antigens were solubilized from ASL1 leukemia cells (H-2^a, Tla^a) by hypotonic salt extraction of intact cells. DEAE-cellulose ion exchange chromatography separated these solubilized antigens into distinct fractions, as evidenced by

Table 3.   Molecular interrelationships between the five TL antigens and other sur~~ antigens on mouse thymocytes and leukemia cells determined by co-capping

Antigens Labeled First[a]	% Cells		Antigens Labeled Second—% Cells Co-capped[b]				
Specificities	Labeled	Capped	TL.1,2,3,5	TL.1,3,5	TL.2	TL.3,5	TL.2,3,5
C57BL/6/TL + Thymocytes							
—	—	—	5	3	0	4	6
TL.1,2,3,5	64	85	—	100	100	100	100
TL.1,3,5	65	78	91	—	100	95	95
TL.2	65	63	68	55	—	56	63
TL.3,5	59	85	94	93	88	—	96
TL.2,3,5[c]	65	85	100	100	100	100	—
$H-2^b(D)$[d]	77	52	5				
$H-2^b(K)$[d]	68	31	5				
$Thy-1.2$[e]	97	27	15				
$Ly-1.1$[f]	54	22	8				
$Ly-2.2$[g]	97	20	4				

ERLD Leukemia Cells			TL.1,2		TL.2		T
—	—	—	3		1		
TL.1,2	63	67	—		100		
TL.2	56	76	57		—		
TL.4	47	53	67		31		

a. Cells were incubated with the appropriate mouse alloantiserum (see Table 1 for TL antisera) for 30 min at 37°C, washed in the cold, then incubated with fluorescein isothiocyanate-conjugated goat anti-mouse IgG antib (green fluorescence) for 30 minutes at 37°C. Antibody concentrations were adjusted to those predetermined to af maximum cap formation. TL alloantisera were preabsorbed *in vitro* with thymocytes from the host strain, and sp cells from the donor strain, to remove possible autoantibody or *H(Tla)* histocompatibility antibodies, respectiv No cross-reactivity of any alloantiserum was demonstrable by cytotoxicity or immunofluorescence.

b. Cells were incubated for 30 minutes at 0°C with alloantibody directly conjugated to tetramethylrhodan isothiocyanate (red fluorescence), washed, and then examined by fluorescence microscopy. Cells with correspon~~ red and green fluorescent caps of label were considered co-capped.

c. Mixture of TL.2 and TL.3,5 alloantisera (see Table 1).

d. $(C57BL/6/H-2^i \times A)F_1$ anti-EL4 antiserum, absorbed with HTI $[H-2^b(K)/H-2^i(D)]$ or HTH $[H-2^i(K)/H-2^b$ strain spleen and lymph node cells, leaving $H-2^b(D)$ and $H-2^b(K)$ specificities, respectively (168).

e. $(A/Thy-1.1 \times AKR/H-2^b)F_1$ anti-ASL1.

f. C3H/An anti-CE thymocytes.

g. $(C3H \times C57BL/6/Ly-2.1)F_1$ anti-ERLD.

Interpretation: On thymocytes, anti-TL.1,3,5 co-caps TL.2, anti-TL.3,5 co-caps TL.1 and TL.2, anti-TL.2 co-caps TL.1, and anti-TL.2 partially co-caps TL.1, TL.3, and TL.5. Capping of $H-2$, Thy–1 or Ly antigens does co-cap TL antigens to a significant extent. On ERLD cells, anti-TL.1,2,3,5 co-caps TL.4, anti-TL.4 partially co-~ TL.1 and TL.2, and anti-TL.2 co-caps TL.4 slightly. Therefore, despite relatively poor co-capping induced by anti-~ and anti-TL.4 (probably reflecting relatively low ratios of antibody-bound antigens to unbound antigens, since ~ antisera are weak compared to the other antisera), TL.1, TL.2, TL.3, TL.4 and TL.5 antigens probably reside ~ common molecule, distinct from molecules bearing $H-2$, Thy–1 or Ly antigens.

the ability of the fractions to specifically absorb cytotoxic activity from appropriate antisera. When H-2^b-specified antigens and TL.1,2,4 antigens were solubilized from the C57BL/6 strain leukemia ERLD (the TL antigens being expressed anomalously), TL and H-2 antigens were again separable (53). In these studies, TL antigens appearing anomalously could not be distinguished from antigens appearing on leukemia cells arising in a strain that normally expresses TL antigens. Furthermore, there were indications that all TL specificities resided within the same fraction.

Subsequent investigations of solubilized cell surface antigens by radioimmunoprecipitation (136, 137, 225, 239) verified that TL and H-2D antigens, as well as H-2K and Thy-1 antigens, are confined to separate molecular entities. Similar results have been obtained by differential antibody-induced redistribution of one antigen into "caps" followed by labeling a second antigen under conditions minimizing capping: considerable co-capping of separate antigen specificities was observed (Table 3), the expected result if the different specificities resided on the same molecule (162, 196).

Perhaps just as interesting as these findings that TL and H-2 antigens reside on separate molecules was the realization that the two molecules are remarkably similar (223, 224). Because of this similarity and the considerably greater information available on the molecular structure of H-2 antigens, these antigens will be discussed prior to TL antigens.

Solubilization characteristics of H-2 antigens indicate that they are large glycoproteins (molecular weight > 100,000) integrated at one end into the lipid bilayer of the plasma membrane with the glycosylated portion and antigenic sites exposed to the external environment (90, 137, 138, 182, 227). Papain solubilization of the externally exposed portions of H-2 antigens from spleen lymphocytes and lymphoma cells produces two distinct glycopolypeptides, with molecular weights of about 35,000–38,000, that seem to correspond to separate H-2D and H-2K molecules (92, 137, 138). Antigenic sites are located on the polypeptide chains, not on the saccharide groups (183). Solubilization of H-2 antigens by detergent disruption of the cell surface membrane produces two glycoproteins with molecular weights of about 44,000, each noncovalently associated with a small (11,000–12,000 molecular weight) nonglycosylated polypeptide chain (166, 187, 225). A close homology between this small polypeptide and the $C_H 3$ constant region of mouse IgG$_{2a}$ immunoglobulin, and to β_2-microglobulin associated with HLA histocompatibility alloantigens on human lymphoid cells (47, 82) has been demonstrated (9).

Henning et al. (90) have proposed that within the cell surface each H-2 molecule consists of one 46,000 molecular weight polypeptide subunit (heavy, or H, chain) associated noncovalently with a β_2-microglobulin-like light (L) chain. Detergent-solubilized H-2 antigens consisted of dimers (H_2L_2) linked by disulfide bonds between the H chains in a manner analogous to an immunoglobulin molecule, but dimer formation was considered a solubilization artifact. Other investigators favor an H_2L_2 configuration to native H-2 antigens (226), or even larger oligomers (182). However, Vitetta et al. (227) point out the difficulty of determining the exact molecular configuration, and the possibility that monomers and dimers may both occur on certain cell types. Integration of H-2 antigens into the lipid bilayer occurs at the COOH terminus of the H chain (90).

TL antigens solubilized from mouse leukemia cells by papain digestion possess biochemical properties quite similar to papain-solubilized H-2 antigens in that both are glycosylated polypeptides with molecular weights of approximately 35,000 (136). Detergent solubilization results in a glycosylated polypeptide of molecular weight approximately 45,000 (224). The carbohydrate moieties of the TL molecule (molecular weight 4500) are somewhat larger than those of the H-2 molecules (molecular weight 3500) (136). Associated with the glycopolypeptide of TL antigens (H chain) is a smaller polypeptide (L chain, molecular weight 12,000) similar to β_2-microglobulin and the polypeptide associated with H-2 antigens (155, 225).

The number of H and L chains comprising individual TL antigens is unknown and may depend upon the method of solubilization. For example, Anundi et al. (4) have proposed an H_2L_2 configuration for EDTA-extracted TL antigens, while detergent solubilization produces antigens composed of single H chains (227). The H and L chains of TL antigens co-electrophorese with the H and L chains of H-2 antigens (225). All five TL antigen specificities appear to be associated with the same molecules on the basis of co-modulation (26, 29, 150; C. Stackpole and J. Jacobson, unpublished observations), radioimmunoprecipitation (125, 241), and co-capping (Table 3).

Vitetta and Uhr (223) have noted the remarkable biochemical similarities between H-2 antigens, TL antigens, and cell surface immunoglobulins. All three molecules are composed of heavy and light polypeptide chains, and the β_2-microglobulin-like light chain associated with H-2 and TL antigens is structurally similar to a portion of the immunoglobulin molecule. It may be that the H-2 and Tla loci (and perhaps other loci; see below) in linkage group IX and immunoglobulin-determining genes are derived from the same ancestral gene by duplication.

As biochemical analysis of murine cell surface antigens progresses, it is becoming apparent that antigens other than TL that are specified by genes residing on linkage group IX in close proximity to, or within, the H-2 complex also show molecular similarities to H-2 antigens.

A cell surface antigen identified on mouse F9 primitive teratocarcinoma cells, cleavage-stage mouse embryos, and mature sperm, and designated F9 (11), appears to be specified by a gene at the T/t locus, which is closely linked to H-2 on linkage group IX (10, 12). The cells on which F9 antigen have been identified are lacking demonstrable H-2 antigens. Radioimmunoprecipitation analysis of F9 antigen reveals a molecular composition similar to H-2 and TL antigens: a 44,000 molecular weight polypeptide and a noncovalently associated 12,000–14,000 molecular weight β_2-microglobulin-like polypeptide (226). As in the case of H-2 antigens, individual heavy chains, each with an associated light chain, may be linked by disulfide bonds to form dimers or oligomers, although the precise molecular configuration has not been determined. Appella et al. (9) have shown that the small chain of F9 antigen is not antigenically identical to the small chain of H-2 antigens, although structurally and/or functionally they may be similar.

C. Mechanism of TL Antigenic Modulation in Vitro

The phenomenon of TL antigenic modulation was, of course, initially described in vivo, and modulation in the animal is obviously the process of primary interest with regard to mechanisms utilized by tumor cells to escape immunological destruction. As is so often the case, however, analysis of modulation in vitro has proven a more valuable system for investigating the underlying mechanism. Just how comparable the processes of modulation occurring in vivo and in vitro are will be discussed in Section II, D.

1. FACTORS INFLUENCING MODULATION. The rate and extent of modulation of TL antigenicity obtainable depends upon a number of factors, including temperature, immunoglobulin class represented by TL antibody, antibody concentration and specificity, source of complement, cell type, method of assay, and availability of serum factors. The role of each of these factors in modulation will be considered separately.

a. Temperature. In their initial investigations of in vitro modulation of TL antigenicity on RADA1 leukemia cells, Old et al. (150) found that modulation of TL.1, TL.3 and TL.5 antigens was completed within 1–2 hours at 37°C, was incomplete within that time period at 22°C, and occurred to a negligible extent at 0°C. Failure of cells incubated with TL antiserum at 0°C to modulate was clearly not due to incomplete sensitization with TL antibody, since cells incubated at 0°C with antibody were fully sensitive to lysis by guinea pig complement.

The effect of low temperature on modulation has quite logically been attributed to the depressed metabolic activity of cells maintained under those conditions. Recent experiments, however, indicate that such a conclusion is no longer valid (204). First of all, when RADA1 cells were saturated with TL.1,2,3,5 antibody at 0°, then washed and further incubated under modulating conditions for 1 hour at 37°, no modulation occurred unless normal mouse serum was added during the second incubation. Also, while the degree of modulation was related to temperature in virtually linear fashion (except for a significant decrease in modulating capacity at 18°), exactly the same relationship was obtained when cells were modulated under normal conditions at 37° with heat-inactivated (56° for 1 hour) TL antiserum (which retains practically no modulating capacity—see Sections II, C, 1h and II, C, 7) plus normal mouse serum preincubated at various temperatures between 0° and 37° (204). These results indicate that temperature is affecting the serum factor(s) in TL antiserum and normal mouse serum that are involved in the modulation process (see Sections II, C, 1h and II, C, 7). The specific modulating factor affected by temperature appears to be the third component (C3) of mouse complement, since modulation-promoting activity of the analogous complement component, human C3, has precisely the same thermosensitive characteristics (including marked lability at 18°) as modulating activity in mouse serum (204).

b. Immunoglobulin Class Represented by TL Antibody.   TL antibody in hyperimmune antisera consists predominantly of 7S IgG_{2a} immunoglobulin (66; C. Stackpole and S. Galuska, unpublished observations). When TL− (C57BL/6 × A/TL−)F_1 mice are initially challenged with a large number (15–30 × 10^6) of RADA1 leukemia cells (Tla^a), however, most TL.1,2,3,5 antibody produced within the first week consists of 19S IgM immunoglobulin (C. Stackpole, unpublished observations). This antibody is cytotoxic on appropriate TL+ cells but fails to induce modulation of TL antigens on RADA1 cells either in vitro or in vivo (see Section II, C, 10 for further discussion). In antisera containing both IgG and IgM antibody, modulating capacity is directly proportional to the amount of IgG antibody present.

c. Antibody Concentration.   Old et al. (150) found that TL.1, TL.3 and TL.5 antigens on RADA1 cells were completely modulated by TL.1,3,5 antiserum [(BALB/c × C3H)F_1 anti-ASL1—see Table 1] after 60 minutes of incubation in vitro at 37°C with an antiserum dilution of 1/320 and guinea pig complement (the titer, or 50% dilution end-point, of that antiserum in a direct cytotoxicity test was 1/256). At antiserum dilutions of 1/10 and 1/640, modulation was completed in 90 minutes and 120 minutes, respectively. Thus, the optimum antiserum concentration for modulation was less than required to achieve lysis of 50% of the cells in the presence of complement; sensitization of cells to complement lysis was also not necessary, since some modulation occurred even with antiserum diluted to 1/2560, although no lysis by complement was evident. This observation suggested that not all TL antigens on the cell surface need be bound by antibody in order to achieve modulation. In these experiments, 5% normal mouse serum was added in tests involving weak antiserum dilutions.

Subsequent investigations of TL modulation on RADA1 cells by Stackpole *et al.* (203) employing higher-titered TL.1,2,3,5 antisera [(C57BL/6 × A/TL−)F$_1$ anti-ASL1 or (C57BL/6 × A/TL−)F$_1$ anti-A thymocytes—see Table 1] in the absence of supplemental normal serum failed to confirm the relationship between antibody concentration and modulation suggested by Old *et al.* (150). Modulation was essentially complete after 60 minutes of incubation with 1/10 to 1/100 dilutions of antiserum with a titer of 1/3000 on RADA1 cells. However, at an antiserum dilution of 1/1000, modulation was only about 25% complete after 120 minutes, even though cells were completely lysed by guinea pig complement in cytotoxicity tests with antiserum at that dilution.

These discrepancies may be accounted for by the recent finding that the modulating capacity of a high-titered TL antiserum is limited not by the amount of antibody available as much as by the content of heat-labile serum factors essential for modulation (204; see Sections II, C, 1h and II, C, 7); thus, addition of normal mouse serum to low concentrations of TL antiserum (dilutions greater than 1/100) enhances modulation of RADA1 cells and A/J thymocytes (Fig. 1).

Provided that antibody is present in considerable excess and sufficient serum factors are available, modulation of TL antigenicity on RADA1 cells is relatively insensitive to TL antiserum concentration. Under the same conditions, however, modulation of A/J thymocytes is reduced significantly at extremely high TL antiserum concentrations (dilutions less than 1/100), as is cap formation on the cell surface (Fig. 1). When serum factors in these high concentrations of antiserum were destroyed by heating at 56° (antibody was not affected by heating) and replaced with constant 1/100 dilutions of normal serum, a comparable "prozone" effect was obtained, indicating that excess TL antibody and not excess serum factors suppresses modulation of thymocyte TL antigenicity. On thymocytes, but not on RADA1 cells, modulation exhibits exactly the same antibody concentration dependence as capping of TL antigens (Fig. 1). The relevance of these observations to the mechanism of modulation on RADA1 cells and thymocytes *in vitro* will be considered in detail in Section II, C, 5.

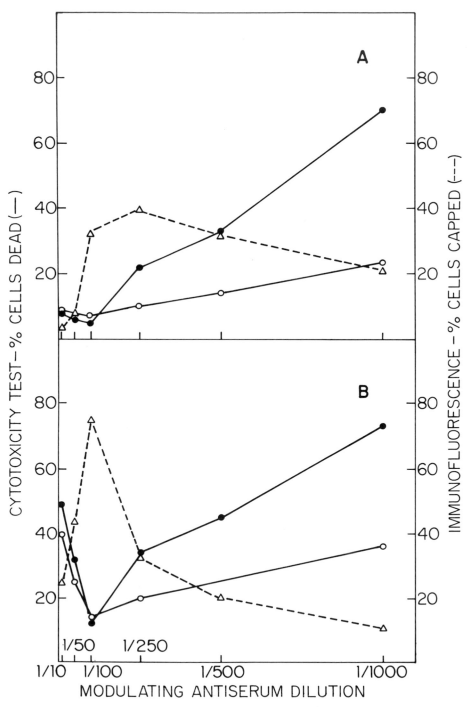

d. Antibody Specificity. All five recognized TL antigen specificities appear to reside on the same basic cell surface molecule (see Section II, B, 4), so that modulation of one specificity can co-modulate other specificities, both *in vivo* and *in vitro* (26, 29, 150). For example, TL.1,3,5 antiserum modulates TL.2 as well as TL.1, TL.3 and TL.5 antigens, TL.3,5 antiserum modulates TL.1 and TL.2 antigens in addition to TL.3 and TL.5, and TL.4 antiserum modulates TL.1 and TL.2 antigens as well as TL.4. Curiously, however, TL.2 antiserum (C57BL/6 anti-129 thymocytes—see Table 1) failed to modulate TL.2 or the other TL specificities *in vitro*.

In the studies of Old *et al.* (150), modulation of RADA1 cells with TL.1,2,3,5 antiserum (C57BL/6 anti-ASL1—see Table 1) occurred to a lesser extent (or more slowly) than modulation with TL.1,3,5 antiserum. This difference was considered to be due to the presence of TL.2 antibody in the TL.1,2,3,5 antiserum, since removal of that antibody from the antiserum by absorption with TL.2+ thymocytes *in vitro* rendered the antiserum comparable to TL.1,3,5 antiserum in modulating capacity.

We have reinvestigated the modulating capacity of TL.2 antibody, since in comparing the modulating capacity of TL.1,2,3,5 and TL.1,3,5 antiserum prepared in the *same* mice [(C57BL/6 × A/TL−)F_1—Table 1], no differences in rate or extent of modulation of TL antigens induced by the two antisera were apparent. Furthermore, while TL.2 antiserum did modulate TL.2, TL.1,2,3,5 and TL.1,2,4 specificities poorly, addition of normal (C57BL/6 × A/TL−)F_1 mouse serum during modulation rendered TL.2 antiserum as effective as any other TL antiserum in promoting modulation (C. Stackpole and J. Jacobson, unpublished observations). The poor capacity for TL.2 antiserum, as well as TL.1,2,3,5 antiserum prepared in C57BL/6 mice, to modulate is, therefore, not due to peculiarities

---

Fig. 1.   Effect of TL antibody and heat-labile serum factor(s) concentrations on modulation and capping of TL antigens on (A) RADA1 leukemia cells and (B) A/J thymocytes. 5×10^6 cells were incubated in 1 ml of medium 199 supplemented with 2% gammaglobulin-free fetal bovine serum at 37° for 2 hours with various dilutions of (C57BL/6 × A/TL−)F_1 anti-ASL1 (anti-TL.1,2,3,5) serum (●), or anti-TL serum preheated at 56° for 1 hour plus a constant 1/100 dilution of (C57BL/6 × A/TL−)F_1 normal mouse serum (○). Residual cytotoxicity was determined with fresh anti-TL serum and guinea pig serum diluted 1/3, each point representing the percent cell lysis at an antiserum dilution of 1/100. Unheated and heated antisera had the same titer on RADA1 cells and on thymocytes, but heated antiserum retained no modulating capacity. Modulation induced by this high-titered antiserum is thus limited more by the availability of serum factor(s) than by TL antibody concentration. Similar results were obtained with other TL antisera. For determination of capping, modulated cells were labeled with fluorescein isothiocyanate-conjugated goat anti-mouse IgG antibody at 0°.

of TL.2 antibody or TL.2 antigens, but rather to heat-labile serum factor(s) in mouse serum responsible for modulation; C57BL/6-strain serum has unusually poor modulating capacity compared with serum from most mice (see Section II, C, 7).

Also of considerable concern in studies of TL modulation is the possible presence of contaminating antibodies in antisera supposedly prepared against TL antigens specifically. Yu and Cohen (239) have, for example, found that TL.1,3,5 antiserum prepared in (BALB/c × C3H)F₁ mice against ASL1 contained antibodies to two additional antigens present on ASL1 cells that were distinct from antibodies formed against TL.1, TL.3, and TL.5 antigens. Reaction of these antibodies with ASL1 surface components was ascertained by radioimmunprecipitation of detergent-solubilized membrane proteins previously labeled enzymatically with ¹²⁵I. The major contaminant antibody appeared to detect a leukemia-specific antigen not present on normal lymphoid cells. The minor contaminant antibody might have formed due to histoincompatibility between (BALB/c × C3H)F₁ and A strain mice, or might represent autoantibody (239).

We have also found that supposedly TL.1,2,3,5-specific antiserum raised in (C57BL/6 × A/TL−)F₁ mice against ASL1 cells contains additional antibody cross-reactive with RADA1 cells but not with A/J or C57BL/6/TL+ thymocytes (J. Jacobson and C. Stackpole, unpublished observations). This contaminant antibody is not cytotoxic under normal conditions, but is demonstrable by immunofluorescence and absorption. Esmon and Little (66) have purified TL.1,2,3,5 antiserum (A/TL− anti-ASL1) by DEAE-cellulose chromatography and starch-block electrophoresis and have obtained fractions that are noncytotoxic or weakly cytotoxic to ASL1 and RADA1 cells. Nevertheless, antibodies in these fractions bound to the cell surface specifically and to a degree equivalent to cytotoxic antibodies in other purified fractions.

Interestingly, none of the contaminant antibodies present in TL antisera prepared by immunization with ASL1 cells appears to participate in, or interfere with, modulation by TL antibodies (67, 97, 203, 240).

A TL.1,2,3,5 antiserum prepared by immunization with thymocytes, (C57BL/6 × A/TL−)F₁ anti-A/J thymocytes, has so far been found free of contaminant antibodies (C. Stackpole and J. Jacobson, unpublished observations).

e. Source of Complement.   In all of the studies on modulation of TL antigenicity by Boyse, Old, and their colleagues (22, 25, 26, 114, 150), modulation was demonstrated as a loss of sensitivity of cells to the lytic action of guinea pig complement in the presence of fresh TL antiserum. This source of complement was provided by pooled whole guinea pig serum. At effective concentrations (dilutions of 1/3 to 1/4), this serum was generally toxic to mouse lymphoid cells (presumably due to heteroantibody), especially thymocytes (180), and had to be rendered nontoxic by absorption with cells from mouse leukemias or tumors such as the sarcoma Meth A.

More recently, modulation has been studied with comparable concentrations of guinea pig serum that is inherently: (1) nontoxic to leukemia cells but toxic to normal mouse lymphoid cells (toxic guinea pig complement), or (2) nontoxic for both leukemia cells and lymphoid cells (nontoxic guinea pig complement) (203). On leukemia cells, toxic and nontoxic complement give comparable results, but toxic serum is slightly more sensitive. Other investigators have employed reconstituted lyophilized whole guinea pig serum obtained commercially, either unabsorbed (124, 125, 240, 241) or absorbed with indubiose agarose (67).

These variations in guinea pig complement might account for differences in cytotoxic sensitivity of TL+ cells to TL antisera noted by various investigators. For example, Yu et al. (241), Liang and Cohen (124) and Esmon and Little (67) have failed to obtain cytolysis of TL+ RADA1 cells in the in vitro cytotoxicity test using various TL antisera and guinea pig complement, although rabbit complement could induce cell lysis (67). These results are particularly puzzling, since Boyse, Old, and their colleagues, and Stackpole and his associates have consistently found that RADA1 cells are highly sensitive to cytolysis by TL antisera and guinea pig complement (22, 150, 203).

To determine whether these differences are due to the particular complement used, we have prepared guinea pig complement as described by several investigators and compared their cytolytic effects on unmodulated and modulated RADA1 cells (Fig. 2). Nontoxic, Meth A-absorbed toxic, and indubiose-absorbed reconstituted complements gave comparable results, while the reconstituted complement obtained from the same source as that employed by Cohen and his colleagues (240) was quite toxic and failed to demonstrate complete modulation. Failure of investigators to utilize standard sources of complement could, therefore, lead to considerable differences in apparent rate and extent of modulation. Nevertheless, the differences in source of complement do not seem to explain the cytotoxic resistance of RADA1 cells observed by some investigators (67, 124) and extreme sensitivity noted by others (22, 150, 203). Possibly, variants of RADA1 cells are being propagated that differ in cytotoxic sensitivity to TL antibody and guinea pig complement.

It is interesting to note that cells modulated by the criterion of acquired resistance to TL antiserum and guinea pig complement remain sensitive to the lytic effects of rabbit serum used at comparable concentrations (203; Fig. 2). Rabbit serum so used is quite toxic to mouse lym-

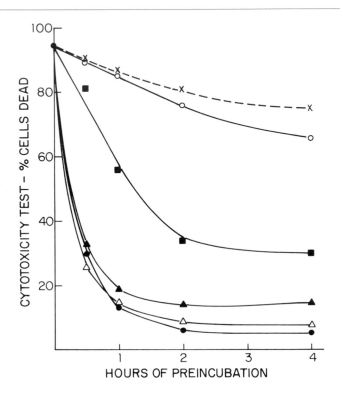

Fig. 2. Effects of different sources of guinea pig complement on modulation of TL.1,2,3,5 antigenicity on RADA1 cells. Cells were preincubated at 37° with a 1/100 dilution of (C57BL/6 × A/TL−)F₁ anti-A thymocyte (anti-TL.1,2,3,5) serum, washed, and then residual antigenicity was determined by cytotoxicity of fresh TL antiserum and the various complements described below. Results are expressed as percent cells lysed at an antiserum concentration of 1/100. ●, nontoxic whole pooled guinea pig serum, stored at −80° and used at a dilution of 1/4, as described by Stackpole *et al.* (203); ▲, reconstituted lyophilized guinea pig serum, obtained from Colorado Serum Co., Denver, Colorado, absorbed with dry indubiose agarose (80 mg/ml) for 1 hour on ice, diluted with an equal volume of phosphate-buffered saline, centrifuged, and stored at −80°, as described by Esmon and Little (67), and tested at a final dilution of 1/10; ■, reconstituted lyophilized guinea pig serum, obtained from Beckman Diagnostics, Chamblee, Georgia, stored at −80°, as described by Yu and Cohen (239), but used at a dilution of 1/5 rather than concentrated (239), since undiluted serum was extremely cytotoxic; ○, highly toxic whole guinea pig serum, unabsorbed, stored at −80° and used at a dilution of 1/3; △, the same serum, but absorbed with cells of the BALB/c sarcoma Meth A, as described by Old *et al.* (150) prior to storage at −80°, and used at a dilution of 1/3; ×, rabbit serum absorbed with mouse lymphoid cells in the presence of EDTA (31), stored at −80°, and used at a dilution of 1/4, as described by Stackpole *et al.* (203). Differences in extent of modulation are due to inherent cytotoxicity of some complement sources for RADA1 cells.

phoid cells and must be absorbed extensively with these cells in the absence of free divalent cations to render the serum free of toxicity but extremely high in complement activity (31).

f. Cell Type. While modulation of TL antigenicity on RADA1 cells occurs rapidly, other leukemia cells, such as ASL1, and normal thymocytes generally modulate more slowly (67, 125, 150, 203, 240). The suggestion has been made that these differences in rate of modulation reflect the metabolic activity and growth characteristics of the cells (26, 150). Whether that conclusion is valid or not has not been ascertained, but there does seem to be a positive correlation between rate of modulation and degree of lateral mobility exhibited by TL antigens within the cell surface membrane (see Section II, C, 5).

The tendency for leukemia cells and thymocytes to modulate does not appear to play an important role in the capacity for such cells to elicit antibody formation during immunization. In this regard, thymocytes and leukemia cells such as ASL1 that modulate slowly effectively stimulate antibody production when inoculated into TL− mice, but so do rapidly modulating leukemias such as RADA1 and ERLD (97).

g. Method of Assaying Cytolysis. In all of the studies on modulation of TL antigenicity discussed in this review (22, 25, 26, 67, 97, 114, 125, 150, 168, 203, 204, 240, 241), modulation was judged as acquisition of resistance to cytolysis, indicated by uptake of trypan blue dye. This method depends upon lysis of the cell surface membrane sufficiently to enable the dye to enter the cell. As Boyse *et al.* (24) pointed out, many cells that appear microscopically to be obviously lysed do not incorporate trypan blue, perhaps because they are too severely disrupted. However, there is another group of cells that appears to be lysed by a more subtle criterion of membrane disruption and also does not take up trypan blue. This is especially true in cytotoxicity tests with guinea pig complement and antisera to TL antigens or monospecific H-2 antisera (168); in contrast, multispecific H-2 antisera generally effect cytolysis that results in trypan blue uptake by nearly all cells (Figs. 3 and 4). For this reason, the degree of cytolysis in the TL system is routinely judged by a combination of those cells incorporating trypan blue *plus* cells that appear to be lysed microscopically; that is, the cell surface membrane appears to have lost its integrity. This is the criterion on which modulation studies by Boyse, Old and colleagues, and in our laboratory, are based.

But how do we know that cells failing to incorporate trypan blue dye but displaying subtle microscopic signs of lysis are actually dead? One way is to correlate the microscopic appearance of cells with the capacity for a similarly treated sample of cells to proliferate in tissue culture (Figs.

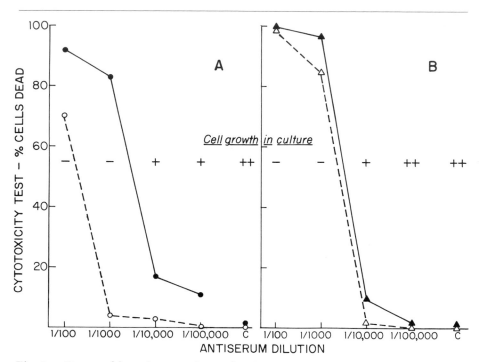

Fig. 3. Trypan blue dye uptake and microscopic appearance as criteria for cytolysis in the *in vitro* cytotoxicity test applied to the TL and H-2 antigen systems. *A*, RADA1 cells incubated at 37° for 45 minutes with varying dilutions of (C57BL/6 × A/TL−)F₁ anti-A thymocytes (anti-TL.1,2,3,5) serum and guinea pig serum, diluted 1/4. Cytolysis was assessed by trypan blue uptake and microscopic indication of cell membrane disruption (●) or trypan blue uptake alone (○). *B*, similar test on RADA1 cells, but with C57BL/6 anti-Meth A (H-2^b vs. H-2^d) serum; cytolysis determined by trypan blue uptake and microscopic appearance (▲) or trypan blue uptake alone (△). In both cases, *C* represents a complement cytotoxic control with antiserum omitted. See Fig. 4 for the microscopic appearance of cells from tests A and B. Cell growth in culture was determined by washing cells from samples prepared identically, but to which trypan blue was not added, with sterile medium (RPMI-1640 plus 8% fetal bovine serum, penicillin, and streptomycin) and incubating each sample at 37° under suspension culture conditions for 48 hours, at which time cells were enumerated.

3 and 4). Use of this method permits accurate microscopic assessment of cytolysis, an assessment that should be as precise as possible because it is the only criterion by which modulation is measured.

h. Serum Modulating Factor(s). Stackpole *et al.* (203) observed that heating TL.1,2,3,5 antiserum at 56° for 1 hour immediately before

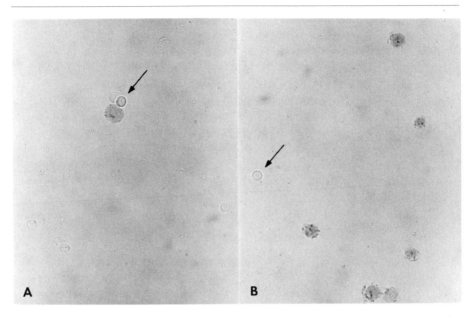

Fig. 4. Microscopic appearance of RADA1 cells from the cytotoxicity tests described in Fig. 3. *A*, representative cells from the TL cytotoxicity test at a TL.1,2,3,5 antiserum dilution of 1/1000. An identical sample of cells failed to grow in culture. Only one cell has incorporated trypan blue dye. Several cells are obviously lysed but have not taken up dye, while several others are considered lysed because they do not appear refractive and fully spherical as do typical untreated cells and the one cell considered viable in this field (*arrow*). *B*, cells from the H-2 cytotoxicity test, at an antiserum dilution of 1/100. These cells also did not grow in culture. The only cell considered viable (*arrow*) has not incorporated dye. × 700.

testing profoundly reduced (by about 70%) the capacity of this antiserum to modulate RADA1 leukemia cells. However, the original modulating capacity of heated TL antiserum could be restored by adding normal mouse serum during sensitization of the cells with TL antibody. Thus, some heat-labile factor or factors in TL antiserum and mouse serum in general appeared to be "blocking" the lytic interaction between guinea pig complement and cell-bound TL antigen-antibody complexes. As noted previously in this section, serum modulating factors (SMF) rather than TL antibody seem to be limiting in terms of modulating capacity of high-titered TL antisera.

Several investigators have studied TL antigenic modulation using TL antisera previously heated at 56° for 30 minutes (67, 240, 241). In view of the results obtained by Stackpole *et al.* (203), it might be expected that these antisera would be incapable of promoting modulation and yet some modulation was achieved. However, those investigators employing heated antiserum froze the sera before use. Since Stackpole et al. (204) have demonstrated that freeze-thawing heated serum restores considerable SMF activity, then antiserum that is heated and freeze-thawed should still retain some modulating capacity. In fact, Esmon and Little (67) have found no differences between the modulating capacities of unheated and heated (and freeze-thawed) TL antisera on TL+ thymocytes.

2. DYNAMICS OF TL ANTIGENS WITHIN THE CELL SURFACE MEMBRANE.

In 1971, Taylor et al. (216) demonstrated by immunofluorescence that attachment of bivalent antibody to Ig molecules on the surfaces of viable mouse lymphocytes under physiological conditions resulted in rapid lateral displacement of uniformly distributed molecules into extensive aggregates or "patches"; on many cells these patches subsequently coalesced into a single aggregate or "cap." Patch and cap formation were temperature-dependent processes occurring primarily at room temperature or higher. In addition, formation of caps required cellular metabolic activity and was followed by rapid and virtually complete internalization of the aggregated complexes by pinocytosis. Capping was subsequently shown to occur over the Golgi region of the cell (54).

Innumerable investigations have since established the generality of lateral displacement and aggregation of surface receptors for a wide variety of bivalent and multivalent ligands on most cells not confined to a rigid tissue matrix, by a process that presumably reflects the dynamic disposition of integral membrane proteins within a fluid lipid matrix (64, 139, 140, 181, 188, 189, 198). While the proposal has been made that lateral displacement of cell surface receptors into patches requires cross-linking of the receptors by multivalent ligands (54), cross-linking may not be essential in certain cases (201, 203); ligands might promote aggregation of receptors as a consequence of perturbing some sort of electrostatic balance at the cell surface responsible for maintaining molecular separation under physiological conditions (198).

Antibody-induced redistribution of TL and other surface antigens on mouse thymocytes and leukemia cells has been examined by a number of investigators (55, 128, 200–203), and the general results are particularly interesting with regard to TL modulation. Comparative studies of TL, H-2, and Thy-1 (θ) antigens on thymocytes by immunofluorescence (128, 202) and immunoelectronmicroscopy (55, 200) tend to indicate that TL antigens are more susceptible to redistribution into patches and caps than the other antigens. When A/J thymocyte antigens were labeled indirectly with mouse alloantisera for 30 minutes followed by fluoresceinated rabbit anti-mouse IgG antibody for 30 minutes, both at 37°, TL caps formed on a maximum of 80% of the cells, while H-2 (D and K) and Thy-1 antigens capped on only 25% and 40% of the cells, respectively (202). Capping of TL antigens also occurred more rapidly at 37° than capping of the other antigens and was less susceptible to inhibition by sodium azide, an agent that suppresses cellular metabolic activity. Likewise, TL antigens on thymocytes were more readily aggregated into patches than H-2 and Thy-1 antigens when labeled with specific alloantisera followed by ferritin-conjugated anti-mouse IgG antibody and examined by electron microscopy (55).

Redistribution of surface antigens on mouse thymocytes and RADA1 leukemia cells into patches and caps generally proceeds more slowly and is less extensive when cells are incubated at 37° with mouse alloantiserum alone, but on both cell types redistribution of TL antigens occurs more rapidly and extensively than other detectable antigens (C. Stackpole, unpublished observations).

Surprisingly, examination of TL caps on thymocytes and leukemia cells by electron microscopy revealed that the caps usually formed over the pole of the cell that was opposite from the position of the Golgi complex (200, 203); furthermore, the caps remained for hours without evidence of appreciable internalization by pinocytosis. Long-term retention of TL caps on thymocytes and leukemia cells has also been observed by Loor et al. (128) and Esmon and Little (67). This type of cap formation was quite distinct from the general occurrence of capping over the Golgi region of the cell followed by rapid internalization (54, 216, 221).

Further analysis demonstrated that capping opposite the Golgi region was a characteristic of thymocytes and thymus-derived leukemia cells rather than being peculiar to TL antigens. Capping on lymphocytes usually occurred over the Golgi region. While both types of capping seemed to require cellular metabolic activity, capping over the Golgi region was inhibited dramatically by cytochalasin B, while cap formation opposite the Golgi region was unaffected. Since cytochalasin B has a disruptive effect on the functioning of contractile cytoplasmic microfilaments in general (230), microfilaments might be responsible for "driving" cap formation on lymphocytes, while another mechanism must be operative in cap formation opposite the Golgi region (198, 200).

3. FATE OF MODULATED TL ANTIGEN-ANTIBODY COMPLEXES.

As noted previously, analysis of TL modulation *in vitro* suggested to Old et al. (150) that modulated TL antigen-antibody complexes were lost from the cell surface by a process requiring cellular metabolic activity. Loss of these complexes could presumably occur either by shedding from the cell surface or by internalization via pinocytotic vesicles. The modulated cell surface was considered to be denuded of TL antigens since antigenicity could not be demonstrated by cytotoxicity with guinea pig complement, modulated cells failed to absorb TL antibody from antiserum, and blocking TL antibody could not be demonstrated by immunofluorescence.

Yu and Cohen (240) favored pinocytosis as a mechanism for the apparent loss of all modulated TL antigens from ASL1 leukemia cells, even though considerable amounts of antigens remained on the surfaces of modulated cells. These investigators labeled the surface proteins of ASL1 cells with ^{125}I by use of lactoperoxidase and then incubated the cells at 37° for 20 hours with TL antiserum or normal mouse serum as a control. After 10 and 20 hours, the cells were extracted with the nonionic detergent NP-40 and the specific activity of antigens precipitated with fresh TL antiserum was determined. By this criterion, after 10 hours and with modulation virtually complete, about 55% of the original amount of antigen remained on modulated ASL1 cells compared with about 80% on control modulated cells. Even after 20 hours the amount of antigen remaining on modulated cells was almost 50% of the original amount.

However, analysis of the antigens remaining on modulated cells by electrophoresis revealed that virtually all of these remaining antigens were recognized by contaminant antibodies in the TL antiserum and thus were not TL antigens. It should be pointed out, however, that if TL antigens were aggregated within the cell surface membrane by antibody during modulation, then such aggregates might escape detection by failing to solubilize completely in the presence of NP-40 and, therefore, might be lost in the insoluble "nuclear" pellet (222).

Stackpole et al. (203) examined modulation of TL antigenicity on RADA1 leukemia cells and A/J thymocytes by immunofluorescence and immunoelectronmicroscopy, as well as by cytotoxicity employing guinea pig and rabbit complement. Most modulated TL antigen-antibody complexes remained bound to the cell surface but displaced laterally and aggregated within the membrane, while a smaller proportion of complexes was internalized by pinocytosis. Cells were modulated with TL.1,2,3,5 antisera raised in (C57BL/6 × A/TL−)F$_1$ mice against either ASL1 cells or A thymocytes (see Table 1).

The fate of bivalent and monovalent (Fab) TL antibody during modulation was visualized by direct or indirect immunofluorescence. In both cases considerable antibody remained bound to the cell surface when modulation was completed (1–2 hours for RADA1 cells, 4 hours for thymocytes). Bivalent antibody was displaced into conspicuous patches or caps while monovalent antibody was only slightly aggregated on the cell surface. Internalization of fluoresceinated bivalent TL antibody by pinocytosis was visualized with pinocytized label ultimately coalescing within the Golgi region of the cell. Capping generally occurred over the pole of the cell opposite from the Golgi region (see the previous section), which may explain the lack of extensive pinocytosis of modulating bivalent antibody. Since modulation with monovalent antibody occurred without patch or cap formation, gross topographical displacement of TL antigen-antibody complexes is apparently not required for modulation. The lack of extensive lateral aggregation of TL antigen-Fab antibody fragments may also explain the relative lack of internalization of these complexes. Pinocytosis may require a certain amount of ligand-induced aggregation of receptors on the cell surface (77), and Fab antibody may not induce sufficient aggregation to stimulate this process. A subtle "microaggregation" may be the requirement for modulation.

Further indication that TL antibody is retained on RADA1 cells following modulation was obtained by incubating 10^8 cells with excess TL.1,2,3,5 antiserum at 37° for 4 hours, then thoroughly washing the cells prior to testing a sample for degree of modulation and incubating the remainder in undiluted normal mouse serum at 37° for 1 hour. Although the cells were completely modulated, significant amounts of antibody were released in cytolytically active form into the serum (C. Stackpole and J. Jacobson, unpublished observations). A similar approach has been used to demonstrate retention of TL antibody on cells modulated in vivo (97; see Section II, D).

Evidence that modulated TL antigen, and not just TL antibody, remains on the cell surface was provided by the retention of sensitivity of modulated cells to the lytic action of rabbit complement (203).

Esmon and Little (66, 67) have employed an indirect radioimmunoassay to study TL modulation on RADA1 and ASL1 cells and C57BL/6/TL+ thymocytes. TL antigen-antibody complexes bound to the cell surface were assayed by cell binding of ^{125}I-labeled rabbit anti-mouse Ig antibody. Although ASL1 cells and thymocytes were modulated with TL.1,2,3,5 antiserum (A/TL− anti-ASL1—see Table 1) within 5–7 hours at 37°, and a progressive decrease in binding of anti-Ig to the cells occurred during this time, nevertheless, considerable amounts of anti-Ig antibody continued to bind to the cells specifically (67). Therefore, a significant portion of the original amount of TL antigens bound to modulating antibody must have remained on the surfaces of modulated cells. In fact, the greatest decrease in binding of secondary antibody often occurred after modulation was essentially complete. Similar results were obtained with RADA1 cells, although these cells could not be tested for modulation serologically because of an inherent resistance of these cells to complement lysis in the presence of TL antisera (see Section II, C, 1e).

A similar progressive but incomplete decrease in binding of the secondary antibody was observed when RADA1 cells were modulated with Fab fragments of TL antibody (67). Indirect immunofluorescence confirmed that some modulating TL antibody remained cell-bound. In addition, Esmon and Little (67) confirmed the observations of Stackpole *et al.* (203) that (1) the extent of lateral displacement of bound TL antibody into patches and caps paralleled the degree of modulation, and (2) Fab antibody fragments induced only subtle aggregation of TL antigens at the cell surface and virtually no capping while modulating cells nearly as effectively as bivalent antibody.

Esmon and Little (67) also demonstrated, by modulating cells with ^{131}I-labeled TL antibody and labeling secondarily with ^{125}I anti-Ig antibody, that most TL antibody lost from the cell surface during modulation was internalized by the cells and that negligible amounts of antibody were shed into the medium surrounding the cells.

While the indirect radioimmunoassay of Esmon and Little (66, 67) might be expected to provide quantitative data on the amount of TL antibody retained on the cell surface following modulation, severe technical limitations indicate that such information is not likely to be very accurate. In several experiments in which $1-2 \times 10^6$ RADA1 cells were incubated under modulating conditions with excess TL.1,2,3,5 antiserum or normal serum, then washed and labeled with ^{125}I-rabbit anti-mouse IgG antibody, only 5–12% of the total available radioactivity (counts per minute, cpm) was bound to cells incubated with TL antiserum, while 2–7% of the total cpm labeled cells incubated with normal serum. The sensitivity of the procedure is therefore very low, there was considerable variation from one experiment to another, and the absorption ratios (cpm bound to cells incubated with TL antiserum/cpm bound to normal serum-treated cells) were quite low (1.8 to 3.2). This procedure also requires that all antibodies in TL antisera that react with TL+ cells are TL antibodies, and studies by Esmon and Little (66) indicate that their antisera contained antibodies reactive with RADA1 cells that could not be removed by extensive absorption with TL.1,2,3,5+ thymocytes.

Evidence for retention of considerable numbers of TL antigen-antibody complexes on the surfaces of cells modulated *in vitro* for several hours has been obtained by several different approaches and seems to have been established. It is nevertheless possible that longer-term modulation would result in a complete loss of complexes from the cell surface. However, following continuous modulation of RADA1 cells *in vitro* for 24 hours with excess antiserum, cell surface-bound antibody remained demonstrable by cytotoxicity with rabbit complement and by immunofluorescence, and active TL antibody was released from these cells by incubation in normal serum at 37° (J. Richards and C. Stackpole, unpublished observations). Therefore, modulation ensues despite retention of TL antigen-antibody complexes on the cell surface, and these complexes persist long after modulation has been completed. For reasons discussed above, accurate data on the quantity of modulating TL antibody retained on the cell surface, shed into the medium, and internalized by the cells have not been obtained (67).

The failure of Boyse and his colleagues (22, 26, 150) to absorb TL antibody from antiserum using modulated cells is most likely due to saturation of modulated TL antigens by antibody prior to absorption, rather than to a lack of antigens on the cell surface. Absorption would therefore not appear to be an appropriate technique for demonstration of presence or lack of cell surface antigens following modulation since blocked antigens cannot be recognized.

4. METABOLISM OF TL ANTIGENS DURING MODULATION.

The initial studies of TL modulation *in vivo* and *in vitro* (22, 26, 150) demonstrated that antibody-induced loss of TL antigenicity from the cell surface was reversible. The normal TL+ phenotype was restored to *in vivo*-modulated leukemia cells within one transplant generation of about two weeks (22) or in 5–7 days in culture (150). It was subsequently demonstrated that leukemia cells modulated *in vivo* can acquire a normal TL+ phenotype within 24 hours after inoculation into unimmunized mice (97). Modulation of RADA1 cells *in vitro* is totally reversible within a comparable length of time, 24–48 hours (150). This delay in restoration of the normal TL+ phenotype is likely to reflect the time required for newly synthesized antigens to be incorporated into the cell surface membrane to the initial level, rather than reversal of the aggregated state of the modulated antigens.

Yu and Cohen (240) have analyzed synthesis and turnover of TL antigens by leukemia cells and thymocytes relative to modulation using radioimmunoprecipitation of antigens metabolically labeled with ^{3}H-fucose as an assay system. ASL1 cells and A/J thymocytes both incorporated radioisotope into molecules that could be solubilized by NP-40 and specifically precipitated with TL.1,3,5 antiserum. At the same time, spleen cells from A/J mice and TL− C57BL/6 thymocytes failed to incorporate label into cellular material precipitable with TL antiserum. Unfortunately, the antiserum used also contained contaminant antibodies (see Section II, C, 1d) so that in most experiments the metabolism of TL antigens specifically may at best be inferred; in certain experiments, effects contributed by contaminant antibodies were separated from those attributable to TL antibodies.

When ASL1 cells in culture were incubated for 5 hours in medium containing ^{3}H-fucose and then incubated for up to 28 hours in medium supplemented with unlabeled fucose, considerable radiolabel was detected in material precipitated with TL antiserum throughout this period, although most label was incorporated during the first 4 hours (240). Thus, the turnover of TL and/or "contaminant antigens" within ASL1 cells appears to be relatively slow, although the rate of turnover of TL antigens alone was not ascertained. At the same time radiolabel was progressively shed from the cells into the surrounding medium after labeling with ^{3}H-fucose, although once again the specific contribution made by TL antigens is not clear.

Yu and Cohen (240) found that these cultured ASL1 cells modulated quite slowly, loss of sensitivity to guinea pig complement being virtually complete by 10 hours. Within this time period, no significant differences were detected between modulating and nonmodulating cells in the amount of radiolabel incorporated into TL and/or contaminant antigens, although by 16 hours almost 50% less incorporation occurred in modulated cells. In order to determine the rates of synthesis of TL and associated antigens, to cells modulated for 20 hours and control unmodulated cells incubated for the same length of time ^{3}H-fucose was added for the last 5 hours of incubation, and total incorporation was determined by radioimmunoprecipitation (240). Results indicated that the rate of synthesis of these antigens was comparable in modulated and unmodulated cells.

Yu and Cohen (240) have thus demonstrated that modulation of ASL1 cells has no effect on intracellular synthesis of TL antigens or on metabolic shedding of antigen from the cell surface. It would therefore seem that even during modulation TL antigens are continually being incorporated into the cell surface, presumably to be modulated almost immediately by antibody. If that were the case, then upon removal of unbound antibody from the vicinity of modulated cells, new TL antigens should begin appearing on the cell surface immediately.

Regarding this point, Loor et al. (128) found that following antibody-induced redistribution of TL antigens on RADA1 cells under conditions that would be expected to simulate modulation, new TL antigens appeared on the cell surface within 2 hours after culturing in antibody-free medium was initiated. These new antigens, demonstrated by immunofluorescence, were expressed maximally by 24 hours. In contrast, A/J thymocytes treated similarly demonstrated only a slight reappearance of TL antigens during the first 6 hours of culturing, but thereafter a progressive loss of antigens was observed until by 24 hours no new antigens were evident on the cell surface. It is important to note, however, that unmodulated thymocytes cultured similarly spontaneously lost much of their TL antigenicity (80% of the cells were TL+ initially, but this was reduced to 30% TL+ cells after 48 hours). These results may, therefore, more reflect a deteriorating population of thymocytes that are notoriously difficult to maintain in culture.

We have similarly found that new TL antigens are detectable by immunofluorescence on RADA1 cells within two hours, but are not evident on thymocytes until several hours later (C. Stackpole, unpublished observations). However, using the high resolution afforded by serial-sectioning immunoelectronmicroscopy (197, 199), the appearance of new TL antigens on modulated thymocytes is evident within 2 hours after removal of TL antiserum and culturing at 37° (Fig. 5). This technique affords unique views of modulated TL antigen-antibody complexes occupying caps opposite from the Golgi region of the cell. Moreover, new antigen appears to be emanating from the vicinity of the Golgi complex to subsequently spread over the rest of the cell surface.

Another indication that TL antigens continue to be synthesized and released onto the cell surface during modulation has come from studies of the consequences of long-term modulation of RADA1 cells in culture (J. Richards and C. Stackpole, unpublished observations). When cells were incubated for 24 hours in medium containing excess TL antiserum (a 1/100 dilution of antiserum with a titer of 1/50,000 on RADA1 cells) added initially, modulation was complete within 1 hour and was still complete after 8 hours. After 24 hours, however, modulation was only 60% complete compared with 8 hours, and very little residual TL antibody was detectable in the culture medium. On the other hand, when fresh TL antiserum was added after 6, 12, and 18 hours, cells were completely modulated after 24 hours. Since there was negligible degradation of TL antibody when added to culture medium alone for 24 hours, there must be a continuous appearance of nascent TL antigen on the cell surface during modulation, resulting in gradual removal of antibody from the culture medium. A significant population of TL antigen-antibody complexes remained on cells modulated for 24 hours, probably reflecting an imbalance in rate of formation of new complexes on the cell surface and rate of removal from the cell surface by internalization and/or shedding, formation outpacing removal.

5. INHIBITION OF MODULATION.

Evidence is currently accumulating that suggests the existence of restraints on lateral mobility of at least some cell surface receptors (64). Based primarily on inhibitory effects of drugs such as colchicine and cytochalasin B on ligand-induced lateral displacement of surface receptors, cytoplasmic microtubules and microfilaments have been implicated in the control of receptor mobility (63, 139, 181, 198). If a control system of this sort does in fact exist, it might serve to establish and maintain topographical differentiation within a fluid membrane.

Since modulation of TL antigenicity seems to involve a subtle topographical displacement of antigens that is readily detectable serologically, we have used this sensitive system to test a variety of agents reported to affect the mobility of cell surface receptors in other systems.

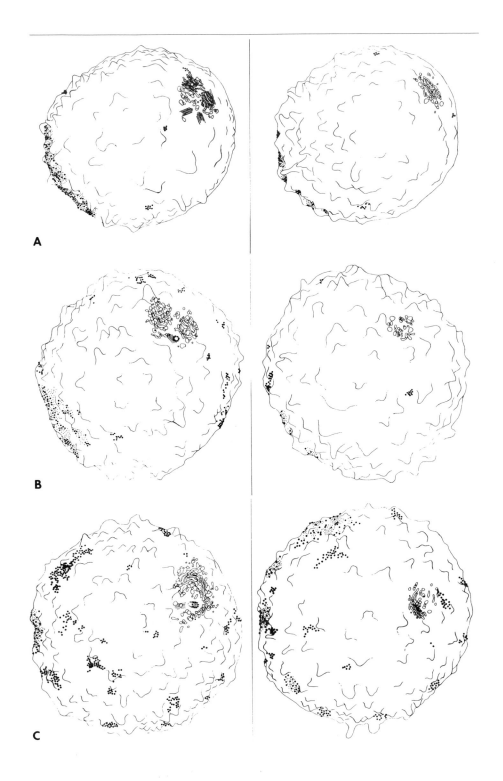

Preliminary results have been reported elsewhere (198), but because of the importance of this sort of information for determining the mechanism(s) underlying TL modulation, more recent experiments will be discussed in detail.

A variety of agents partially inhibited modulation of TL.1,2,3,5 antigenicity by (C57BL/6 × A/TL−)F$_1$ anti-ASL1 serum on RADA1 leukemia cells and A/J thymocytes *in vitro* when cells were preincubated with the agents for 1 hour at 37° (Table 4). Inhibitory effects were generally more pronounced on thymocytes than on RADA1 cells. In all cases, agents were used at maximum concentrations compatible with cell viability of at least

---

Fig. 5. Reconstruction of serial-section electron micrographs of three A-strain thymocytes showing the reappearance of TL antigens on the cell surface following modulation. Cells were initially "modulated" by sequentially incubating with TL.1,2,3,5 antiserum, hybrid rabbit anti-mouse IgG/anti-ferritin antibody, and ferritin (200), each for 30 minutes at 37°; cells treated similarly were totally refractive to lysis by fresh TL antiserum and guinea pig complement. Cells were then further incubated for 0 hours (A), 2 hours (B), or 4 hours (C) at 37° before labeling new TL antigens at 0° with TL antiserum, hybrid anti-mouse IgG/anti-southern bean mosaic virus (SBMV), and SBMV (200), each for 30 minutes. The cells were processed for serial-section electron microscopy, and the labeled cell surface reconstructed as described previously (197, 199) from 70–80 serial sections.

In these diagrams, only the cell surface and Golgi regions (with associated centrioles) are indicated, with small dots representing ferritin markers, and larger dots SBMV. The top half of each cell is at the left, the lower half at the right, oriented so that the complete cell would be obtained if the top half were slid directly over the lower half. "Modulated" caps of TL antigen-antibody complexes reside opposite the Golgi region (modulated complexes also label with SBMV, but antigens appearing after modulation are labeled only with SBMV). The appearance of SBMV label in patches represents a labeling artifact due to antibody-induced lateral displacement of TL antigens, but this change was allowed to occur since otherwise the small number of nascent antigens would not label efficiently. However, the overall topographical distribution of nascent antigens should be accurate. The capped configurations of ferritin/SBMV label is, of course, a consequence of modulation.

Over the 4-hour period, capped TL antigen-antibody complexes remain on the cell surface with very little erosion by endocytosis evident, although the caps do disperse to some extent. SBMV label dispersed on the cell surface at 0 hours may represent nascent antigens, but more likely is the background level of nonspecific labeling inherent in this procedure. Nascent TL antigens are evident at 2 hours and appear to emanate from the hemisphere of the cell occupied by the Golgi region. By 4 hours, new antigens are generally dispersed over the cell surface, but the smallest patches are within the Golgi-containing cell hemisphere. These cells represent typical results obtained from a limited number of cells (5–10) serially sectioned at each time period. × 10,000.

Table 4.   Inhibitory effects of various agents on TL antigenic modulation

	Concentration		Inhibition of Modulation[a] (% ± SE)	
Agent	M	μg(μl)/ml	RADA1	Thymocytes
Actinomycin D	8×10^{-6}	10	46 ± 2	76 ± 5
Dimethyl sulfoxide	6.5×10^{-1}	50	30 ± 5	48 ± 7
Persantin (1×10^{-1} M ethanol)	2×10^{-5}	10	28 ± 3	37 ± 8
Cytochalasin B (4.5×10^{-1} M ethanol)	1×10^{-4}	50	23 ± 4	38 ± 6
Colchicine	2.5×10^{-5}	10	27 ± 3	36 ± 6
Colchicine + Cytochalasin B	$2.5 \times 10^{-5}/1 \times 10^{-4}$	10/50	29 ± 2	54 ± 5
Vincristine	5×10^{-4}	50	23 ± 2	41 ± 8
Vinblastine	1×10^{-5}	10	22 ± 5	44 ± 7
Vinblastine + colchicine	$1 \times 10^{-5}/2.5 \times 10^{-5}$	10/10	28 ± 3	46 ± 3
Podophyllotoxin (2×10^{-2} M ethanol)	2.5×10^{-5}	10	15 ± 2	38 ± 5
Lumicolchicine	2.5×10^{-5}	10	12 ± 3	18 ± 3
N,N-dimethyl formamide	1×10^{-1}	10	14 ± 3	26 ± 6
Ethanol	4.5×10^{-1}	20	9 ± 2	14 ± 3
Sodium azide	1×10^{-4}	6	< 5	15 ± 2

a. 5×10^6 RADA1 cells or A/J strain thymocytes were incubated for 1 hour at 37°C in 1 ml of medium 199 containing 2% gamma globulin-free fetal bovine serum (control modulation) plus the appropriate agent (test and sham modulations). Then, a 1/100 dilution of TL.1,2,3,5 antiserum [(C57BL/6 × A/TL−)F$_1$ anti-ASL1; titer on RADA1 1/3000, and on thymocytes 1/5000] was added (antiserum was omitted from shams), and the cells were modulated for 1 hour (RADA1) or 2 hours (thymocytes) at 37°C. Residual TL antigenicity was measured by cytotoxicity with fresh TL antiserum and guinea pig complement (203), with figures obtained at an antiserum dilution of 1/100 being used to calculate the percent inhibition of modulation (assuming that 100% modulation represents the difference between percent cells killed in control and sham modulations):

$$\% \text{ inhibition} = \frac{\% \text{ cells dead (test)} - \% \text{ cells dead (control)}}{\% \text{ cells dead (sham)} - \% \text{ cells dead (control)}} \times 100$$

Inhibitory effects of ethanol have been subtracted from the appropriate figures. Persantin (dipyridamole) was a gift from Boehringer Ingelheim Ltd., Elmsford, N. Y. Lumicolchicine was prepared according to Mizel and Wilson (134). Cytochalasin B and podophyllotoxin were obtained from Aldrich Chemical Co., Milwaukee, Wis., vincristine sulfate (Oncovin) and vinblastine sulfate (Velban) from Eli Lilly and Co., Indianapolis, Ind.; dimethyl sulfoxide and sodium azide from Fisher Scientific Co., Fair Lawn, N. J. and all other reagents from Sigma Chemical Co., St. Louis, Mo.

90% at the end of the cytotoxicity test. Actinomycin D, an inhibitor of DNA-directed RNA synthesis (167) that had previously been shown to inhibit modulation (150), was the most effective agent tested. Dimethyl sulfoxide (DMSO), which has diverse effects on cells (236); Persantin, an inhibitor of transmembrane nucleoside transport (160); cytochalasin B, which disrupts microfilament functioning (230), and colchicine and related plant alkaloids (vincristine, vinblastine and podophyllotoxin) that prevent assembly of tubulin dimers into functional microtubules (130, 229) were also partially effective in inhibiting modulation. Lumicolchicine, which does not interact with microtubules (134), was considerably less inhibitory than colchicine on RADA1 cells and thymocytes. Dimethyl formamide, a solvent with properties similar to DMSO (16), also slightly inhibited modulation, while sodium azide, which may suppress cell movements by blocking intracellular ATP formation (132), had only a slight inhibitory effect on thymocytes and no effect on RADA1 cells.

Several investigators have found that treatment of cells with both cytochalasin B *and* colchicine (or colchicine-like drugs) has a greater effect on reducing ligand-induced lateral movement of cell surface receptors than either agent alone. We have failed to observe such a cumulative effect of colchicine plus cytochalasin B on RADA1 cells, although an additive inhibitory effect is evident on modulation of thymocytes (Table 4). Colchicine plus vinblastine had no greater inhibitory effect on either cell type than each agent alone. Colchicine plus DMSO and cytochalasin B plus DMSO also had no cumulative inhibitory effects on modulation of RADA1 cells. These drug combinations were toxic to thymocytes, while cytochalasin B plus vinblastine (or vincristine) was toxic to both cell types.

Griseofulvin, an antimitotic agent that may not affect microtubules (83), had no effect on modulation of either RADA1 cells or thymocytes at concentrations as high as 3×10^{-4} M. Other reagents that did not inhibit modulation (less than 5% inhibition) following preincubations of 1–2 hours included: deuterium oxide, a microtubule stabilizer (172), as a replacement for 25% or 75% of the water in the modulating medium; 10^{-3}–10^{-6} M N^6,O^2-dibutyryl adenosine 3′:5′ cyclic monophosphoric acid (dibutyryl cyclic AMP) alone or in combination with 10^{-3}–10^{-6} M theophylline, two agents that might stabilize or promote assembly of microtubules (163); strychnine (10^{-3}–10^{-6} M), a membrane-perturbing agent (96); and glycerol (10^{-4}–10^{-6} M), which shares some properties with DMSO (165).

Old et al. (150) had previously determined that the antimetabolites puromycin (20 μg/ml), chloramphenicol (100 μg/ml), p-fluorophenylalanine (1 mg/ml), cycloheximide (20 μg/ml), deoxyadenosine (0.5 mg/ml), 5-fluorodeoxyuridine (1 μg/ml), cytosine arabinoside (20 μg/ml), and hydrocortisone-21-phosphate (1 mg/ml) did not inhibit modulation (at maximum concentrations compatible with normal cell viability). We have confirmed these results and have additionally found that 2,4-dinitrophenol, sodium cyanide, sodium fluoride, oligomycin, 2-deoxy-D-glucose, 5-bromo-2′-deoxyuridine, antimycin A, and valinomycin at concentrations of $10^{-3}-10^{-6}$ M were ineffective. Iodoacetamide, previously shown to be effective in inhibiting modulation (150), was toxic to both RADA1 cells and thymocytes at a concentration of 3×10^{-5} M, and had no inhibitory effect at lower concentrations. Ineffective agents thus include inhibitors of cellular DNA, RNA, and protein synthesis, as well as suppressors of cellular utilization of energy sources for metabolic purposes.

All of the agents that inhibited modulation were at least 80% as effective following a 15-minute preincubation with cells at 37° as after a 1-hour preincubation, with the exception of actinomycin D. Modulation of RADA1 cells was only 9% inhibited after a 15-minute preincubation, and 17% inhibited after a 30-minute preincubation with actinomycin D (see also ref. 150).

There also was no difference in degree of inhibition when cells were preincubated with agents at 0° rather than at 37°, or when cells that are

Table 5.   Reversibility of inhibition of TL antigenic modulation

Inhibitor	Presence (+) or Absence (−) of Inhibitor during			Inhibition of Modulation (%)	
	Preinc.	Mod. I[a]	Mod. II[b]	RADA1	Thymocytes
Actinomycin D	+	+		47	75
			−	45	90
Dimethyl sulfoxide	+	+		33	44
			−	9	43
Persantin	+	+		32	41
			−	8	4
Cytochalasin B	+	+		20	33
			−	8	11
Colchicine	+	+		23	40
			−	10	25
Vinblastine	+	+		26	42
			−	12	20

a. RADA1 cells were modulated 1 hour, thymocytes 2 hours (see Table 4 for inhibitor concentrations and other details).

b. Following preincubation and modulation in the presence of inhibitor, cells were washed and reincubated at 37°C for 1 hour in fresh medium and antiserum, but without inhibitor.

normally washed at 0° and stored on ice before preincubation were washed and maintained at 37° prior to and during the entire test.

With the exception of actinomycin D (both cell types) and DMSO (thymocytes), inhibition by all agents was at least partially reversed following removal of the inhibitor and further incubation at 37° (Table 5).

In control experiments, in which cells were incubated for up to 2 hours at 37° with inhibiting agents, alone or together with normal mouse serum, and then the cytotoxicity titer of TL.1,2,3,5 antiserum on these cells was determined, treated cells were no more or less susceptible to lysis in the presence of TL antiserum and guinea pig complement than untreated cells. Thus, the cells are not simply being rendered more vulnerable to TL antibody and complement by pretreatment with these agents, nor is inhibition of modulation due to restriction of uptake of TL antibody by the treated cells.

a. Effects of Modulation Inhibitors on the Fate of TL Antigen-Antibody Complexes.

RADA1 cells were preincubated for 1 hour at 37° with inhibitors or in medium alone (control), then modulated with either (a) TL antiserum directly conjugated to fluoresceinyl thioureido caproic acid (203) (anti-TL/FTC), or (b) unconjugated antiserum for 1 hour. Cells were subsequently washed, and one aliquot was tested for residual TL antigenicity while the other aliquot was fixed and prepared for examination by fluorescence microscopy, either (a) directly, or (b) following incubation with fluorescein isothiocyanate-conjugated anti-mouse IgG antibody (anti-Ig/FITC) at 0°. Results obtained by direct and indirect immunofluorescence were comparable, but the increased intensity afforded by indirect labeling was advantageous because of the relative paucity of TL antigens on the cell surface compared to other surface receptors (202).

About 50% of control-modulated RADA1 cells typically displayed caps of label over one pole of the cell with surface label on the remainder of cells distributed in very large patches (Fig. 6, Table 6). Cells modulated in the presence of 2% ethanol, the vehicle for cytochalasin B, were labeled similarly. Label was distributed in large discrete patches on most cells modulated in the presence of cytochalasin B (Fig. 7), with capping occurring on less than 10% of the cells (Table 6). Labeling on cells modulated in the presence of colchicine was in smaller patches and aggregates more uniformly distributed over the cell surface (Fig. 8), while label was uniform or only slightly aggregated on the surfaces of cells treated with DMSO (Fig. 9). Results with Persantin were similar to those with DMSO. A uniform surface labeling of cells modulated in the presence of actinomycin D was apparent on more than 85% of the cells, the remainder exhibiting very slight aggregation (Fig. 10). Uniform labeling was only obtained when cells were fixed with 2% paraformaldehyde–0.5%

glutaraldehyde prior to incubation with anti-Ig/FITC; fixation with 2% paraformaldehyde alone permitted some aggregation of label to occur on all cells.

A sample of cells modulated with anti-TL/FTC in the presence of DMSO was modulated for an additional 1 hour with fresh anti-TL/FTC in the absence of DMSO to test reversibility. Modulation of DMSO-treated

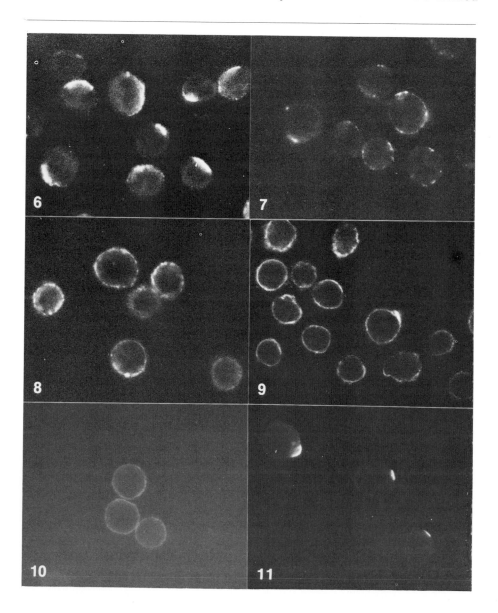

cells (30% inhibition) following removal of inhibitor was markedly reversed (11% inhibition), and all label was concentrated into dense caps on more than 90% of the cells (Fig. 11).

Results of a quantitative colorimetric assay for internalized horseradish peroxidase tracer (205) during modulation confirmed that considerable endocytosis occurred in cytochalasin B- and DMSO-treated cells, compared with control cells, while only 48% and 25% of the control level of HRP incorporation occurred in colchicine- and actinomycin D-treated cells, respectively (Table 7).

The effects of modulation inhibitors on the surface distribution of TL antigen-antibody complexes on thymocytes was strikingly different from the effects of the same agents on RADA1 cells. More than 70% of control-modulated thymocytes exhibited small dense caps of label, the remaining cells being labeled in large patches (Fig. 12, Table 6). Modulation inhibitors had only a slight effect on this labeling pattern in that the proportion of capped cells to patchy cells was altered, and a variable population of uniformly labeled cells was observed (Fig. 13); the proportion of uniformly labeled cells increased as the inhibitory effect became more pronounced (Table 8). Actinomycin D, DMSO, and Persantin inhibited capping to an extent approximately proportional to the degree of inhibition of modulation, while cytochalasin B, colchicine and vinblastine actually *increased* the percentage of capped cells (Table 6).

Indirect immunofluorescence microscopy of RADA1 cells preincubated for 1 hour with inhibitors, modulated for 1 hour with TL.1,2,3,5 antiserum in the presence of inhibitors, fixed for 30 minutes at 0° with 2% paraformaldehyde—0.5% glutaraldehyde, and labeled with anti-Ig/FITC antibody for 30 minutes at 0°. ×1500 (Figs. 6–10).

Fig. 6. Control modulated cells. Label on most cells is in a capped configuration, or is in large patches.

Fig. 7. Cells modulated with 1×10^{-4} M cytochalasin B, with surface label distributed in large patches.

Fig. 8. Cells modulated with 2.5×10^{-5} M colchicine. Label is distributed fairly uniformly over the cell surface in small patches or aggreates.

Fig. 9. Cells modulated with 6.5×10^{-1} M DMSO. Surface label is either uniform or slightly aggregated.

Fig. 10. Cells modulated with 8×10^{-6} M actinomycin D. Label is uniformly distributed over the cell surface.

Fig. 11. Direct immunofluorescence of RADA1 cells modulated with a 1/10 dilution of anti-TL/FTC antibody (approximate titer: 1/80) in the presence of DMSO for 1 hour at 37°, washed, and then incubated for 1 hour at 37° with fresh anti-TL/FTC in the absence of DMSO. Label is exclusively in dense caps.

Table 6. Effect of modulation inhibitors on capping of TL antigens on RADA1 cells and thymocytes[a]

	Percent Cells Capped	
Inhibitor[b]	RADA1	Thymocytes
—	48	72
Actinomycin D	<1	49
Dimethyl sulfoxide	5	62
Persantin	18	57
Cytochalasin B	8	85
Colchicine	10	84
Colchicine + cytochalasin B	< 1	44
Vinblastine	14	81
Vinblastine + colchicine	9	80

a. RADA1 cells were modulated 1 hour and thymocytes 2 hours with TL antiserum, then fixed for 30 minutes at 0°C with 2% paraformaldehyde–0.5% glutaraldehyde in medium 199, pH 7.4, and labeled with fluoresceinated rabbit anti-mouse IgG antibody for 30 minutes at 0°C in medium 199 containing 5% fetal bovine serum.

b. Concentrations as in Table 4.

Capping even occurred on nearly half of the cells treated simultaneously with colchicine and cytochalasin B.

It has been established that cap formation is a secondary consequence of TL antigen-antibody interactions leading to modulation (203), even though the two processes may appear virtually indistinguishable (Fig. 1). Furthermore, from the present results it is evident that capping of TL antigens by antibody does not necessarily render the cells insensitive to a subsequent exposure to lytic guinea pig complement; for example, about 75% of thymocytes modulated in the presence of actinomycin D were killed by fresh antibody and guinea pig complement even though half of the cells had already capped.

To determine the effects of modulation inhibitors on the surface distribution of TL antigen-antibody complexes on thymocytes in which capping was reduced, sodium azide was administered to cells together with the inhibitor. The maximum concentration of sodium azide compatible with 90% cell viability only partially suppressed capping (Fig. 14), but nevertheless a correlation is evident between the extent of inhibition of modulation and the percentage of cells displaying a uniform surface label (Fig. 15, Table 8). Interestingly, cells treated with sodium azide plus

Table 7. Effect of modulation and modulation inhibitors on incorporation of horseradish peroxidase (HRP) by RADA1 cells[a]

Inhibitor[b]	Incorporation of HRP per mg Cell Protein (ng ± SE)
None	92.6 ± 8.2
Actinomycin D	22.9 ± 3.5
Dimethyl sulfoxide	125.0 ± 7.9
Persantin	66.7 ± 8.6
Cytochalasin B	92.0 ± 7.6
Colchicine	44.1 ± 5.3

a. Following a 1-hour preincubation with or without inhibitor, HRP was added to cell suspensions to a final concentration of 1 mg/ml; TL antiserum was added at the same time. After modulation for 1 hour, cells were washed five times with cold medium 199, resuspended in 0.25 mg/ml trypsin in medium 199, and incubated for 15 minutes at 37°C to remove any cell surface-bound HRP (205). After washing, cells were dissolved in 0.1% sodium dodecyl sulfate in distilled water. Cell lysates were analyzed colorimetrically for HRP immediately following addition of 10^{-4} mM o-dianisidine and 10^{-3} mM hydrogen peroxide in 0.1 M phosphate buffer, pH 5.0.

b. Concentrations as in Table 4.

either cytochalasin B or colchicine capped to a greater extent than cells treated with azide alone.

Modulation of TL antigenicity from RADA1 cells and thymocytes by univalent (Fab) fragments of TL.1,2,3,5 antibody is accompanied by a slight aggregation of TL antigens on the cell surface (203). Although capping does not occur on RADA1 cells modulated for 2 hours with 200 μg/ml Fab fragments, caps form on about 10–15% of thymocytes modulated in the same manner. While aggregation was barely perceptible on RADA1 cells (and undoubtedly accentuated by labeling with anti-Ig/FITC), uncapped thymocytes presented a uniform surface label. Therefore, TL antigen-univalent antibody complexes can be aggregated more readily on RADA1 cells than on thymocytes, although capping occurs only on thymocytes.

RADA1 cells preincubated for 1 hour with actinomycin D, modulated for 2 hours with Fab antibody fragments in the presence of actinomycin D, then fixed and labeled with anti-Ig/FITC displayed a uniform surface label. These results indicate that actinomycin D prevents visible aggregation of TL antigen-univalent antibody complexes.

b. Effects of Modulation Inhibitors on Cellular Incorporation of Thymidine, Uridine, and Leucine. The ability of RADA1 cells modulated in

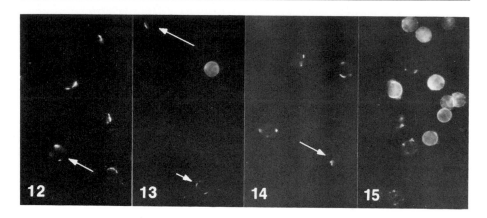

Indirect immunofluorescence microscopy of A/J thymocytes preincubated for 1 hour with inhibitors, modulated for 2 hours with TL.1,2,3,5 antiserum together with inhibitors, then fixed and labeled with anti-Ig/FITC antibody at 0°. × 900 (Figs. 12–15).

Fig. 12.   Control modulated cells. Four cells are capped and one cell is labeled in large discrete patches (*arrow*).

Fig. 13.   Cells modulated in the presence of 8×10^{-6} M actinomycin D. Three distinct labeling patterns are evident: uniform, patchy (*short arrow*) and capped (*long arrow*).

Fig. 14.   Cells modulated in the presence of 10^{-4} M sodium azide. Three cells are labeled in large patches, and one cell is capped (*arrow*).

Fig. 15.   Cells modulated in the presence of 8×10^{-6} M actinomycin D and 10^{-4} M sodium azide. Cells are labeled uniformly or in patches.

the presence of inhibitors to incorporate ^{3}H-thymidine, ^{3}H-uridine and ^{3}H-leucine was compared with incorporation by sham- and control-modulated cells. In all cases, control-modulated cells incorporated these radioisotopes nearly as effectively as sham-modulated cells. Cells treated with actinomycin D were virtually incapable of incorporating uridine and relatively ineffective in incorporating thymidine and leucine as well (15% and 56% of control levels, respectively) (see also Ref. 150). DMSO-treated cells had a slightly depressed capacity for uptake of both uridine and leucine (86% and 70% of control levels, respectively). Persantin slightly depressed cellular incorporation of thymidine (80% of control) without affecting uptake of other radioisotopes. Cytochalasin B, colchicine, and vinblastine similarly affected incorporation by treated cells, slightly depressing uptake of thymidine and leucine (75–85% of control levels).

Table 8. Effects of sodium azide on inhibition of modulation and surface distribution of TL antigen-antibody complexes on thymocytes[a]

Inhibitor	Sodium Azide (10^{-4} M)	Inhibition of Modulation (%)	Percent Cells		
			Capped	Patchy	Diffuse
—	—	—	78	22	0
	+	15	35	65	0
Actinomycin D	—	74	49	41	10
	+	72	19	23	58
Dimethyl sulfoxide	—	53	62	30	8
	+	49	23	30	47
Cytochalasin B	—	39	85	13	2
	+	46	47	48	5
Colchicine	—	34	84	13	3
	+	37	48	40	12

a. Thymocytes were preincubated for 1 hour at 37°C with or without inhibitors (concentrations as in Table 4). During this incubation, sodium azide was added to some samples (+) to a final concentration of 10^{-4} M. Cells were then modulated for 2 hours and prepared for fluorescence microscopy as indicated in Table 6.

c. Effects of Modulation Inhibitors on Tubulin and Actin Polymerization. Since several of the agents effective as inhibitors of modulation have primary effects on microtubule or microfilament assembly, the effects of modulation inhibitors on polymerization of isolated tubulin and actin preparations were tested. Tubulin was isolated and purified from porcine brain, while actin was prepared from rabbit skeletal muscle. Polymerization of tubulin and actin preparations was effected by short-term incubations and assessed by negative staining electron microscopy.

Colchicine, vinblastine and vincristine were the only inhibitors that completely prevented tubulin polymerization into microtubules. Podophyllotoxin only partially inhibited tubulin polymerization, possibly reflecting the lesser extent of modulation inhibition by this agent compared with colchicine, vinblastine and vincristine. Polymerization of actin into filaments was inhibited only by cytochalasin B.

Considering the extraordinary ease and rapidity with which TL antigens can be laterally displaced and aggregated following binding of antibody to the cell surface at 37° (202), it is not surprising that inhibition of TL antigenic modulation is at best only partially effective. Since loss of sensitivity to guinea pig complement-mediated cytolysis seems to occur following "microaggregation" of TL antigen-antibody complexes (203), the cell surface would presumably have to be "frozen" for modulation to be suppressed completely. While actinomycin D virtually abolishes visible aggregation of complexes on the surfaces of RADA1 cells, considerable microaggregation might still occur since less than 50% inhibition of modulation is achieved with this agent. Nevertheless, immunofluorescence results with RADA1 cells and thymocytes tend to indicate that the extent of inhibition of modulation is directly proportional to the degree of restriction of lateral mobility of TL antigen-antibody complexes, despite the strong tendency for thymocytes to cap these complexes.

The generally greater inhibition of modulation of thymocytes compared to RADA1 cells presumably reflects the slower rate at which modulation occurs on thymocytes (203). These results indicate that caps can form on thymocytes in the absence of localized aggregation and cross-linking of TL antigens, as may occur in other systems (169), and that capped TL antigen-antibody complexes are not necessarily resistant to guinea pig complement lysis. Nevertheless, the close correlation between TL antibody concentration and both capping and modulation of thymocyte TL antigens (Fig. 1) indicates that forces driving capping are the same as the forces driving modulation. This is clearly not the case in modulation of RADA1 cells (Fig. 1). Localized aggregation of TL antigens that occurs more readily on RADA1 cells and is consequently more difficult to inhibit on this cell type is clearly the mobility characteristic directly bearing on modulation. The difference in tendency for TL antigens to aggregate on RADA1 cells and thymocytes could be due to differences in membrane fluidity, quantity of antigens, or disposition of antigens within the cell surface.

These observations might help to explain apparent inconsistencies in results from other laboratories. For example, Edidin and Henney (65) have demonstrated a loss of susceptibility of mouse mastocytoma cells to guinea pig complement-mediated lysis following capping of target H-2 antigens. A similar loss of sensitivity of mouse L cells to lysis by guinea pig complement parallels capping of H-2 antigens (213). Further indications that restricted lateral mobility of surface antigens enhances cell lysis by complement have come from experiments on antigens incorporated into model membrane liposomes, in which complement fixation increases as the rigidity of the membrane is increased by addition of cholesterol (93). On the other hand, Boyle et al. (17) have failed to find a correlation between enhanced sensitivity of metabolic inhibitor-treated guinea pig hepatoma cells to rabbit antibody and guinea pig complement and restriction of antigen movement (cap formation). Results obtained in a particular cell system may depend on the tendency for the surface antigen to be aggregated, irrespective of capping.

Restriction of TL antigen mobility by modulation inhibitors could enhance complement-mediated cytolysis in a variety of ways: (1) antibody and/or complement may bind more efficiently to dispersed antigens than to clustered antigens; (2) cell lysis by complement may be more efficient when antigen-antibody complexes remain dispersed; or (3) the cell surface membrane may be rendered more susceptible to the lytic action of complement. Recent information indicates that inhibition of modulation by suppressing "microaggregation" of TL antigen-antibody complexes may result from failure of mouse complement component C3 to intercalate into the complexes and block guinea pig complement-mediated lysis (204; see Section II, C, 7).

Although inhibitors of TL modulation have in common the tendency to restrict antibody-induced lateral aggregation of TL antigens to at least some extent, restriction seems to be effected in several ways, either by disrupting cytoplasmic microtubules or microfilaments, blocking cellular metabolism, or interacting directly with the cell surface membrane. The possible mechanisms involved and the relationship between inhibition of TL modulation and regulation of the organization of the cell surface have been discussed extensively by Stackpole (198).

6. RESISTANCE TO MODULATION. The rate at which TL modulation proceeds is highly variable, depending upon the cell type. For example, RADA1 leukemia cells may be modulated completely within 30 minutes under optimum conditions (203), while ASL1 leukemia cells require more than 10 hours to achieve the same state (240). But are there any cells on which TL antigens cannot be modulated at all?

Liang and Cohen (125) have formed somatic hybrids between ASL1 cells (TL.1,2,3,5) and LM(TK)⁻ cells, a thymidine kinase-deficient mutant of mouse LM cells (TL⁻), that expressed approximately half of the amount of TL antigens present on ASL1 cells. When these hybrid cells were exposed to TL.1,2,3,5, TL.1,3,5 or TL.2 antisera under conditions that resulted in total modulation of the parental ASL1 cells within about 10 hours, essentially no modulation occurred even in 30 hours. The hybrid cells resisted the modulating effects of TL antisera even when TL antibody-sensitized cells were further incubated with anti-mouse Ig antibody for 20 hours at 37°. Susceptibility of TL antigens to modulation, therefore, is highly variable and seems to be very much dependent on the particular cell type on which the antigens reside, for reasons that are unclear.

7. ROLE OF MOUSE COMPLEMENT IN MODULATION. In Section II, C, 1, the dependence of TL modulation on a heat-labile factor, or factors, present in TL antisera and in normal mouse serum (serum modulating factor(s), or SMF) was noted. Since these initial observations (203), the nature of this apparent "blocking" of guinea pig complement lytic interaction with cell-bound TL antigen-antibody complexes on RADA1 cells and A/J thymocytes has been investigated more extensively, and these studies implicate the C3 component of mouse complement as the responsible "blocking" factor (204).

Analysis of SMF activity in sera from 33 mouse strains, congenic stocks, and F_1 hybrids indicated that not all sera (from mice 2 months of age or older) were equally effective in restoring modulating activity to heated (56° for 1 hour) TL antiserum (204). In all cases, female sera possessed significantly more activity than male sera. Restoring activity was extremely low (10–15% restoration) in C57BL/6 strain and C57BL/6/TL+ congenic stock sera, and moderately low (45–55% restoration) in AKR strain and AKR/H-2^b congenic stock sera, compared with all other sera tested (male: 70–90% restoration; female: 80–100% restoration).

In addition to heat-lability, SMF activity was destroyed by treating sera with zymosan, an immune complex, and cobra venom factor, and activity could be restored partially to heated serum by freeze-thawing. Modulation was almost completely (90–95%) restored to cells treated with heated TL antiserum and cobra venom factor-pretreated normal serum by washing and incubating cells with 100 CH_{50} units of purified human C3. A slight (30–35%) restoration was achieved with human C4, but all other human complement components and guinea pig complement components C1–9 were ineffective. Human serum genetically deficient in C3 was also incapable of restoring modulation. A comparable near-linear sensitivity of modulating activity of human C3 and mouse serum to temperatures from 37° to 0° (with an abrupt increase in sensitivity at 18°) indicated that the mouse complement component analogous to human C3, mouse C3, was required for modulation.

The capacity for genetically C2-deficient human serum to restore modulation to cells presensitized with heated TL antiserum and cobra venom factor-pretreated normal serum, and the susceptibility of SMF to treatment of sera with zymosan, immune complexes, and cobra venom factor, indicated involvement of the alternative pathway of complement activation (81) in TL modulation (204).

All modulating activity in mouse serum and in human C3 preparations could be absorbed by RADA1 cells and thymocytes in the absence of TL antibody and could be eluted from cells with 1 mM sodium ethylenediaminetetraacetic acid, pH 8.0 (204). Immunofluorescence analysis of mouse or human C3 binding to the cell surface indicated specific binding only under conditions promoting modulation.

Unlike mouse SMF activity, human C3 modulating activity was not susceptible to heating at 56°, and modulation of RADA1 cells and thymocytes could be achieved with the purified IgG fraction of TL.1,2,3,5 antiserum and heated human C3, in the absence of any factor B (204). These results suggested that cells undergoing modulation contributed factor B or factor B-like C3 cleaving activity resulting in deposition of C3 (probably C3b) onto the cell surface. Both deposition of C3 and "microaggregation" of TL antigen-antibody complexes (Section II, C, 5) are, therefore, requirements for TL modulation. While not explicitly demonstrated, intercalation of C3 into aggregated antigen-antibody complexes may sterically hinder guinea pig complement attachment to the cell surface or activation of the complete lytic sequence (see Section II, C, 10).

8. UNIVALENT ANTIBODY-INDUCED MODULATION. The basic features of TL antigenic modulation on RADA1 cells using univalent Fab fragments of TL antibody have been determined by Lamm et al. (114), Stackpole et al. (203), and Esmon and Little (67) using cytotoxicity, immunofluorescence, and an indirect radioimmunoassay, and have been noted in Sections I, B, 7; II, C, 3, and II, C, 5. There are potential problems regarding interpretation of the results that should be pointed out, however.

Lamm et al. (114) and Stackpole et al. (203) ascertained that Fab fragments of TL antibody modulated TL antigenicity by the same criterion used for assessment of modulation by bivalent antibody, that is, acquisition of resistance by univalent antibody-sensitized cells to a subsequent exposure to bivalent TL antibody and guinea pig complement. But how is such an assay possible, since cell-bound TL antigen-Fab antibody complexes lacking Fc portions of antibody molecules cannot bind or activate complement? Presumably, bivalent antibody added during the cytotoxicity test can also attach to these complexes, perhaps by displacing the Fab fragments. This is the likely explanation on the basis of results obtained by Lamm et al. (114) in attempting to modulate H-2 antigens on RADA1 cells with Fab fragments of H-2 antibody: presensitization of the cells with these Fab fragments did not reduce the cytotoxic effects of bivalent antibody and complement added subsequently. Inhibition of Fab antibody-induced modulation of TL antigens by treatment of the cells with 10 μg/ml actinomycin D for 1 hour at 37° (114) also suggests that bivalent antibody can attach to antigens already bound by univalent antibody, since most cells were lysed despite saturation of antigens with univalent antibody.

Esmon and Little (67) claim that an indirect radioimmunoassay (66) is more effective in demonstrating Fab antibody-induced modulation of TL antigens on RADA1 cells than is a cytotoxicity assay. While these investigators draw similar conclusions regarding the capacity for Fab fragments to modulate TL antigens and induce a simultaneous aggregation of antigens within the cell surface membrane as do Lamm et al. (114) and Stackpole et al. (203; see also Section II, C, 5), they have not determined that modulation has actually occurred. Nevertheless, the results of all investigators are compatible, so Fab antibody probably does in fact modulate TL antigenicity, at least on RADA1 cells, the only cell type studied.

It is possible that modulation of TL antigenicity by Fab antibody fragments occurs in the same manner as modulation by bivalent antibody. While preparation of Fab fragments of antibody destroys SMF activity in the original TL antiserum, modulation only occurred when normal mouse serum was added during the modulation incubation (114, 203). These observations implicate mouse C3 in Fab antibody-induced TL modulation, but additional investigation will be necessary to ascertain the precise mechanism involved.

9. INTERRELATIONSHIP BETWEEN TL AND H-2D ANTIGENS.

The peculiar reciprocal relationships that exist between TL and H-2D antigens in terms of cell surface expression, as indicated by altered capacity of cells to absorb specific antibody, have been discussed in Sections I, B, 7 and II, A, 3. With regard to TL modulation in vitro, the following observations were made by Old et al. (150): (1) during modulation of TL.1,2,3,5 antigens on RADA1 cells, which was essentially complete after 1 hour of preincubation with TL antiserum at 37°, the relative absorption capacity of these cells for antibody directed against H-2D antigens increased nearly 1.5 times, while the absorptive capacity of the same cells for antibody to H-2K specificities remained at 1.0; and (2) over the next 3.5 hours of preincubation with TL antiserum, the relative absorptive capacity of the cells for H-2D antibody increased linearly to approximately 2.2, then leveled off, while again H-2K antibody-absorbing capacity was unchanged. The net result after 4.5 hours was more than a twofold increase in H-2D antigens available to antibody. This is just opposite from the effect occurring when thymocytes acquire the TL.1,2,3,5 (Tla^a) phenotype, that is, a net decrease in H-2D antigens available to antibody (26, 27).

Does this quantitative change in H-2D antigenicity (1) reflect an alleviation of steric hindrance to antibody attachment inherently existing between TL and H-2D antigens at the cell surface, (2) enhance the appearance of new H-2D antigens concomitant with TL modulation or the disappearance of these antigens upon acquisition of TL antigens, or (3) represent some other mechanism? Unfortunately, that question cannot be answered at the present time, simply because there is not enough information available. The possibility that TL and H-2D antigens (as well as Ly-2 antigen) reside on the cell surface in some configuration such as a supramolecular complex of loosely associated molecules has been extensively reviewed by Stackpole (198). If such a preferential molecular association does exist, despite general indications that cell surface membrane proteins are for the most part free to diffuse laterally within a fluid lipid matrix (64), then the steric hindrance hypothesis would be strengthened. On the other hand, perturbing TL antigens with antibody may somehow specifically stimulate increased appearance of new H-2D antigens. Such a concept is not likely to explain the significant increase in H-2D antigens occurring during the first hour of modulation, however. It is not inconceivable, of course, that the overall increase in H-2D antigens results from an initial alleviation of steric hindrance followed by an enhanced appearance of nascent antigens.

10. A MODEL FOR TL MODULATION IN VITRO. Figure 16 summarizes diagrammatically our current conception of the mechanism of TL antigen modulation on leukemia cells and thymocytes, on the basis of experimental results discussed in previous sections. This model considers only bivalent antibody-induced modulation and the populations of TL antigens remaining bound to the cell surface. Modulation now appears to be a dynamic process that entails some removal of antigen-antibody complexes by endocytosis (shedding of complexes into the surrounding medium appears to be negligible and essentially inconsequential), that removal being more than offset by the appearance of nascent antigens on the cell surface. Nascent antigens are presumably engaged by antibody almost immediately and modulated very rapidly.

It is not known at present why guinea pig complement fails to lyse modulated cells. Since rabbit complement lyses modulated and unmodulated cells to a comparable extent, modulation does not render the cells insensitive to complement lysis. We therefore assume that the differences in behavior of guinea pig and rabbit complement may relate to differences in requirements for attachment of the initial ligand, C1q, to antigen-antibody complexes. Since activation of guinea pig complement appears to depend upon the close approximation of two IgG antibody molecules on the cell surface whereas rabbit complement requires only a single attachment site, this might account for failure of the modulation process to block rabbit complement lysis (204). The C1q component of guinea pig complement, in contrast to rabbit C1q, may not be able to attach to IgG molecules of modulating TL antibody because of steric im-

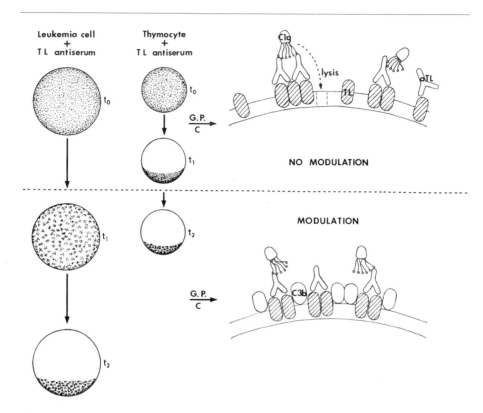

Fig. 16. Diagram illustrating how modulation of TL antigenicity may occur on leukemia cells and thymocytes *in vitro*. Stippling on cells represents the topography of TL antigen-antibody complexes at various time intervals $(t_0 - t_2)$ during incubation of cells with antiserum at 37°. Modulation precedes capping on RADA1 cells but may follow capping on thymocytes. According to this hypothesis (*see text*), cytolysis by guinea pig complement (G.P.C) occurs only when the C1q molecule attaches to two IgG antibody molecules (a-TL), and on the modulated cell that attachment is prevented by steric hindrance imposed by C3b molecules intercalated within antigen-antibody aggregates.

positions by intercalated mouse C3b molecules, or guinea pig C1q may be otherwise prevented from initiating an effective lytic complement cascade sequence.

IgM molecules of TL antibody are incapable of promoting modulation but are able to induce lateral redistribution and aggregation of antigens in the same manner as IgG antibody molecules (C. Stackpole and J. Jacobson, unpublished observations). Presumably, IgM antibody affords a configuration such that a single molecule may be necessary for guinea pig complement activation. According to our model, it should not be possible to modulate TL antigenicity when IgM antibody is substituted for IgG antibody, or when rabbit complement is substituted for guinea pig complement. To date, it has not been possible to obtain modulation under these conditions even after extended incubations *in vitro*.

D. Modulation In Vivo

What indications do we have that modulation of TL antigenicity *in vitro* as outlined in the previous section has any relevance to the phenomenon of modulation described initially *in vivo*?

Jacobson et al. (97) have recently found that *in vivo* modulation as originally described by Boyse and his colleagues (22) does in fact occur in basically the same manner as modulation *in vitro*. These studies were done primarily with RADA1 cells and (C57BL/6 × A/TL−)F$_1$ mice (TL−) hyperimmunized with either ASL1 leukemia cells or A/J thymocytes (both TL.1,2,3,5). Most experiments were done with animals immunized with thymocytes because of the presence of noncytotoxic contaminating antibodies in anti-ASL1 serum that cross-react with RADA1 cells (see Section II, C, 1d). Despite these contaminating antibodies, results with anti-ASL1 serum were similar to those obtained with antithymocyte serum, indicating that, as in modulation *in vitro*, the contaminating antibodies did not contribute to, or interfere with, the process of TL modulation.

In one series of experiments (Fig. 17), RADA1 cells were inoculated into immunized or unimmunized mice and removed after 1, 2, 3, and 4 days. The number of cells inoculated (30 × 10^6) was the optimum number determined by preliminary tests to afford adequate cell recovery by day 1, since considerable cell loss occurred in that time period. Residual TL.1,2,3,5 antigenicity was assessed by cytotoxicity, using guinea pig or rabbit complement, and the presence and topographical distribution of cell surface-bound TL antibody was determined by indirect membrane immunofluorescence. The titer of TL.1,2,3,5 antibody in the serum of each mouse before inoculation, and immediately prior to sacrifice, was determined by cytotoxicity on A/J thymocytes.

Cells inoculated into immunized mice were almost completely modulated (TL.1,2,3,5 → TL−) after 1 day by the criterion of acquired resistance to TL antiserum and guinea pig complement-mediated cytolysis, although reactivity to antiserum plus rabbit complement was only slightly diminished (about 10%) even after 4 days. Moreover, each day 75–85% of the cells recovered were labeled with TL antibody, as determined by immunofluorescence, with the percentage of cells displaying patchy and capped configurations increasing progressively. Consistent with indications from *in vitro* modulation of a requirement for "microaggregation" of TL antigen-antibody complexes rather than patchiness or capping (see Section II, C, 5), very few cells were patchy or capped after 1 day. The sera from all mice retained very high titers of TL.1,2,3,5 antibody at the time of sacrifice.

Cells inoculated into unimmunized mice and also removed at days 1–4 showed no evidence of modulation as judged by guinea pig or rabbit complement (Fig. 17), although the sera from these animals contained progressively more TL antibody as the experiment continued, indicating the beginning of an immune response. The presence of small amounts of circulating TL antibody was also evident from immunofluorescence of cells removed at days 3 and 4, but labeling was extremely weak compared to experimental animals. Antibody appearing in control mice was predominantly 19S IgM immunoglobulin that had no modulating capacity (see Sections II, C, 1b and II, C, 10).

In comparable experiments, Jacobson et al. (97) have demonstrated that RADA1 cells modulated in vivo for one to several weeks still retained TL antibody on the cell surface, demonstrable by rabbit complement-mediated cytotoxicity and immunofluorescence; similar results were obtained when A/J thymocytes (TL.1,2,3,5) were modulated for 7 days in mice passively immunized with TL.1,2,3,5 antiserum, and when ERLD leukemia cells (TL.1,2,4) were modulated in TL.1,2,3,5-immunized mice for 11 days. In all cases, when modulated and extensively washed cells were injected intraperitoneally into unimmunized mice, specific TL antibody was released into the serum within 24 hours, and this antibody was shown to originate from the surfaces of modulated cells. Under these conditions, modulation of RADA1 cells (7 days) was completely reversible within 24 hours, so the released antibody was not capable of re-modulating those cells or fresh RADA1 cells in vitro, for reasons that are unclear.

Short-term in vivo experiments demonstrated that RADA1 cells injected intraperitoneally could become sensitized with TL antibody within 3 hours, but no modulation was evident by that time (97); cells were almost totally modulated 16 hours after injection, however.

The process of in vivo modulation of leukemia cells and thymocytes appears to require the same heat-labile SMF activity as does in vitro modulation, according to the results of preliminary experiments (97; J. Jacobson, S. Galuska and C. Stackpole, in preparation). RADA1 cells could be modulated in male C57BL/6 mice passively immunized with unheated TL antiserum [(C57BL/6 × A/TL−)F$_1$ anti-ASL1] but remained unmodulated when heated TL antiserum was introduced into these animals; (C57BL/6 × A/TL−)F$_1$ serum contains high SMF activity, but male C57BL/6 serum is extremely low in such activity (204; see Section II, C, 7). Thus, modulation occurred in C57BL/6 mice only when unheated SMF was present. Similar requirements were demonstrated for modulation of

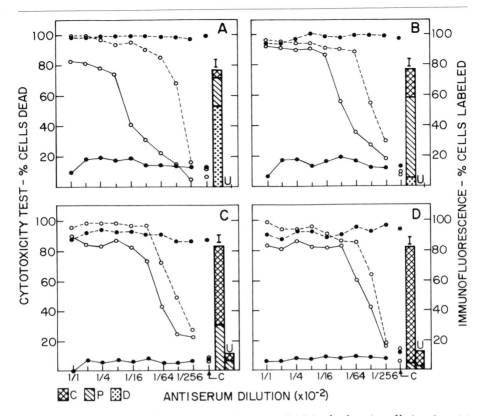

Fig. 17. Modulation of TL.1,2,3,5 antigens on RADA1 leukemia cells *in vivo*. 30 × 10⁶ RADA1 cells were inoculated intraperitoneally into (C57BL/6 × A/TL−)F₁ mice that had been hyperimmunized against A thymocytes (TL.1,2,3,5) or into unimmunized mice. Immunized and unimmunized mice were sacrificed after 1 day (*A*), 2 days (*B*), 3 days (*C*), and 4 days (*D*) and cell surface TL antigenicity was assessed by cytotoxicity of (C57BL/6 × A/TL−)F₁ anti-A thymocyte antiserum plus guinea pig complement (*solid lines*) or absorbed rabbit complement (*broken lines*), and by indirect immunofluorescence (*bars*). Cells recovered from immunized mice are indicated by solid dots or I; cells from unimmunized mice by open circles or U. C, complement cytotoxic controls with TL antiserum omitted. The cell surface labeling patterns ascertained by immunofluorescence are designated D, diffuse or slightly aggregated; P, patchy; or C, capped.

On all days, RADA1 cells from unimmunized mice were essentially completely modulated, while reactivity to rabbit complement remained high. Meanwhile, the percentage of positively-labeled cells in immunofluorescence tests labeled in patches and caps increased. At 1 day, most modulated cells were labeled diffusely or in small aggregates. Some labeling of cells in unimmunized mice was apparent by immunofluorescence after 3 and 4 days, and apparently represents TL antibody present in the sera of these animals and formed against the inoculated RADA1 cells. The cytotoxicity titer of TL.1,2,3,5 antibody in immunized mice remained the same at sacrifice as at the time of inoculation (approximately 1/64,000) (97).

C57BL/6/TL+ thymocytes; that strain is also extremely low in SMF activity, and modulation was achieved only when mice were passively immunized with unheated TL antiserum.

While the experiments of Jacobson et al. (97; in preparation) suggest that TL modulation in vivo involves localized aggregation of TL antigens by antibody and intercalation of mouse complement component C3, as occurs in vitro (see Section II, C, 10), it is difficult to envision how such a mechanism could permit leukemia cells to escape immune destruction. Intercalation of mouse C3 into TL antigen-antibody aggregates in vitro may prevent guinea pig complement-mediated lysis, but if mouse complement is lytic in vivo, then attachment of C3 should set the alternative pathway of complement activation in motion, resulting in cell lysis. This obviously does not occur, nor are RADA1 cells that have been introduced into passively immunized C57BL/6 mice destroyed, even though very little modulation occurs.

Attachment of mouse C3 to leukemia cells during in vivo modulation, if it in fact occurs, may be irrelevant with regard to escape of these cells from destruction within the animal. Intercalation of C3 into aggregated TL antigen-antibody complexes is necessary to effect blockage of guinea pig complement cytolysis, but "microaggregation" of complexes on the cell surface may be sufficient to prevent lysis by mouse complement in vivo. In that case, C3 attachment, like capping, may be a secondary consequence of modulation. Unfortunately, considerably more information regarding in vivo modulation of TL antigenicity must be gathered before this or any other hypothesis can be seriously entertained.

III. MODULATION OF OTHER CELL SURFACE ANTIGENS

Is modulation of TL antigens unique, or are other cell surface antigens also susceptible to this type of alteration? If other antigens can be modulated, does phenotypic suppression occur in the same manner as in TL modulation? Modulation-like changes have been reported for a variety of cell surface molecules recognizable as antigens, and we will review these reports with the purpose of comparing the results with those obtained for TL antigenic modulation. In this way, we might be able to establish either the generality of antigenic modulation or the uniqueness of TL modulation.

A. Histocompatibility Antigens

1. H-2 ANTIGENS.   There is considerable confusion regarding the capacity for cell surface antigens determined by the major histocompatibility locus in the mouse, the *H-2* complex, to be modulated. Lamm *et al.* (114) and Stackpole *et al.* (203) failed to modulate H-2 antigens on RADA1 cells, as did Schlesinger and Chaouat (176) on thymocytes and lymphocytes. However, there have been reports of H-2 modulation on peritoneal cells and myeloma cells that seem comparable to TL modulation (120, 121, 176). Also, exposure of lymphocytes or leukemia cells to H-2 antiserum followed by anti-mouse IgG serum has been found to render those cells resistant to subsequent lysis by complement alone (117, 214) or complement plus fresh H-2 antiserum (84, 85, 118). And finally, Richards *et al.* (168) have recently demonstrated H-2 modulation on normal peritoneal cells under certain conditions, while no modulation occurred on thymocytes, lymphocytes, or any malignant cell type examined.

Takahashi (214) first reported "modulation" of H-2 antigens on the surfaces of leukemia cells by further incubating H-2 antibody-presensitized cells with rabbit anti-mouse IgG serum. Previous attempts to modulate H-2 antigens on cells that undergo rapid TL antigenic modulation (RADA1 leukemia cells) directly with H-2 antiserum or univalent Fab fragments of H-2 antibody had been unsuccessful (114). Takahashi (214) was employing indirect sensitization of cells with H-2 antiserum and anti-Ig serum in an attempt to enhance the susceptibility of cells to lytic complement but unexpectedly observed just the opposite effect: diminution of complement lysis.

In the studies of Takahashi (214), cells of the C57BL/6 leukemia EL4 were initially sensitized for 45 minutes at 0° with varying concentrations of antiserum raised against H-2^b haplotype antigens. Cells were then washed free of excess antibody and further incubated at 0° or 37° with a constant concentration of anti-Ig serum. After varying lengths of time, cells were washed and sensitivity to guinea pig complement (pooled whole guinea pig serum) was assessed by incubation at 37°, cell lysis being measured by trypan blue dye uptake. When EL4 cells were sensitized with 1/200 to 1/400 dilutions of H-2 antiserum (approximate titer: 1/800) followed by incubation with anti-Ig serum at 37° for 45 minutes, complement sensitivity was totally lost. Loss of sensitivity did not occur at 0° and was progressively less dramatic as H-2 antiserum concentration was increased beyond a 1/200 dilution. Neither H-2 antiserum nor anti-Ig serum alone induced resistance to complement lysis.

Similar loss of complement sensitivity was observed by Lengerová *et al.* (117) on EL4 cells and normal bone marrow cells using H-2 antisera recognizing haplotypes or individual antigen specificities and anti-mouse Ig antibody. H-2 antigen-antibody-anti-Ig complexes were demonstrated on the surfaces of modulated and nonmodulated cells by immunofluorescence, and internalized complexes were detected by ultrastructural histochemistry, employing peroxidase-labeled antibodies. A positive corre-

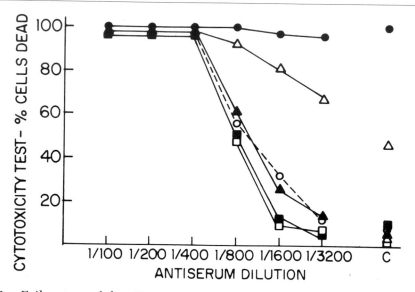

Fig. 18. Failure to modulate H-2 antigens on RADA1 leukemia cells (H-2^{dk}) indirectly, by sensitizing cells with excess H-2^d antiserum for 60 minutes at 0°, then washing the cells free from unbound H-2 antibody and further incubating with various dilutions of rabbit anti-mouse IgG serum for 90 minutes at 37°. Each sample consisted of 10^7 cells in 1 ml of medium 199 supplemented with 2% fetal bovine serum. The cells were finally washed, and the cytotoxicity of fresh H-2^d antiserum and toxic guinea pig complement (1/4) was determined by trypan blue dye uptake. The H-2 antiserum, C57BL/6 anti-Meth A (H-2^b vs. H-2^d), had a titer of approximately 1/800 on RADA1 cells and was used at a dilution of 1/200. The anti-IgG serum was diluted 1/10 (□), 1/25 (■), 1/50 (▲) and 1/100 (△), or was omitted (●). In one sample (○), both H-2 and anti-IgG sera were omitted. C, cytotoxic control with H-2 antiserum omitted.

While "modulation" is suggested by the loss of complement sensitivity of cells treated with H-2 antiserum plus 1/10–1/50 dilutions of anti-IgG serum, the cells retained essentially as much reactivity to H-2 antiserum and complement as cells incubated with no antiserum. Similar results were obtained when the concentration of presensitizing H-2 antiserum was varied (168).

lation was noted between loss of complement sensitivity, capping, and internalization of complexes. Other investigators have noted a similar correlation (65, 213).

Richards et al. (168) have attempted to "modulate" H-2^d antigenicity on RADA1 leukemia cells (H-2^a = H-2^{dk}) in the same manner as Takahashi (214) and Lengerová et al. (117). While similar results were obtained in terms of loss of sensitivity to guinea pig complement, "modulated" cells retained essentially the same sensitivity to fresh H-2 antiserum and complement as untreated cells, even after exposure to optimum concentrations of anti-Ig serum for 90 minutes at 37° (Fig. 18). In these cases, therefore, loss of complement sensitivity, which could result simply from steric interference imposed by the anti-Ig antibody (203), detachment of cell-bound antibody from antigen (3, 38, 40), or internalization of antigen-antibody complexes followed by appearance of new antigen at the cell surface, does not satisfy the criterion of modulation applicable to TL antigens; that is, loss of sensitivity to fresh antiserum plus guinea pig complement. Results obtained by Richards et al. (168) indicate that resistance to complement lysis is probably the consequence of steric hindrance.

Despite these indications that H-2 antigens on EL4 and RADA1 leukemia cells do not modulate in the same manner as TL antigens, even when an indirect sensitization procedure is employed, there have been reports of direct modulation of H-2 antigens on other murine cell types.

Schlesinger and Chaouat (176) observed that sensitization of peritoneal cells from various mouse strains with excess multispecific H-2 antiserum at 37° for 2 hours could render the cells partially resistant to the cytotoxic effects of fresh H-2 antiserum and guinea pig complement, supplied in the form of agar-absorbed whole guinea pig serum (a decrease from 85% lysis to approximately 20% lysis). Spleen and lymph node cells, however, did not modulate. Modulation of H-2 antigens on peritoneal cells was restricted to specificities to which sensitizing antisera were directed. The process did not proceed at 0° and was completely inhibited by preincubation with the antimetabolites sodium azide (10^{-4} M), iodoacetate (10 μg/ml) and 2,4-dinitrophenol (10^{-4} M), the corticosteroid hormones cortisol phosphate and succinate (1 mg/ml), colchicine (10^{-4} M), and cytochalasin B (10 μg/ml), for 1 hour at 37° (177). Agents that did not inhibit modulation following a 2-hour preincubation included: puromycin (20 μg/ml), cytosine arabinoside (10 μg/ml), chloramphenicol (10 μg/ml) and cycloheximide (10 μg/ml). Actinomycin D (20 μg/ml) totally inhibited modulation of cells pretreated for 3 hours, but exerted no inhibitory effect within shorter time periods. When modulated cells were washed free from H-2 antiserum and incubated at 37° in medium supplemented with normal mouse serum, complete cytotoxic sensitivity to H-2 antisera was restored within 2 hours.

The characteristics of H-2 antigenic modulation on mouse peritoneal cells observed by Schlesinger and Chaouat (176, 177) seem quite similar in many respects to those exhibited by TL modulation. Both processes can be inhibited by actinomycin D (after a lag phase), colchicine and cytochalasin B, while inhibitors of DNA and protein synthesis have little effect (see Section II, C, 5). However, corticosteroid hormones, 2,4-dinitrophenol, and sodium azide inhibited H-2 modulation but not TL modulation. These discrepancies in inhibitor effects may either be due to the differences in cell type used in the respective investigations or to inherent differences in the processes of modulation that are reflected in distinct metabolic requirements. Unfortunately, Schlesinger and Chaouat (176) did not determine the fate of modulated H-2 antigen-antibody complexes, information that would have been valuable for comparison of H-2 and TL modulation. On the basis of inhibitor effects, they presumed that modulated antigens were interiorized by pinocytosis (177).

Lesley and Hyman (120) have also obtained modulation of H-2 antigens (H-2^d haplotype) on BALB/c mouse myeloma (S194) cells maintained in suspension culture. Loss of sensitivity of these cells to guinea pig complement (agar-absorbed pooled whole guinea pig serum) alone, or H-2 antiserum plus complement, resulted from presensitization with excess H-2 antiserum for 1 hour at 0° followed by further incubation with antiserum for 2–3 hours at 37°, all in the absence of lytic complement. The fate of modulating antibody was assessed by use of H-2 antibody and rabbit anti-mouse IgG antibody, both radiolabeled with ^{125}I. By the time modulation was complete, approximately 30–40% of modulating H-2 antibody was lost from the cell surface by internalization (as indicated by the difference between total ^{125}I-labeled H-2 antibody detectable and the amount of ^{125}I-labeled anti-Ig antibody bound to the cell surface). A modulated state could be maintained for 24 hours by periodic addition of H-2 antiserum to restore antibody lost as a result of internalization, but a consistent 60–70% of the initial amount of H-2 antibody bound to the cells remained on the cell surface. Removal of H-2 antiserum and further culturing permitted restoration of the H-2 phenotype within 3 hours.

Modulation of H-2^d antigenicity on S194 cells occurred only when absorbed guinea pig complement was employed, not when unabsorbed complement was used (120). This difference was attributed to the presence of heteroantibody in unabsorbed complement that was reactive with the myeloma cells, but Budzko and Kierszenbaum (35) have shown that agar absorption of serum does not remove heteroantibody but significantly diminishes lytic complement by promoting activation of the alternative pathway. Therefore, while H-2 modulation was obtained, this condition may partially reflect the relative insensitivity of agar-absorbed complement.

H-2 antigen modulation studied by Lesley and Hyman (120) was completely inhibited at 0°, and at 37° in the presence of 2.5 × 10^{-3} M 2,4-dinitrophenol or 100 μg/ml concanavalin A [which may restrict mobility of the antigens (237)]. Partial inhibition was achieved with 4 × 10^{-4} M colchicine, 10^{-2} M sodium cyanide, 10^{-5} M iodoacetamide, 5 × 10^{-3} M sodium fluoride, 3 × 10^{-2} M sodium azide, 60 μg/ml oligomycin, and 100 μg/ml cytochalasin B, although the latter five agents were slightly cytotoxic.

In related studies, Lesley et al. (121) attempted to correlate H-2 antigen density on the surfaces of various cultured myeloma, lymphoma and mastocytoma cell lines with cell sensitivity to H-2 antibody and complement-mediated lysis and tendency for the cells to undergo H-2 antigenic modulation. Cell lines expressing one-half or less of the density of H-2 antigens on S194 myeloma cells (120; see above discussion) were relatively insensitive to lysis by H-2^d antiserum and guinea pig complement. However, loss of sensitivity to H-2 antiserum and complement resulting from presensitization of cells with H-2 antiserum (modulation) was achieved when the density of H-2 antigens was reduced to about 0.6–0.8 of the H-2 density on unmodulated S194 myeloma cells. These observations suggested to Lesley et al. (121) that a certain minimum density of H-2 antigens is necessary for successful antibody- and complement-mediated cell lysis, below which a cell is either inherently resistant to lysis or has been modulated. Presumably, then, modulation could be achieved when that threshold level of antigen density is reached as a result of antigen loss by internalization.

Unfortunately, this hypothesis fails to account for antibody-induced lateral displacement and aggregation of H-2 antigens within the cell surface membrane, a phenomenon of critical importance in TL modulation (203; see Sections II, C, 3–5). Undoubtedly, some lateral displacement and aggregation occurred during H-2 modulation as well, and that would have the effect of increasing local H-2 antigen density. Since local antigen density is a more crucial factor in antibody- and complement-mediated cytolysis than overall surface density (213), then it is unlikely that overall H-2 antigen density is of much consequence with regard to modulation.

The energy requirements for H-2 antigenic modulation observed by Schlesinger and Chaouat (176, 177) and Lesley and Hyman (120) are sufficiently distinct from the requirements for TL modulation (see Section II, C, 5) that a different mechanism could be operative in H-2 modulation. Inhibition of H-2 modulation is, in fact, more suggestive of a requirement for capping and extensive internalization (54, 216). If capping on these cells occurs over the Golgi region, as is likely but not established, then modulation may result more from internalization of capped antigen-antibody complexes than in the case of TL modulation (see Section II, C, 3). H-2 modulation would, therefore, be more sensitive to inhibitors of capping than TL modulation. The rapid appearance of new H-2 antigens following modulation suggests that new antigens may also be appearing at the cell surface during modulation (120). As in TL modulation, these nascent antigens would undoubtedly be modulated almost immediately, and such a process could account for retention of H-2 antigen-antibody complexes on modulated cells despite constant and extensive internalization.

Richards *et al.* (168) have attempted to modulate H-2 antigens on cultured RADA1 leukemia cells directly with H-2 antisera against the H-2^d (D and K), H-2^d (D) and H-2^d (K) group, and H-2.4, specificities. These investigators failed to obtain the slightest indication of true modulation under a variety of conditions, even after 24 hours in culture, as long as excess antiserum was maintained in the culture medium by periodic addition (Fig. 19). Misleading results were obtained if the antiserum level was permitted to become depleted. During this time period, considerable redistribution of H-2 antigen-antibody complexes into aggregates, patches and caps was noted by immunofluorescence, although capping occurred on relatively few cells (< 10% to 25–35%, depending upon the antiserum used). There were indications of considerable endocytosis of H-2 antibody (i.e., constant depletion of H-2 antiserum from the culture medium), probably because relatively little capping occurred (unlike the situation during TL modulation), but no extensive net loss of antibody from the cell surface was evident. These results, like those of Lesley and Hyman (120), indicate that endocytosis of H-2 antigen-antibody complexes is largely offset by the appearance of nascent antigens on the cell surface.

This failure of H-2 antigens to modulate on RADA1 cells on which TL antigens are so readily modulated seems puzzling in light of the rapid modulation of H-2 antigens obtained by other investigators (120, 121, 176) on different cell types. Moreover, Richards *et al.* (168) were also unable to modulate multiple, group, or individual H-2 antigen specificities on any other malignant cell type tested, including the TL+ leukemias ASL1 (H-2^a) and RL♂ 1 (TL.1,2; H-2^d), the TL− leukemia EL4 (H-2^b), the sarcoma Meth A (H-2^d), and the H-2^d myelomas MOPC-70A (IgG$_1$-producing) and S194 (non-Ig-producing). This inability to modulate S194 cells, which were modulated by Lesley and Hyman (120), appears to be related to the nature of the guinea pig complement used in the two studies. Lesley and Hyman (120) succeeded in modulating that cell type only when *absorbed* complement was employed, and their results suggest that absorbed complement is insufficiently sensitive to distinguish a modulated from a nonmodulated condition, at least in this case. Generally, studies of TL modulation have been done using the most sensitive guinea pig complement available, and therefore the ultimate criterion for modulation may be acquisition of resistance to lysis by the most sensitive source of guinea pig complement. Nevertheless, the possibility that tumor cells may "modulate" at all, regardless of the sensitivity of the complement, is fascinating and deserves more detailed examination.

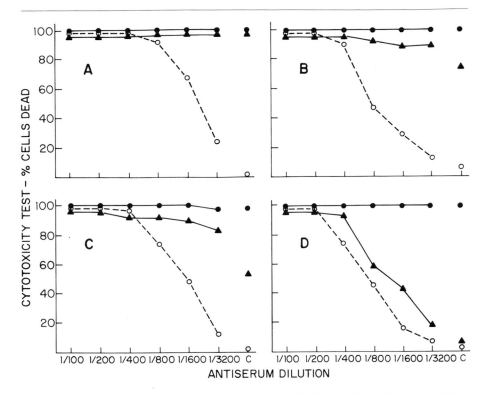

Fig. 19. Failure of H-2 antigens to modulate on RADA1 cells cultured in RPMI-1640 medium supplemented with 8% fetal bovine serum for 6 hours (*A*), 12 hours (*B*), 18 hours (*C*), and 24 hours (*D*). H-2^d antiserum (C57BL/6 anti-Meth A) was added to a final dilution of 1/100 initially only (▲) or initially and also at 6, 12, and 18 hours (●), or inappropriate H-2^b antiserum (1/100) was added at 0, 6, 12, and 18 hours (○); each sample consisted of 2×10^7 cells in 20 ml of medium. The cells were then washed, and the cytotoxic effect of fresh H-2^d antiserum and toxic guinea pig complement (1/4) was determined by tryptan blue uptake. C, complement cytotoxic control with H-2 antiserum omitted.

No modulation of H-2 antigens was evident even after 24 hours when antiserum was periodically added to the culture medium; these cells also failed to lose complement sensitivity (C control). When H-2 antiserum was added only initially, presensitizing antibody was gradually lost from the cell surface (and also from the medium) until at 24 hours, presensitized cells reacted like unsensitized cells. This loss of sensitizing antibody was not due to conditions of incubation, but presumably reflects endocytosis of H-2 antigen-antibody complexes by the cells. The same results were also obtained when (C57BL/6 × A/TL−)F₁ normal serum was added every 6 hours, indicating that serum factors essential for TL modulation are not effective in the H-2 system (168).

Using unabsorbed and highly sensitive guinea pig complement, Richards et al. (168) were able to demonstrate modulation of group (H-2D or H-2K) or individual H-2 antigen specificities on approximately two-thirds of normal peritoneal cells from several mouse strains within 2 hours at 37°. Under similar conditions, thymocytes and lymphocytes failed to modulate. Modulation did not occur when peritoneal cells were incubated with antisera directed against entire H-2 antigen haplotypes. Modulated cells remained sensitive to lysis by rabbit complement and retained considerable antibody on the cell surface detectable by indirect immunofluorescence, indicating that as in TL modulation, modulation of H-2 antigens does not entail net large-scale removal of H-2 antigen-antibody complexes from the cell surface. There was also no correlation between modulation and capping of H-2 antigens, which occurred on only 10–30% of affected cells.

Modulation of H-2 antigenicity on peritoneal cells required the presence of cobra venom factor-sensitive serum components that could be replaced by human C3 (168). Apparently, H-2 modulation requires deposition of mouse C3 onto the cell surface, as does TL modulation (204; see Section II, C, 7). While mouse C3 and the appropriate activating or cleaving enzyme (factor B?) had to be provided exogenously for TL modulation of thymocytes and leukemia cells, that was not true for H-2 modulation of peritoneal cells. Presumably, peritoneal macrophages contributed the necessary factors directly, possibly by synthesis of C3 and/or factor B (168).

Modulation of H-2 antigens on (C57BL/6 × A/TL⁻)F_1, BALB/c, and A/J peritoneal cells could be achieved when H-2 antiserum was supplemented with normal mouse serum with high TL-modulating (SMF) activity, human C3-sufficient serum (but not C3-deficient serum), or purified human C3 (168). These supplements failed to promote modulation of C57BL/6 peritoneal cells, however. These peculiarities of cells from C57BL/6 mice are consistent with the low SMF activity in sera from that strain (204). It is possible that peritoneal cells from that strain produce H-2 modulation-suppressing factor(s) which may be the same as TL-suppressing factor(s) that indirect evidence suggests is present in C57BL/6 serum (204).

Why H-2 antigens failed to modulate on malignant cells when unabsorbed complement was used (168) has not been ascertained but it may relate to an innate difference between the normal and malignant cell surface membrane that is reflected in more efficient lysis of the malignant cell by guinea pig complement. In this regard, it is curious that TL antigens generally modulate more rapidly and effectively on leukemia cells than on thymocytes.

To summarize, individual and group H-2 antigen specificities can be significantly modulated in vitro on normal mouse peritoneal cells, apparently in basically the same manner as outlined for TL modulation in vitro (see Section II, C, 10). Malignant cells, thymocytes, and lymphocytes appear to be completely resistant to modulation, even when an indirect sensitization procedure is employed, provided that unabsorbed guinea pig serum is used as the source of complement. The reason for this significant difference between TL and H-2 modulation is unclear.

2. HLA ANTIGENS. Miyajima et al. (133) have found that human peripheral lymphocytes sensitized with HLA antisera for 30 minutes at 37° become almost totally resistant to lysis by rabbit complement when incubated with complement alone for 1–5 hours at 37°. As in the related situations of loss of complement sensitivity by cells presensitized with H-2 antisera (117, 214), this "escape" from sensitization appeared to require cellular metabolic activity, since almost complete inhibition was achieved with 15 μg/ml actinomycin D, and partial inhibition with 100 μg/ml puromycin. Miyajima et al. (133) postulated that HLA antigen-antibody complexes were either actively shed from the cell surface or internalized by pinocytosis. Cells that had escaped complement sensitivity could nevertheless by lysed by fresh HLA antiserum plus rabbit complement, indicative that true modulation as in the TL and H-2 systems had not occurred. Considerable amounts of HLA antigens remained on the cells after incubation with complement, therefore, possibly representing antigens from which bound antibody has been shed, or newly synthesized antigens replacing molecules lost by endocytosis.

Sadeghee et al. (170) have obtained what appears to be true modulation of HLA antigens on human peripheral leukocytes by incubating cells with rabbit anti-HLA serum for several hours at room temperature or passing cells through columns coated with anti-HLA serum. Cells were resistant to the lytic effects of antiserum and guinea pig complement in a subsequent cytotoxicity test. In that test, cells were incubated at 37° for 1 hour with HLA antiserum prior to addition of complement, so modulation may have proceeded during that incubation as well. Modulated cells probably retained considerable amounts of HLA-anti-HLA complexes on the cell surface, since they exhibited a suppressed capacity to stimulate responder cells in the mixed leukocyte reaction, indicative of shedding antigen-antibody complexes.

B. Surface Immunoglobulins

In Section II, C, 2, the unusual susceptibility of TL antigens to antibody-induced lateral displacement and cap information was documented. This tendency for TL antigens to be aggregated seems to be

critical to the process of modulation. In this light, it is particularly interesting to examine the tendency for cell surface Ig molecules to
modulate, since these molecules are as susceptible to lateral displacement
within the cell surface membrane as are TL antigens (127, 202, 216, 237).
As might be expected, surface Ig modulates readily on a variety of cell
types (94, 109, 214, 215).

Modulation of κ-chain Ig on mouse lymph node cells, and κ and $\gamma 1$
chains on IgG$_1$-producing MOPC-70A myeloma cells, was achieved by
Takahashi (214) and Takahashi et al. (215) in essentially the same manner
as modulation of TL antigenicity. Cells were incubated at 37° for varying
lengths of time with excess rabbit anti-κ or anti-$\gamma 1$ serum, then washed
free of unbound antibody and tested for cytotoxicity of fresh antiserum
and guinea pig complement, cell lysis being assessed by uptake of trypan
blue dye. When cells were preincubated for 45 minutes at 0° with optimum concentrations of anti-κ serum, or for 45 minutes at 37° with normal rabbit serum, approximately 50% of lymph node cells and 70–80% of
MOPC-70A cells were killed. Preincubation of lymph node cells for 45
minutes at 37° with anti-κ serum resulted in complete loss of sensitivity to
fresh antiserum and complement; under the same conditions, myeloma
cells were totally modulated within 20 minutes. Cytotoxic sensitivity of
these cells to antisera directed against other cell surface receptors (H-2
and PC antigens) was undiminished following Ig modulation, indicating
that the $\kappa +\ \rightarrow\ \kappa -$ phenotypic change was highly specific.

Modulation of κ chains on lymph node cells was inhibited by preincubation with 50 μg/ml actinomycin D for 1 hour at 37°, suggesting that
cellular energy utilization was necessary, as with TL and H-2 modulation.
Curiously, however, actinomycin D exerted no inhibitory effect on κ
modulation on myeloma cells.

The $\gamma 1$ Ig chain on MOPC-70A cells was modulated similarly (214,
215). Furthermore, modulation of either κ or $\gamma 1$ chains separately resulted
in phenotypic suppression of both chains ($\kappa +\gamma 1+\ \rightarrow\ \kappa -\gamma 1-$). This result
is similar to the situation in TL modulation, with antisera to individual TL
specificities also modulating the other specificities residing (presumably)
on the same molecule (25, 26, 150). By the same criterion, κ and $\gamma 1$ chains
must reside on the same molecule on the surfaces of MOPC-70A cells.

It is likely that Lesley et al. (122) were observing the effects of
modulation when they examined κ-chain Ig on murine thymus-derived
lymphocytes. These investigators found that washing κ antiserum-
sensitized cells free from unbound antibody and incubating for 15 minutes at 37° resulted in a loss of sensitivity of these cells to the lytic effects
of κ antiserum and guinea pig complement.

Knopf and colleagues (109) also reported modulation of Ig from the
surfaces of IgG-secreting P3 (Ig+) myeloma cells in culture. The fate (i.e.,

cellular retention or shedding) of rabbit anti-mouse IgG_1 antibody used to modulate the cells was ascertained by radiolabeling that antibody with ^{125}I. Double labeling with ^{125}I-anti-mouse Ig and ^{131}I-labeled sheep anti-rabbit Ig antibody was used to distinguish cell surface-bound anti-Ig from interiorized antibody. Cells were sensitized with anti-Ig serum for 15 minutes at 0°, washed free from unbound antibody, and incubated at 0°, 24° or 37° for various lengths of time before determining the cytotoxic effect of fresh antiserum and guinea pig complement at 37°. Cells incubated at 0° for up to 60 minutes following sensitization remained susceptible to cytolysis, and very little ^{125}I-labeled anti-Ig antibody bound to the cells was lost, either by shedding or internalization. There was also negligible antibody loss after incubation for 80 minutes at 24°, but the cells had become totally resistant to antibody- and complement-mediated cytolysis (a decrease from about 70% to less than 20% lysis). Virtually all of this label proved to be interiorized by the cells. At 37°, modulation was essentially complete within 10 minutes and was accompanied by a 20–25% decrease in the amount of ^{125}I-labeled antibody detectable on the cell surface. More antibody was progressively lost from the cell surface over the next 70 minutes until only about 25% of the original amount was detectable. The considerable loss of anti-Ig antibody during the first several minutes was attributed to shedding into the medium, the remainder to internalization by the labeled cells followed by degradation of the antibody molecules. Modulated cells remained refractory to lysis by anti-Ig antibody and complement for at least 1 hour after washing cells free from sensitizing antibody and incubating at 37° in fresh medium.

The modulation results obtained by Knopf et al. (109) and others probably can be explained by the unusual tendency for labeled surface Ig to be capped over the Golgi region of the cell and rapidly interiorized at 37° (54, 202). Capping and internalization would also be anticipated at 24°, but to a lesser extent than at 37°. Shedding of surface Ig into the surrounding medium should also be considered as a reasonable explanation for modulation of some molecules. Surface Ig seems to have an unusual tendency to shed from the cell surface as a consequence of ligand binding (45, 98, 232, 238).

That there is a virtually complete loss of modulated Ig molecules and modulating antibody from the cell surface by internalization is supported by the following observations: (1) when MOPC-70A myeloma cells were modulated with rabbit anti-IgG_1 serum, all cells that became resistant to fresh antiserum and guinea pig complement also resisted lysis by rabbit complement; (2) modulated cells displayed no cell-bound antibody by immunofluorescence; (3) negligible antibody was shed into fresh medium following modulation; and (4) the modulating activity of antiserum was not altered by preheating at 56° (C. Stackpole, unpublished observations).

Modulation of surface Ig appears, therefore, to result from a loss of those molecules from the cell surface, most likely by rapid capping followed by internalization of Ig-anti-Ig complexes, as is certainly not the case in TL or H-2 antigenic modulation.

Raff et al. (164a) have also found that anti-μ chain antibodies cause reversible modulation and loss of IgM molecules from the surfaces of mouse B lymphocytes. However, when 14–15 day fetal liver explants were cultured with antiserum for several days, the development of IgM+ lymphocytes was irreversibly suppressed, even with 10-fold less antiserum than required for modulation of adult IgM+ cells. Thse results indicate that antigen suppression occurs by a different mechanism than antigen modulation. Both processes also occurred with univalent (Fab) antibody fragments as does TL modulation (see Section II, C, 8).

Modulation of surface Ig may also have been achieved on cultured human lymphoid cells (94), but the criterion for modulation was not strictly satisfied. In these studies, complement sensitivity was not assessed. Instead, loss of antibody reactivity to κ or μ Ig chains following presensitization with anti-κ or anti-μ serum at 37° was determined by a mixed antiglobulin reaction (based on rosette formation between Ig-sensitized red blood cells and anti-Ig coated lymphoid cells). Exposure of cells to anti-κ serum for 2 hours resulted in loss of reactivity for both anti-κ and anti-μ serum, while modulation with anti-μ serum had no effect on κ chains. Modulation was not achieved at 0° or when univalent anti-κ antibody was employed at 37°, and was inhibited by 5×10^{-2} M sodium azide, but not by 50 μg/ml actinomycin D, puromycin or cycloheximide. Restoration of κ and μ phenotypes occurred within 3–12 hours after removal of sensitizing antisera. The failure of univalent antibody to "modulate" these molecules, and the sensitivity of the process to azide is suggestive of capping/internalization or capping/shedding as the most likely mechanism.

C. Oncogenic Virus-Related and Tumor-Specific Cell Surface Antigens

While TL antigens are not tumor-specific (with the possible exception of TL.4), TL antigenic modulation occurs most dramatically on leukemia cells, possibly because of differences between malignant cells and their counterparts in terms of metabolic activity, organization of the cell surface, membrane fluidity, etc. In contrast, modulation of H-2 antigens may not occur on tumor cells and certainly does not occur on neoplastic cells under conditions promoting modulation of normal peritoneal cells (see Section III, A, 1). It is difficult to predict, therefore, whether tumor-specific or oncogenic virus-related antigens on the surfaces of tumor cells and infected normal cells might be particularly susceptible to antigenic modulation. While the evidence is fragmentary and imprecise at present, there are indications that modulation of some of these antigens does occur.

1. VIRUS-RELATED ANTIGENS.   a. Gross MuLV-Related Surface Antigens (GCSA and G_{IX}).

Aoki and Johnson (5) found that when the C57BL/6 mouse strain leukemia E♂G2, which was induced by Passage A Gross MuLV, was transplanted into C57BL/6 mice that had been hyperimmunized against the AKR spontaneous leukemia K36, a group of Gross virus-related cell surface antigens (GCSAa) on E♂G2 cells underwent antigenic suppression, or "modulation." Specifically, the cytotoxic titer of GCSAa typing serum with guinea pig complement dropped from 1/64 to less than 1/2, but was completely restored upon a single passage of these cells into unimmunized C57BL/6 mice. The two other groups of Gross virus-related antigens on E♂G2 cells (GCSAb and G_{IX}) as well as H-2 antigens, were unaffected by suppression of GCSAa antigens. There was a corresponding decrease in the amount of GCSAa antigenicity demonstrable on suppressed cells by immunoelectronmicroscopy, but the degree of labeling returned to normal levels following transplantation into unimmunized animals. No GCSAa antigens were detectable on modulated cells by immunofluorescence.

There are two notable differences between GCSAa antigen suppression observed by Aoki and Johnson (5) and TL modulation that may be significant:

1. Transplantation of E♂G2 cells into immunized hosts delayed growth of the transplants to a degree proportional to the extent of immunization and degree of antigen suppression. Normally, E♂G2 transplants (1.5×10^5 cells intraperitoneally) produce palpable splenomegaly within 7–8 days in unimmunized hosts, with death ensuing by 10–12 days. In transplants into *actively* immunized mice, GCSAa antigen suppression was only partial (the titer of test antiserum on these cells was reduced to 1/4 to 1/16), splenomegaly was not palpable until days 10–13, and death did not occur until days 15–22. Suppression was complete in hosts immunized both *actively and passively* (by injection of GCSAa typing serum), but spleen enlargement was delayed until days 12–16, and hosts did not succumb to leukemic growth until 17–25 days. Modulation of TL antigenicity *in vivo*, by contrast, is normally not accompanied by any change in the growth rate of the leukemic transplants (22, 25, 26).

2. There was no indication that GCSAa antigen suppression could occur during exposure of cells to GCSAa antiserum *in vitro* for 2–3 hours, while TL modulation occurs rapidly *in vitro*.

Suppression or "modulation" of GCSAa antigenicity on E♂G2 cells *in vivo* by specific antibody may have relevance to growth of Gross MuLV-induced leukemias under natural conditions. While it is obvious that tumors might escape destruction by "modulation" in intentionally hyperimmunized animals, escape might also occur as a result of natural immunization of certain hosts to GCSA antigens, since antibodies to these antigens have been detected in animals bearing Gross MuLV-induced leukemias (6). In this regard, a similar reversible suppression of Gross MuLV-related cell surface antigens has been observed on rat lymphoma cells transplanted into unimmunized but intolerant mature rats (95). At the same time, other Gross MuLV-related surface antigens show no evidence of "modulation," so that immunization in these cases may actually be protective against leukemic growth (149, 171).

Obata *et al.* (143) have noted a modulation-like phenomenon affecting G_{IX} antigens on mouse thymocytes *in vivo*. G_{IX} antigen as expressed on the thymocytes of certain mouse strains is a type-specific antigenic constituent of gp70 glycoprotein, the major envelope component of MuLV (58, 142, 220). In the prototype G_{IX}^+ strain, 129, G_{IX}-gp70 is expressed independently of virus production as a mendelian character, and is demonstrable by *in vitro* cytotoxicity, with rabbit serum as a source of lytic complement. Expression of G_{IX} antigen in this strain depends on genes at two loci, one (*Gv-1*) showing quasi-linkage with *H-2* on chromosome 17, the other (*Gv-2*) on chromosome 7 (207, 208, 210). Like TL antigens, G_{IX} expression occurs primarily in the thymus (it is also present on testicular cells and sperm).

Part of the G_{IX}-gp70 molecule bears MuLV group-specific antigens, but these are normally inaccessible to antibody at the intact thymocyte surface, although they may be released upon membrane disruption (220). Only the G_{IX} antigen determinant is accessible to antibody. Cells producing MuLV, regardless of tissue type or inherited G_{IX} genotype, may express G_{IX} antigenicity concomitantly with group-specific antigenicity.

Until recently, all attempts to produce antiserum to G_{IX} antigen in mice had failed, and thus, G_{IX} could only be demonstrated with a rat typing serum (208). However, Obata *et al.* (143) found that an F_1 hybrid between a G_{IX}^+ congenic mouse stock (C57BL/6/G_{IX}^+, obtained by transfer of the G_{IX}^+ allele from the 129 strain onto a G_{IX}^- C57BL/6 background—ref. 209) and 129 spontaneously produces G_{IX} antibody, suggestive of an autoimmune syndrome. Of interest to the present discussion is the finding that as production of G_{IX} antibody increases with age (1–14 months), there is a progressive decrease in expression of G_{IX} antigenicity on the surfaces of thymocytes taken from these mice, until antigen is no longer detectable. Quantitative expression of TL and H-2 antigens on the same cells was not affected by this change in G_{IX} antigenicity.

This phenotypic alteration $(G_{IX}^+ \rightarrow G_{IX}^-)$ may represent antigenic modulation, and in fact similar phenotypic loss of G_{IX} antigenicity has been demonstrated with both rat and mouse antisera during short-time incubations *in vitro* under conditions comparable to those employed to demonstrate TL modulation (Y. Obata and E. Stockert, personal communication). The alternate possibility, that G_{IX}^+ thymocytes were destroyed by specific antibody, leaving a G_{IX}^- population of cells to proliferate in the thymus, was not supported by experimental evidence. In that case, medullary thymocytes (G_{IX}^-) would have been selected, and these cells have characteristically different profiles of surface antigens than the G_{IX}^+ cortical thymocytes. However, G_{IX}^- thymocytes recovered from hybrid mice with G_{IX} antibody had the typical antigen profile of cortical thymocytes (143).

It will be of great interest to determine whether G_{IX} antigen on MuLV-producing leukemia cells are unusually sensitive to suppression by specific antibody.

b. Moloney MuLV-Related Cell Surface Antigens.

Several investigators have shown that Moloney MuLV-transformed mouse lymphocytes established in continuous culture undergo changes in susceptibility to the lytic effects of viral antibody and complement during the cell cycle (41, 43, 119). Maximum sensitivity to complement-mediated cytolysis occurs during the G_1 phase, and minimum sensitivity during the S phase. Cell cycle-related fluctuations in complement sensitivity have been observed with a variety of other cell types as well (80, 157, 184, 217), suggesting that it is a general phenomenon.

In their studies on Moloney MuLV-transformed YCAB lymphoma cells, Lerner et al. (119) observed that cytolytic sensitivity to MuLV antiserum and guinea pig complement was confined to the G_1 phase of the cell cycle. No differences were noted between sensitive and resistant phases in terms of viral antigen expression on the cell surface, accessibilty of antigen to antibody, or capacity of the cells to activate complement and bind complement components C3 and C4.

Subsequent analysis by Cooper et al. (46) indicated that resistance of YCAB cells to antibody-dependent complement-mediated lysis during the S, G_2, and M phases of the cell cycle did not result from failure to activate the complement effector system, lack of binding of terminal complement components to the cells, or absence of ultrastructural lesions in the cell surface membrane that are indicative of terminal complement component activation.

This phenomenon of acquired resistance to complement lysis during portions of the cell cycle may be related to TL modulation. The underlying mechanism is unclear, but it is possible that cells in the G_1 phase are less capable of rapidly healing membrane lesions induced by complement than cells in the remainder of the cell cycle, or that complement lysis is being "blocked" during resistant phases of the cycle.

c. Friend MuLV-Related Cell Surface Antigens. Lilly (126) has found that on spleen cells of BALB/c mice infected with Friend MuLV, virus-related (FMR) cell surface antigens appear during the first 2 weeks after infection, but thereafter begin to decrease in quantity progressively. The likelihood is that this observation does not constitute an example of antigenic modulation, since Lilly (126) also found a simultaneous decrease in H-2.31 antigen specified by the K region of the H-2 locus.

Genovesi et al. (76a) have found that antigenic modulation may explain suppression of a rapidly fatal Friend MuLV-induced erythroleukemia in DBA/2 mice to a "dormant" state by statolon, an extract of mycophage-infected Penicillium. Serum from mice bearing dormant malignancies contains antibodies that are able to modulate virus-specified cell surface antigens on erythroleukemia cells in vitro. Continued exposure of cells to dormant-immune serum in vitro resulted in nearly complete loss of cell susceptibility to anti-Friend MuLV serum and guinea pig complement within 48 hours, and the process was reversible. After 48 hours, 74% of modulated cells retained antibody demonstrable by immunofluorescence. In contrast to TL modulation, modulation in this case was achieved with heat-inactivated immune serum.

d. Murine Mammary Tumor Virus-Specified Antigens. Calafat et al. (37) have examined antibody-induced redistribution and modulation potential of normal (H-2.8 and Thy-1.2) and murine mammary tumor virus (MuMTV)-specified cell surface antigens on GR strain leukemia cells transplanted serially in ascites form. MuMTV antigens, which are present on viruses budding through the cell surface as well as on the generalized cell surface, could be completely modulated after 2.5 to 3 hours incubation at 37° with excess rabbit anti-MuMTV serum. Modulation was judged by loss of sensitivity to fresh antiserum plus a mixture of guinea pig and rabbit complement. No modulation occurred at 0°, and neither H-2.8 nor Thy-1.2 antigens could be modulated at 37° within 5 hours.

Immunoelectronmicroscopy demonstrated that MuMTV antigens labeled indirectly with rabbit antiserum followed by ferritin-conjugated goat anti-rabbit IgG antibody tended to redistribute into patches and caps more dramatically than H-2 or Thy-1 antigens labeled in corresponding fashion (37). This enhanced lateral displacement was evident at 0° and at 37°. Labeled MuMTV antigens were rapidly shed from the cell surface into the surrounding medium, where antigen-antibody complexes could be demonstrated. Shedding was less apparent in the case of H-2 and Thy-1 antigens.

These results suggested to Calafat *et al.* (37) that modulation of MuMTV antigens *in vitro* occurred principally by shedding of antigen-antibody complexes from the cell surface, and that a similar phenomenon might occur *in vivo* due to naturally occurring antibodies to MuMTV present in certain mice (135).

It would not be surprising to find that virus-related cell surface antigens "modulated" by shedding from the membrane, since much of the antigen is associated with virus particles that are enveloped at the cell surface and constantly "shed" from infected cells. Aside from the indications that MuMTV-related antigens are extremely mobile within the cell surface, and thus may modulate either in the manner of TL and H-2 antigens or in the manner of surface Ig, there is insufficient evidence available to draw any conclusions as to the exact nature of the various examples of virus-related antigen suppression discussed here.

e. Measles Virus Antigens.   Oldstone and his colleagues (99, 151) have examined the interaction between HeLa cells actively or persistently infected with measles virus in culture and measles antibody from convalescent human serum. These investigators have identified and characterized a dramatic case of antigenic modulation which may have relevance to the persistence of measles infections in patients with adequate cellular and humoral immune responses to prevent continued virus infection.

When acutely infected cells (4 days after inoculation with virus) or persistently infected cells (cells surviving acute infection) were cultured with excess measles antibody (immune serum preheated at 56° to inactivate complement) and then the cells were tested for the cytolytic effect of fresh immune serum (containing active complement), there was a progressive decrease in number of cells lysed during the first 12–24 hours (99). Initially, nearly 100% of acutely infected cells were lysed, but by 6 hours less than 40% of the cells could be lysed. The same number of cells was susceptible to lysis after 24 hours, but thereafter the number of susceptible cells increased until by 48 hours control levels were reached. The percentage of persistently infected cells lysed under the same conditions was about 95% initially and 10–15% after 24 hours of culturing with measles antibody. Lytic sensitivity returned to original levels within 24 hours after washing cells free from antibody and culturing in fresh medium. Persistently infected cells remained modulated for as long as excess antibody remained in the medium. Presumably, modulation was more complete on persistently infected cultures because acutely infected cells possessed considerably greater amounts of viral antigens than persistently infected cells.

In these experiments, modulation of measles virus antigens coincided with capping of the antigens and shedding from the cell surface (99), apparently as antigen-antibody complexes (151). After 24 hours of modulation, persistently infected cells were essentially denuded of viral antigens as monitored by immunofluorescence, although 33% of modulating ^{125}I-labeled anti-measles virus antibody (IgG fraction) remained cell-bound (99).

In related experiments, Joseph and Oldstone (99) observed that some persistently infected HeLa cells survived long-term culturing with measles immune serum containing active complement and that the surfaces of these resistant cells were devoid of viral antigens. The length of time required for new viral antigens to appear on the cell surface following washing and culturing with fresh medium depended on the length of exposure to antibody plus complement. After a 24-hour exposure, antigens reappeared on 50% of the cells within 24 hours; after 5 days of exposure, 6 days of recovery were necessary before antigens reappeared on 50% of the cells. When cells were continually exposed to antibody plus complement for 6 weeks, antigens failed to reappear over the next 6 weeks of culture with fresh medium. This suppressive effect of immune serum thus differs from antibody-induced modulation.

Joseph and Oldstone (99) observed that the growth rate of persistently infected HeLa cells, which was considerably slower than the growth rate of uninfected cells, was increased to uninfected cell levels by modulation with measles antiserum devoid of lytic complement. Modulation also promoted normalization of cell morphology and growth characteristics despite the continued production of cytoplasmic virus antigens.

Patients suffering from the chronic measles virus infection, subacute sclerosing panencephalitis, retain both significant levels of circulating virus antibodies and a persistent low-grade measles virus infection, despite the presence of competent cellular and humoral immune responses. This situation may result from a combination of antibody-induced antigenic modulation and antibody/complement-induced antigen suppression (99, 151). Modulation might occur in certain regions of the body that are deficient in lytic complement, such as the brain. Since Joseph and Oldstone (99) demonstrated that modulated virus antigens are largely shed from the cell surface as immune complexes, these complexes may serve to extend modulation by engaging complement components within the general circulation; circulating complexes might also prevent cellular responses from reaching the infected cells (151). Antigen suppression may occur in areas of the body rich in complement, and this phenomenon may serve to contain the progression of disease to complement-deficient body regions.

f. Herpes Simplex Virus-Specified Antigens.   In attempting to ascertain how latent infection of herpes simplex virus (HSV) is maintained in spinal ganglion neurons in the mouse, Stevens and Cook (206) found that exposure of ganglia to the IgG fraction of antiserum to HSV antigens prevented appearance of HSV antigens and initiation of viral DNA synthesis, indicative of an active infection. When ganglia were transplanted into latently infected syngeneic mice, the transplanted tissue remained latently infected. However, when ganglia were cultured in vitro, or transplanted into uninfected mice, active infection developed within several days. Furthermore, latent infection persisted in transplants into mice actively immunized with HSV or passively immunized with rabbit anti-HSV serum or the IgG fraction of that serum. The possibility that anti-HSV IgG was inherently cytotoxic for ganglion neurons bearing HSV antigens on their surfaces could not be eliminated altogether but was unlikely.

The results of Stevens and Cook (206) suggest that modulation of HSV antigens on neuron cell surfaces by anti-HSV IgG may play a role in maintenance of latent infection. However, more detailed examination of this system will be necessary to determine whether antibody is directly affecting cell surface antigens and if so, how suppression of virus DNA and antigen synthesis is achieved and maintained.

2. TUMOR-SPECIFIC ANTIGENS.
There are several examples of antigen suppression by specific antibody involving cells obtained from patients with Burkitt's lymphoma that deserve consideration as possible candidates for modulation.

Smith and his colleagues (191, 193) observed that incubation of cell lines derived from Burkitt's lymphoma cells with sera obtained from patients with that malignancy at 37° for 1–2 hours resulted in a marked decrease in detectable tumor-specific cell surface antigenicity. If the serum was then removed, the cells recovered the ability to specifically bind antibody within 2–3 cell divisions (12–24 hours). This reversible decrease in antigenicity did not occur at 0–4° and was blocked at 37° by agents interfering with cellular utilization of metabolic energy (191).

The P3J cell line, derived from a patient with Burkitt's lymphoma, expresses intracellular and cell surface antigens demonstrable by immunofluorescence and immunoprecipitation with serum from certain healthy patients (Burkitt-positive sera); this is in contrast to the general lack of demonstrable antigens in cells obtained directly from patients (7). When P3J cells were grown in medium supplemented with 15% Burkitt-positive serum, expression of both intracellular and surface antigens was suppressed. Cells grown with Burkitt-negative serum continued to express normal amounts of antigens. Suppression of cell surface antigenicity was not complete in the presence of Burkitt-positive serum, but intracellular antigens were totally lost from all but about 1% of the cells. It may be that cellular synthesis of these antigens was suppressed as a result of interaction of antibody with cell surface antigens (7). Since patients with Burkitt's lymphoma so often have detectable amounts of specific antibody in their sera, suppression in vivo could conceivably account for the undetectable levels of antigens in tumor cells obtained directly from patients. It should be pointed out, however, that TL antigen modulation in vitro does not seem to entail suppression of TL antigen synthesis by modulated cells (240).

Whether antibody suppression of antigen expression in cells of Burkitt's lymphoma in the patient has any relevance to "escape" of the tumor from immune destruction can only be a matter of conjecture at present.

Ortaldo et al. (154) claim to have obtained modulation of fetal antigens on Rauscher MuLV-induced leukemia cells passed in syngeneic C57BL/6 mice. These investigators found a 50–100-fold increase in expression of fetal antigens on cells passed in irradiated mice as compared to cells passed in normal mice, and this change was found to be mediated by humoral antibody. Antigenicity was measured by an antiglobulin method and absorption. Decreased expression of antigens on cells passed in normal mice required from 24 to 48 hours.

Unfortunately, neither in this system nor in the Burkitt's lymphoma systems was antibody-dependent complement-mediated cytolysis assessed, so it is impossible to draw any conclusions regarding the relationship between these phenomena and antigenic modulation. Hopefully, in future efforts, this parameter, as well as the fate of the suppressed antigens, will be examined.

D. Molecular Targets of Autoimmune Attack

Myasthenia gravis (MG), a disorder in man characterized by muscle weakness and fatigability, apparently results from a decrease in accessible acetylcholine receptors at neuromuscular junctions as a consequence of autoimmune attack mediated by antibody directed against receptor molecules (101, 219). Characteristics of the disease state (reduction in amplitude of miniature end-plate potentials and depletion of functional receptors) have been observed in mice receiving passive injection of the IgG fraction of serum from patients with MG (219). Treatment of passively immunized mice with cobra venom factor significantly lessened amplitude reduction, suggesting that complement component C3 enhances development of the MG syndrome.

Kao and Drachman (101) have further demonstrated that MG immune serum IgG enhances degradation of acetylcholine receptors on cultured rat skeletal muscle cells, assayed as label released into the medium from ^{125}I-labeled α-bungarotoxin bound to the receptors. Compared with a control degradation rate of about 4% per hour, addition of patients' serum IgG resulted in a degradation rate of 8.5% per hour. Accelerated degradation persisted throughout the 40-hour duration of these experiments. Apparently, many labeled receptors were lost from the cell surface by internalization, resulting in release of ^{125}I from metabolic degradation of the labeled receptors within the cells. A considerable population of receptors may have remained exposed on the cell surface but were inaccessible to α-bungarotoxin, although that was not established.

While it is not possible at present to determine whether development of MG involves modulation, the possibility that some acetylcholine receptors remain on the cell surface following interaction with antibody, and that C3 is directly involved, suggests that a process akin to TL modulation may account for some of the loss of functional receptors. Certainly this possibility should be considered in future studies of MG as well as other autoimmune syndromes.

IV. SIGNIFICANCE OF ANTIGENIC MODULATION AS A GENERAL TUMOR ESCAPE MECHANISM

While it should be evident from the preceding discussion that modulation is not unique to antigens of the TL system, there is as yet insufficient information available to ascertain how general the phenomenon may be. It appears that modulation entails varying degrees of antigen loss from the cell surface by internalization or shedding, depending upon the cell type and the antigen system. The important consideration, perhaps, is that antigen need not actually leave the cell surface for the cell to be rendered insensitive to specific antibody and lytic complement.

But does the specific loss of sensitivity of cells exposed to excess antibody in vivo or in vitro to fresh antibody and an exogenous source of complement in an in vitro cytotoxicity test have relevance to the escape of tumor cells from immune onslaught in situ? In the mouse, the answer seems to be yes. Modulation of TL+ or GCSA+ leukemias in animals hyperimmunized against TL or GCSA antigens permits these tumors to progress as in unimmunized hosts, whereas tumors do not generally grow in hosts hyperimmunized against antigens that do not modulate. TL antigens on leukemia cells are able to stimulate antibody production in TL− hosts despite their tendency to undergo modulation (97), so it is conceivable that spontaneously arising tumors bearing antigens capable of modulating can stimulate a host antibody response. A strong host response would probably enhance the chances of tumor escape, since as the number of tumor cells increased, the number of target antigens would multiply and a greater number of antibody molecules would be required to modulate those antigens. In other words, tumor cells would have to be bathed in excess antibody to modulate and escape destruction.

In the mouse, not all virus-related or tumor-specific antigens appear to be susceptible to modulation (18, 149, 171), so escape of tumor cells from destruction by the immune system is not a foredrawn conclusion. It will be important in future research in this area to try to determine why certain antigens can be modulated readily while other antigens (even on the same cells) cannot be modulated under the same conditions. In this regard, efforts must be made to distinguish true modulation from processes such as patch and cap formation, internalization, and shedding, because while these processes may accompany, and perhaps even "drive," modulation, modulation does not necessarily result from such dynamic changes on the cell surface.

Perhaps the most important question that needs to be answered is how exactly does our artificial criterion of modulation translate into tumor cell escape. There are indications that TL+ leukemia cells may escape destruction when all requirements for modulation have not been met (see Section II, D). What are the minimum requirements for escape, and what is the nature of the potentially destructive attack—humoral, cellular, or both? And while this information may be obtained in experimental animal systems, the possibility that modulation occurs on human tumor cells needs to be investigated in a more precise way, since at present we do not know whether modulation represents a significant tumor escape route in man. If it does, we may be able to learn enough about the processes underlying the phenomenon to eventually prevent escape by such a route.

ACKNOWLEDGMENTS

We wish to express our appreciation to Stefan Galuska for excellent assistance in a number of unpublished studies cited, and to Dr. Lloyd J. Old, Dr. Edward A. Boyse, and Dr. Elisabeth Stockert for invaluable ideas, advice and assistance in helping us to better comprehend many subleties in the area of antigenic modulation. Supported by National Cancer Institute grants CA-16168, CA-16889, and CA-08748.

NOTES

1. The term "modulation" is currently being used widely to describe a variety of changes occurring at the cell surface (cf. 63, 153, 211, 228), and should not be confused with the specific phenomenon of *antigenic* modulation so carefully defined and characterized by Boyse, Old, Stockert, and their colleagues during the 1960s. To add to the confusion, changes in cell surface antigens not specifically demonstrated to result in loss of sensitivity to antibody plus complement are often referred to as antigenic modulation (1, 69). Where such changes are likely to have resulted in antigenic modulation, we will use the designation modulation-like phenomenon.

2. The recent discovery by Flaherty *et al.* (76) of the TL.5 specificity and of antibody to that antigen in TL antisera (Table 1) has prompted us to designate the presence of TL.5 in all studies reviewed. In no instance does the presence of this unexpected antigen, or the corresponding antibody, warrant reinterpretation of experimental results.

REFERENCES

1. Akeson, R., and Herschman, H. R. 1974. Modulation of cell-surface antigens of a murine neuroblastoma. *Proc. Natl. Acad. Sci. U.S.* 71: 187–191.

2. Alexander, P. 1974. Escape from immune destruction by the host through shedding of surface antigens: Is this a characteristic shared by malignant and embryonic cells? *Cancer Res.* 34: 2077–2082.

3. Amos, D. B., Cohen, I., and Klein, W. J., Jr. 1970. Mechanisms of immunological enhancement. *Transplant. Proc.* 2: 68–75.

4. Anundi, H., Rask, L., Ostberg, L., and Peterson, P. A. 1975. The subunit structure of thymus leukemia antigens. *Biochemistry* 14: 5046–5054.

5. Aoki, T., and Johnson, P. A. 1972. Suppression of Gross leukemia cell-surface antigens: a kind of antigenic modulation. *J. Natl. Cancer Inst.* 49: 183–192.

6. Aoki, T., Boyse, E. A., and Old, L. J. 1966. Occurrence of natural antibody to the G (Gross) leukemia antigen in mice. *Cancer Res.* 26: 1415–1419.

7. Aoki, T., Geering, G., Beth, E., and Old, L. J. 1971. Suppression of antigen in Burkitt's lymphoma and human melanoma cells grown in selected human sera. In W. Nakahara, K. Nishioka, T. Hirayama, and Y. Ito (eds.), *Recent Advances in Human Tumor Virology and Immunology*, Proc. 1st Int. Symp. Princess Takamatsu Cancer Res. Fund, pp. 425–429. University Park Press, Baltimore.

8. Aoki, T., Chieco-Bianchi, L., Plata, E. J., Sendo, F., Hollis, V. W., Jr., and Kudo, T. 1974. Host immune response to virus-induced tumors. Some recent concepts. *Prog. Exp. Tumor Res.* 19: 23–36.

9. Appella, E., Tanigaki, N., Natori, T., and Pressman, D. 1976. Partial amino acid sequence of mouse β_2-microglobulin. *Biochem. Biophys. Res. Commun.* 70: 425–430.

10. Artzt, K., and Bennett, D. 1975. Analogies between embryonic (T/t) antigens and adult major histocompatibility (H-2) antigens. *Nature (London)* 256: 545–547.

11. Artzt, K., Dubois, P., Bennett, D., Condamine, H., Babinet, C., and Jacob, F. 1973. Surface antigens common to mouse cleavage embryos and primitive teratocarcinoma cells in culture. *Proc. Natl. Acad. Sci. U.S.* 70: 2988–2992.

12. Artzt, K., Bennett, D., and Jacob, F. 1974. Primitive teratocarcinoma cells express a differentiation antigen specified by a gene at the T-locus in the mouse. *Proc. Natl. Acad.Sci. U.S.* 71: 811–814.

13. Baldwin, R. W., Price, M. R., and Robins, R. A. 1972. Blocking of lymphocyte-mediated cytotoxicity for rat hepatoma cells by tumour-specific antigen-antibody complexes. *Nature (London) New Biol.* 238: 185–187.

14. Basch, R. S., and Goldstein, G. 1974. Induction of T-cell differentiation *in vitro* by thymin, a purified polypeptide hormone of the thymus. *Proc. Natl. Acad. Sci. U.S.* 71: 1474–1478.

15. Bennett, D., Boyse, E. A., and Old, L. J. 1972. Cell surface immunogenetics in the study of morphogenesis. *In* L. G. Silvestri (ed.), *Cell Interactions, Third Lepetit Colloq.*, pp. 247–263. North-Holland Publ., Amsterdam.

16. Borenfreund, E., Steinglass, M., Korngold, G., and Bendich, A. 1975. Effect of dimethyl sulfoxide and dimethylformamide on the growth and morphology of tumor cells. *Ann. N.Y. Acad. Sci.* 243: 164–171.

17. Boyle, M. D. P., Ohanian, S. H., and Borsos, T. 1975. Lysis of tumor cells by antibody and complement. III. Lack of correlation between antigen movement and cell lysis. *J. Immunol.* 115: 473–475.

18. Boyse, E. A. 1973. Immunogenetics in the study of cell surfaces: some implications for morphogenesis and cancer. *Curr. Res. Oncol.* 1972: 57–94.

19. Boyse, E. A., and Old, L. J. 1969. Some aspects of normal and abnormal cell surface genetics. *Annu. Rev. Genetics* 3: 269–290.

20. Boyse, E. A., and Old, L. J. 1971. A comment on the genetic data relating to expression of TL antigens. *Transplantation* 11: 561–562.

21. Boyse, E. A., Old, L. J., and Stockert, E. 1962. Immunological enhancement of a leukaemia. *Nature (London)* 194: 1142–1144.

22. Boyse, E. A., Old, L. J., and Luell, S. 1963. Antigenic properties of experimental leukemias. II. Immunological studies *in vivo* with C57BL/6 radiation-induced leukemias. *J. Natl. Cancer Inst.* 31: 987–995.

23. Boyse, E. A., Old, L. J., and Luell, S. 1964. Genetic determination of the *TL* (thymus-leukaemia) antigen in the mouse. *Nature (London)* 201: 779.

24. Boyse, E. A., Old, L. J., and Chouroulinkov, I. 1964. Cytotoxic test for demonstration of mouse antibody. *Methods Med. Res.* 10: 39–47.

25. Boyse, E. A., Old, L. J., and Stockert, E. 1965. The TL (thymus leukemia) antigen: a review. *In* P. Grabar and P. A. Miescher (eds.), *Immunopathology, 4th Int. Symp.*, Monte Carlo, 1965, pp. 23–40. Schwabe & Co., Basel.

26. Boyse, E. A., Stockert, E., and Old, L. J. 1967. Modification of the antigenic structure of the cell membrane by thymus-leukemia (TL) antibody. *Proc. Natl. Acad. Sci. U.S.* 58: 954–957.

27. Boyse, E. A., Stockert, E., and Old, L. J. 1968. Isoantigens of the *H-2* and *Tla* loci of the mouse. Interactions affecting their representation on thymocytes. *J. Exp. Med.* 128: 85–95.

28. Boyse, E. A., Old, L. J., and Stockert, E. 1968. An approach to the mapping of antigens on the cell surface. *Proc. Natl. Acad. Sci. U.S.* 60: 886–893.

29. Boyse, E. A., Stockert, E., and Old, L. J. 1969. Properties of four antigens specified by the *Tla* locus. Similarities and differences. *In* N. R. Rose and F. Milgrom (eds.), *Int. Convoc. Immunol.*, Buffalo, N.Y., 1968, pp. 353–357. Karger-Basel, New York.

30. Boyse, E. A., Old, L. J., and Stockert, E. 1970. Antigenic modulation. *In* H. Peeters (ed.), *Protides of the Biological Fluids, Proc. 17th Colloq.*, Bruges, 1969, pp. 225–227. Pergamon Press, New York.

31. Boyse, E. A., Hubbard, L., Stockert, E., and Lamm, M. E. 1970. Improved complementation in the cytotoxic test. *Transplantation* 10: 446–449.

32. Boyse, E. A., Stockert, E., Iritani, C. A., and Old, L. J. 1970. Implications of TL phenotype changes in an H-2-loss variant of a transplanted H-2^b/H-2^a leukemia. *Proc. Natl. Acad. Sci. U.S.* 65: 933–938.

33. Boyse, E. A., Old, L. J., and Stockert, E. 1972. The relation of linkage group IX to leukemogenesis in the mouse. *In* P. Emmelot and P. Bentvelzen (eds.), *RNA Viruses and Host Genome in Oncogenesis*, pp. 171–185. North-Holland Publ., Amsterdam.

34. Boyse, E. A., Flaherty, L., Stockert, E., and Old, L. J. 1972. Histoincompatibility attributable to genes near *H-2* that are not revealed by hemagglutination or cytotoxicity tests. *Transplantation* 13: 431–432.

35. Budzko, D. B., and Kierszenbaum, F. 1977. Cytotoxic effects of normal sera on lymphoid cells. II. Requirements for inhibition of nonspecific serum cytotoxicity by agarose. *Transplantation* 23: 337–342.

36. Burnet, F. M. 1970. The concept of immunological surveillance. *Prog. Exp. Tumor Res.* 13: 1–27.

37. Calafat, J., Hilgers, J., van Blitterswijk, W. J., Verbeet, M., and Hageman, P. C. 1976. Antibody-induced modulation and shedding of mammary tumor virus antigens on the surfaces of GR ascites leukemia cells as compared with normal antigens. *J. Natl. Cancer Inst.* 56: 1019–1029.

38. Ceppellini, R. 1971. Old and new facts and speculations about transplantation antigens of man. *In* B. Amos (ed.), *Progress in Immunology, 1st Int. Congr. Immunol.*, pp. 973–1025. Academic Press, New York.

39. Cerottini, J-C., and Brunner, K. T. 1974. Cell-mediated cytotoxicity, allograft rejection, and tumor immunity. *Adv. Immunol.* 18: 67–132.

40. Chang, S., Stockert, E., Boyse, E. A., Hämmerling, U., and Old, L. J. 1971. Spontaneous release of cytotoxic alloantibody from viable cells sensitized in excess antibody. *Immunology* 21: 829–838.

41. Cikes, M. 1970. Relationship between growth rate, cell volume, cell cycle kinetics, and antigenic properties of cultured murine lymphoma cells. *J. Natl. Cancer Inst.* 45: 979–988.

42. Cikes, M. 1975. Antigenic changes in cultured murine lymphomas after retransplantation into syngeneic hosts. *J. Natl. Cancer Inst.* 54: 903–906.

43. Cikes, M., Friberg, S., Jr., and Klein, G. 1972. Quantative studies of antigen expression in cultured murine lymphoma cells. II. Cell-surface antigens in synchronized cultures. *J. Natl. Cancer Inst.* 49: 1607–1611.

44. Colten, H. R. 1976. Biosynthesis of complement. *Adv. Immunol.* 22: 67–118.

45. Cone, R. E., Marchalonis, J. J., and Rolley, R. T. 1971. Lymphocyte mem-

brane dynamics. Metabolic release of cell surface proteins. *J. Exp. Med.* 134: 1373–1384.

46. Cooper, N. R., Polley, M. J., and Oldstone, M. B. A. 1974. Failure of terminal complement components to induce lysis of Moloney virus transformed lymphocytes. *J. Immunol.* 112: 866–868.

47. Cresswell, P., Turner, M. J., and Strominger, J. L. 1973. Papain-solubilized HL-A antigens from cultured human lymphocytes contain two peptide fragments. *Proc. Natl. Acad. Sci. U.S.* 70: 1603–1607.

48. Cruse, J. M., Lewis, G. K., Whitten, H. D., Watson, E. S., Fields, J. F., Adams, S. T., Jr., Harvey, G. F., III, Paslay, J. W., and Porter, M. 1974. Mechanisms of immunological enhancement. *Prog. Exp. Tumor Res.* 19: 110–156.

49. Currie, G. 1976. Immunological aspects of host resistance to the development and growth of cancer. *Biochim. Biophys. Acta* 458: 135–165.

50. Currie, G. A., and Sime, G. C. 1973. Syngeneic immune serum specifically inhibits the motility of tumour cells. *Nature (London) New Biol.* 241: 284–285.

51. Davey, G. C., Currie, G. A., and Alexander, P. 1976. Spontaneous shedding and antibody induced modulation of histocompatibility antigens on murine lymphomata: correlation with metastatic capacity. *Brit. J. Cancer* 33: 9–14.

52. Davies, D. A. L., Boyse, E. A., Old, L. J., and Stockert, E. 1967. Mouse isoantigens: separation of soluble TL (thymus-leukemia) antigen from soluble H-2 histocompatibility antigen by column chromatography. *J. Exp. Med.* 125: 549–558.

53. Davies, D. A. L., Alkins, B. J., Boyse, E. A., Old, L. J., and Stockert, E. 1969. Soluble TL and H-2 antigens prepared from a TL positive leukaemia of a TL negative mouse strain. *Immunology* 16: 669–676.

54. de Petris, S., and Raff, M. C. 1972. Distribution of immunoglobulin on the surface of mouse lymphoid cells as determined by immunoferritin electron microscopy. Antibody-induced, temperature-dependent redistribution and its implications for membrane structure. *Eur. J. Immunol.* 2: 523–535.

55. de Petris, S., and Raff, M. C. 1974. Ultrastructural distribution and redistribution of alloantigens and concanavalin A receptors on the surface of mouse lymphocytes. *Eur. J. Immunol.* 4: 130–137.

56. de Vaux Saint Cyr, C. 1969. Variations de l'antigénicité des fibroblastes de hamsters transformés par le SV40 puis clonées (TSV₅CL₂) selon qu'ils sont maintenus en culture de tissu ou propagés chez l'animal. *C. R. Acad. Sci. (D) (Paris)* 269: 1148–1150.

57. de Vaux Saint Cyr, C. 1974. Modulation of expression of virus-induced tumor antigens *in vivo* and *in vitro*. In D. W. Weiss (ed.), *Immunological Parameters of Host-Tumor Relationships*, Vol. 3, pp. 12–21. Academic Press, New York.

58. Del Villano, B. C., Nave, B., Croker, B. P., Lerner, R. A., and Dixon, F. J. 1975. The oncornavirus glycoprotein gp 69/71: a constituent of the surface of normal and malignant thymocytes. *J. Exp. Med.* 141: 172–187.

59. Démant, P., and Graff, R. J. 1973. Transplantation analysis of the *H-2* system. *Transplant. Proc.* 5: 267–270.

60. Doljanski, F., and Kapeller, M. 1976. Cell surface shedding—the phenomenon and its possible significance. *J. Theor. Biol.* 62: 253–270.

61. Dorval, G., Witz, I. P., Klein, E., and Wigzell, H. 1976. Tumor-bound

immunoglobulins: an in vivo phenomenon of masked specificity. *J. Natl. Cancer Inst.* 56: 523–527.

62. Eddy, B. E., Grubbs, G. E., and Young, R. D. 1964. Tumor immunity in hamsters infected with adenovirus type 12 or simian virus 40. *Proc. Soc. Exp. Biol. Med.* 117: 575–579.

63. Edelman, G. M. 1976. Surface modulation in cell recognition and cell growth. *Science* 192: 218–226.

64. Edidin, M. 1974. Rotational and translational diffusion in membranes. *Annu. Rev. Biophys. Bioeng.* 3: 179–201.

65. Edidin, M., and Henney, C. S. 1973. The effect of capping H-2 antigens on the susceptibility of target cells to humoral and T cell-mediated lysis. *Nature New Biol.* 246: 47–49.

66. Esmon, N. L., and Little, J. R. 1976. An indirect radioimmunoassay for thymus leukemia (TL) antigens. *J. Immunol.* 117: 911–918.

67. Esmon, N. L., and Little, J. R. 1976. Different mechanisms for the modulation of TL antigens on murine lymphoid cells. *J. Immunol.* 117: 919–926.

68. Evans, R., and Alexander, P. 1970. Cooperation of immune lymphoid cells with macrophages in tumour immunity. *Nature (London)* 228: 620–622.

69. Faanes, R. B., Choi, Y. S., and Good, R. A. 1973. Escape from isoantiserum inhibition of lymphocyte-mediated cytotoxicity. *J. Exp. Med.* 137: 171–182.

70. Fenyö, E. M., Klein, E., Klein, G., and Swiech, K. 1968. Selection of an immunoresistant Moloney lymphoma subline with decreased concentration of tumor-specific surface antigens. *J. Natl. Cancer Inst.* 40: 69–89.

71. Fenyö, E. M., Grundner, G., Klein, G., Klein, E., and Harris, H. 1971. Surface antigens and release of virus in hybrid cells produced by fusion of A9 fibroblasts with Moloney lymphoma cells. *Exp. Cell Res.* 68: 323–331.

72. Flaherty, L., and Bennett, D. 1973. Histoincompatibilities found between congenic strains which differ at loci determining differentiation antigens. *Transplantation* 16: 505–514.

73. Flaherty, L., and Bennett, D. 1973. The unusual fate of second skin grafts across an H(Tla) barrier. *Transplantation* 16: 682–684.

74. Flaherty, L., and Wachtel, S. S. 1975. H(Tla) system: allelism and linkage studies. *Transplant. Proc.* 7: 143–145.

75. Flaherty, L., and Wachtel, S. S. 1975. *H(Tla)* system: identification of two new loci, *H-31* and *H-32*, and alleles. *Immunogenetics* 2: 81–85.

76. Flaherty, L., Sullivan, K., and Zimmerman, D. 1977. The *Tla* locus: a new allele and antigenic specificity. *J. Immunol.*, 119:571–575.

76a. Genovesi, E. V., Marx, P. A., and Wheelock, E. F. 1977. Antigenic modulation of Friend virus erythroleukemic cells in vitro by serum from mice with dormant erythroleukemia. *J. Exp. Med.* 146: 520–534.

77. Gingell, D. 1973. Membrane permeability change by aggregation of mobile glycoprotein units. *J. Theor. Biol.* 38: 677–679.

78. Goldner, H., Girardi, A. J., Larson, V. M., and Hilleman, M. R. 1964. Interruption of SV_{40} virus tumorigenesis using irradiated homologous tumor antigen. *Proc. Soc. Exp. Biol. Med.* 117: 851–857.

79. Gorer, P. A., and O'Gorman, P. 1956. The cytotoxic activity of isoan-

tibodies in mice. *Transplant. Bull.* 3: 142–143.

80. Götze, D., Pellegrino, M. A., Ferrone, S., and Reisfeld, R. A. 1972. Expression of H-2 antigens during the growth cycle of cultured tumor cells. *Immunol. Commun.* 1: 533–544.

81. Götze, O., and Müller-Eberhard, H. J. 1976. The alternative pathway of complement activation. *Adv. Immunol.* 24: 1–35.

82. Grey, H. M., Kubo, R. T., Colon, S. M., Poulik, M. D., Cresswell, P., Springer, T., Turner, M., and Strominger, J. L. 1973. The small subunit of HL-A antigens is β2-microglobulin. *J. Exp. Med.* 138: 1608–1612.

83. Grisham, L. M., Wilson, L., and Bensch, K. G. 1973. Antimitotic action of griseofulvin does not involve disruption of microtubules. *Nature (Lond.)* 244: 294–296.

84. Hauptfeld, V., and Klein, J. 1975. Molecular relationship between private and public *H-2* antigens as determined by antigen redistribution method. *J. Exp. Med.* 142: 288–298.

85. Hauptfeld, V., Hauptfeld, M., and Klein, J. 1975. Induction of resistance to antibody-mediated cytotoxicity. *H-2*, Ia, and Ig antigens are independent entities in the membrane of mouse lymphocytes. *J. Exp. Med.* 141: 1047–1056.

86. Haywood, G. R., and McKhann, C. F. 1971. Antigenic specificities of murine sarcoma cells. Reciprocal relationship between normal transplantation antigens (H-2) and tumor-specific immunogenicity. *J. Exp. Med.* 133: 1171–1187.

87. Hellström, I., Hellström, K. E., Sjögren, H. O., and Warner, G. A. 1971. Serum factors in tumor-free patients cancelling the blocking of cell-mediated tumor immunity. *Int. J. Cancer* 8: 185–191.

88. Hellström, K. E., and Hellström, I. 1969. Cellular immunity against tumor antigens. *Adv. Cancer Res.* 12: 167–223.

89. Hellström, K. E., and Hellström, I. 1974. Lymphocyte-mediated cytotoxicity and blocking serum activity to tumor antigens. *Adv. Immunol.* 18: 209–277.

90. Henning, R., Milner, R. J., Reske, K., Cunningham, B. A., and Edelman, G. M. 1976. Subunit structure, cell surface orientation, and partial amino-acid sequences of murine histocompatibility antigens. *Proc. Natl. Acad. Sci. U.S.* 73: 118–122.

91. Herberman, R. B. 1974. Cell-mediated immunity to tumor cells. *Adv. Cancer Res.* 19: 207–263.

92. Hess, M., and Davies, D. A. L. 1974. Basic structure of mouse histocompatibility antigens. *Eur. J. Biochem.* 41: 1–13.

93. Humphries, G. M. K., and McConnell, H. M. 1975. Antigen mobility in membranes and complement-mediated immune attack. *Proc. Natl. Acad. Sci. U.S.* 72: 2483–2487.

94. Hütteroth, T. H., Cleve, H., and Litwin, S. D. 1973. Modulation of membrane associated immunoglobulins of cultured human lymphoid cells by specific antibody. *J. Immunol.* 110: 1325–1333.

95. Ioachim, H. L., Dorsett, B., Sabbath, M., and Keller, S. 1972. Loss and recovery of phenotypic expression of Gross leukemia virus. *Nature (London) New Biol.* 237: 215–218.

96. Jacob, H., Amsden, T., and White, J. 1972. Membrane microfilaments of erythrocytes: alterations in intact cells reproduce the hereditary spherocytosis

syndrome. *Proc. Natl. Acad. Sci. U.S.A.* 69: 471–474.

97. Jacobson, J. B., Galuska, S., and Stackpole, C. W. *In vivo* modulation of TL antigens on mouse leukemia cells and thymocytes: modulating antibody remains on the cell surface. *J. Natl. Cancer Inst.* (In press).

98. Jones, G. 1973. Release of surface receptors from lymphocytes. *J. Immunol.* 10: 1526–1531.

99. Joseph, B. S., and Oldstone, M. B. A. 1975. Immunologic injury in measles virus infection. II. Suppression of immune injury through antigenic modulation. *J. Exp. Med.* 142: 864–876.

100. Kaliss, N. 1958. Immunological enhancement of tumor homografts in mice; a review. *Cancer Res.* 18: 992–1003.

101. Kao, I., and Drachman, D. B. 1977. Myasthenic immunoglobulin accelerates acetylcholine receptor degradation. *Science* 196: 527–529.

102. Kassel, R. L., Old, L. J., Carswell, E. A., Fiore, N. C., and Hardy, W. D., Jr. 1973. Serum-mediated leukemia cell destruction in AKR mice. Role of complement in the phenomenon. *J. Exp. Med.* 138: 925–938.

103. Kawashima, K., Ikeda, H., Stockert, E., Takahashi, T., and Old, L. J. 1976. Age-related changes in cell surface antigens of preleukemic AKR thymocytes. *J. Exp. Med.* 144: 193–208.

104. Kim, U., Baumler, A., Carruthers, C., and Bielat, K. 1975. Immunological escape mechanism in spontaneously metastasizing mammary tumors. *Proc. Natl. Acad. Sci. U.S.* 72: 1012–1016.

105. Kirkwood, J. M., and Gershon, R. K. 1974. A role for suppressor T cells in immunological enhancement of tumor growth. *Prog. Exp. Tumor Res.* 19: 157–164.

106. Klein, E., and Klein, G. 1956. Mechanism of induced change in transplantation specificity of a mouse tumor passed through hybrid hosts. *Transplant. Bull.* 3: 136–142.

107. Klein, G. 1975. Immunological surveillance against neoplasia. *Harvey Lect.* 69: 71–102.

108. Klein, J. 1975. *Biology of the Mouse Histocompatibility-2 Complex*, pp. 241–251. Springer-Verlag, New York.

109. Knopf, P. M., Destree, A., and Hyman, R. 1973. Antibody-induced changes in expression of an immunoglobulin surface antigen. *Eur. J. Immunol.* 3: 251–259.

110. Komuro, K., and Boyse, E. A. 1973. *In-vitro* demonstration of thymic hormone in the mouse by conversion of precursor cells into lymphocytes. *Lancet* 1: 740–743.

111. Komuro, K., Boyse, E. A., and Old, L. J. 1973. Production of TL antibody by mice immunized with TL− cell populations. A possible assay for thymic hormone. *J. Exp. Med.* 137: 533–536.

112. Konda, S., Nakao, Y., and Smith, R. T. 1972. Immunologic properties of mouse thymus cells. Identification of T cell functions within a minor, low-density subpopulation. *J. Exp. Med.* 136: 1461–1477.

113. Konda, S., Stockert, E., and Smith, R. T. 1973. Immunologic properties of mouse thymus cells: membrane antigen patterns associated with various cell subpopulations. *Cell. Immunol.* 7: 275–289.

114. Lamm, M. E., Boyse, E. A., Old, L. J., Lisowska-Bernstein, B., and Stockert, E. 1968. Modulation of TL (thymus-leukemia) antigens by Fab-fragments of TL antibody. *J. Immunol.* 101: 99–103.

115. Lance, E. M., Cooper, S., and Boyse, E. A. 1971. Antigenic change and cell maturation in murine thymocytes. *Cell. Immunol.* 1: 536–544.

116. Leckband, E., and Boyse, E. A. 1971. Immunocompetent cells among mouse thymocytes: a minor population. *Science* 172: 1258–1260.

117. Lengerová, A., Pokorná, Z., Viklický, V., and Zelený, V. 1972. Phenotypic suppression of H-2 antigens and topography of the cell surface. *Tissue Antigens* 2: 332–340.

118. Lengerová, A. Pêknicová, J., and Pokorná, Z. 1974. Structural relationships between individual H-2 specificities on the cell surface. *J. Immunogenet.* 1: 239–248.

119. Lerner, R. A., Oldstone, M. B. A., and Cooper, N. R. 1971. Cell cycle-dependent immune lysis of Moloney virus-transformed lymphocytes: presence of viral antigen, accessibility to antibody, and complement activation. *Proc. Natl. Acad. Sci. U.S.* 68: 2584–2588.

120. Lesley, J., and Hyman, R. 1974. Antibody-induced changes in expression of the H-2 antigen. *Eur. J. Immunol.* 4: 732–739.

121. Lesley, J., Hyman, R., and Dennert, G. 1974. Effect of antigen density on complement-mediated lysis, T-cell-mediated killing, and antigenic modulation. *J. Natl. Cancer Inst.* 53: 1759–1765.

122. Lesley, J. F., Kettman, J. R., and Dutton, R. W. 1971. Immunoglobulins on the surface of thymus-derived cells engaged in the initiation of a humoral immune response. *J. Exp. Med.* 134: 618–629.

123. Levy, M. H., and Wheelock, E. F. 1974. The role of macrophages in defense against neoplastic disease. *Adv. Cancer Res.* 20: 131–163.

124. Liang, W., and Cohen, E. P. 1975. Complement sensitivity of somatic hybrids of a complement-resistant murine leukemia cell line. *J. Natl. Cancer Inst.* 55: 309–317.

125. Liang, W., and Cohen, E. P. 1975. Somatic hybrid of thymus leukemia (+) and (−) cells forms thymus leukemia antigens but fails to undergo modulation. *Proc. Natl. Acad. Sci. U.S.* 72: 1873–1877.

126. Lilly, F. 1972. Antigen expression on spleen cells of Friend virus-infected mice. *In* P. Emmelot and P. Bentvelzen (eds.), *RNA Viruses and Host Genome in Oncogenesis*, pp. 229–238. North-Holland Publ., Amsterdam.

127. Loor, F., Forni, L., and Pernis, B. 1972. The dynamic state of the lymphocyte membrane. Factors affecting the distribution and turnover of surface immunoglobulins. *Eur. J. Immunol.* 2: 203–212.

128. Loor, F., Block, N., and Little, J. R. 1975. Dynamics of the TL antigens on thymus and leukemia cells. *Cell. Immunol.* 17: 351–365.

129. MacLennan, I. C. M. 1972. Antibody in the induction and inhibition of lymphocyte cytotoxicity. *Transplant. Rev.* 13: 67–90.

130. Marantz, R., Ventilla, M., and Shelanski, M. 1969. Vinblastine-induced precipitation of microtubule protein. *Science (Washington, D.C.)* 165: 498.

131. Metcalf, D. 1966. Histologic and transplantation studies on preleukemic thymus of the AKR mouse. *J. Natl. Cancer Inst.* 37: 425–442.

132. Mishra, R. K., and Passow, H. 1969. Induction of intracellular ATP synthesis by extracellular ferricyanide in human red blood cells. *J. Membr. Biol.* 1: 214–224.

133. Miyajima, T., Hirata, A. A., and Terasaki, P. I. 1972. Escape from sensitization to HL-A antibodies. *Tissue Antigens* 2: 64–73.

134. Mizel, S. B., and Wilson, L. 1972. Nucleoside transport in mammalian cells. Inhibition by colchicine. *Biochemistry* 11: 2573–2578.

135. Müller, M., Hageman, P. C., and Daams, J. H. 1971. Spontaneous occurrence of precipitating antibodies to the mammary tumor virus in mice. *J. Natl. Cancer Inst.* 47: 801–805.

136. Muramatsu, T., Nathenson, S. G., Boyse, E. A., and Old, L. J. 1973. Some biochemical properties of thymus leukemia antigens solubilized from cell membranes by papain digestion. *J. Exp. Med.* 137: 1256–1262.

137. Nathenson, S. G. 1970. Biochemical properties of histocompatibility antigens. *Annu. Rev. Genet.* 4: 69–90.

138. Nathenson, S. G., and Cullen, S. E. 1974. Biochemical properties and immunochemical-genetic relationships of mouse H-2 alloantigens. *Biochim. Biophys. Acta* 344: 1–25.

139. Nicolson, G. L. 1976. Transmembrane control of the receptors on normal and tumor cells. I. Cytoplasmic influence over cell surface components. *Biochim. Biophys. Acta* 457: 57–108.

140. Nicolson, G. L. 1976. Transmembrane control of the receptors on normal and tumor cells. II. Surface changes associated with transformation and malignancy. *Biochim. Biophys. Acta* 458: 1–72.

141. Nossal, G. J. V. 1974. Principles of immunological tolerance and immunocyte receptor blockade. *Adv. Immunol.* 20: 93–130.

142. Obata, Y., Ikeda, H., Stockert, E., and Boyse, E. A. 1975. Relation of G_{IX} antigen of thymocytes to envelope glycoprotein of murine leukemia virus. *J. Exp. Med.* 141: 188–197.

143. Obata, Y., Stockert, E., Boyse, E. A., Tung, J.-S., and Litman, G. W. 1976. Spontaneous autoimmunization to G_{IX} cell surface antigen in hybrid mice. *J. Exp. Med.* 144: 533–542.

144. Oettgen, H. F. 1974. Serology of cancer. *In* F. H. Bach and R. A. Good (eds.), *Clinical Immunobiology*, Vol. 2, pp. 205–231. Academic Press, New York.

145. Ohno, S., Natsu-ume, S., and Migita, S. 1975. Alteration of cell-surface antigenicity of the mouse plasmacytoma. I. Immunologic characterization of surface antigens masked during successive transplantations. *J. Natl. Cancer Inst.* 55: 569–577.

146. Old, L. J., and Boyse, E. A. 1965. Antigens of tumors and leukemias induced by viruses. *Fed. Proc.* 24: 1009–1017.

147. Old, L. J., Boyse, E. A., Clarke, D. A., and Carswell, E. A. 1962. Antigenic properties of chemically induced tumors. *Ann. N.Y. Acad. Sci.* 101: 80–106.

148. Old, L. J., Boyse, E. A., and Stockert, E. 1963. Antigenic properties of experimental leukemias. I. Serological studies *in vitro* with spontaneous and radiation-induced leukemias. *J. Natl. Cancer Inst.* 31: 977–986.

149. Old, L. J., Stockert, E., Boyse, E. A., and Geering, G. 1967. A study of passive immunization against a transplanted G+ leukemia with specific an-

tiserum. *Proc. Soc. Exp. Biol. Med.* 124: 63–68.

150. Old, L. J., Stockert, E., Boyse, E. A., and Kim, J. H. 1968. Antigenic modulation. Loss of TL antigen from cells exposed to TL antibody. Study of the phenomenon *in vitro. J. Exp. Med.* 127: 523–539.

151. Oldstone, M. B. A. 1977. Role of antibody in regulating virus persistence: modulation of viral antigens expressed on the cell's plasma membrane and analysis of cell lysis. National Institute of Child and Human Development Conference on Development of Host Defenses, May, 1976, Elkridge, Md., in press.

152. Oldstone, M. B. A., Aoki, T., and Dixon, F. J. 1972. The antibody response of mice to murine leukemia virus in spontaneous infection: absence of classical immunologic tolerance. *Proc. Natl. Acad. Sci. U.S.* 69: 134–138.

153. Orly, J., and Schramm, M. 1975. Fatty acids as modulators of membrane functions: catecholamine-activated adenylate cyclase of the turkey erythrocyte. *Proc. Natl. Acad. Sci. U.S.* 72: 3433–3437.

154. Ortaldo, J. R., Ting, C. C., and Herberman, R. B. 1974. Modulation of fetal antigen(s) in mouse leukemia cells. *Cancer Res.* 34: 1366–1371.

155. Ostberg, L., Rask, L., Wigzell, H., and Peterson, P. A. 1975. Thymus leukaemia antigen contains β2-microglobulin. *Nature (London)* 253: 735–737.

156. Owen, J. J. T., and Raff, M. C. 1970. Studies on the differentiation of the thymus-derived lymphocytes. *J. Exp. Med.* 132: 1216–1232.

157. Pellegrino, M. A., Ferrone, S., Cooper, N. R., Dierich, M. P., and Reisfeld, R. A. 1974. Variation in susceptibility of a human lymphoid cell line to immune lysis during the cell cycle. *J. Exp. Med.* 140: 578–590.

158. Perlmann, P., and Holm, G. 1969. Cytotoxic effects of lymphoid cells *in vitro. Adv. Immunol.* 11: 117–193.

159. Perlmann, P., Perlmann, H., and Wigzell, H. 1972. Lymphocyte mediated cytotoxicity *in vitro.* Induction and inhibition by humoral antibody and nature of effector cells. *Transplant. Rev.* 13: 91–114.

160. Plagemann, P. G. W., and Erbe, J. 1972. Thymidine transport by cultured Novikoff hepatoma cells and uptake by simple diffusion and relationship to incorporation into deoxyribonucleic acid. *J. Cell Biol.* 55: 161–178.

161. Prehn, R. T. 1974. Immunological surveillance: pro and con. *In* F. H. Bach and R. A. Good (eds.), *Clinical Immunobiology,* Vol. 2, pp. 191–203. Academic Press, New York.

162. Poulik, M. D., Bernoco, M., Bernoco, D., and Ceppellini, R. 1973. Aggregation of HL-A antigens at the lymphocyte surface induced by antiserum to β_2-microglobulin. *Science* 182: 1352–1355.

163. Puck, T. T., and Jones, C. 1974. Cyclic AMP and microtubular dynamics in cultured mammalian cells. *In* W. Braun, L. M. Lichtenstein, and C. W. Parker (eds.), *Cyclic AMP, Cell Growth, and the Immune Response,* Symp. Marco Island, Florida, 1973, pp. 338–348. Springer-Verlag, New York.

164. Raff, M. C. 1971. Evidence for subpopulation of mature lymphocytes within mouse thymus. *Nature (London) New Biol.* 229: 182–184.

164a. Raff, M. C., Owen, J. J. T., Cooper, M. D., Lawton, A. R. III, Megson, M., and Gathings, W. E. 1978. Differences in susceptibility of mature and immature mouse B lymphocytes to anti-immunoglobulin-induced immunoblobulin suppression *in vitro.* Possible implications for B-cell tolerance to self. *J. Exp. Med.*

142: 1052–1064.

165. Rammler, D. H., and Zaffaroni, A. 1971. Biological implications of DMSO based on a review of its chemical properties. Ann. N.Y. Acad. Sci. 141: 13–23.

166. Rask, L., Lindblom, J. B., and Peterson, P. A. 1974. Subunit structure of H-2 alloantigens. Nature (London) 249: 833–834.

167. Reich, E. 1963. Biochemistry of actinomycins. Cancer Res 23: 1428–1441.

168. Richards, J. M., Jacobson, J. B., and Stackpole, C. W. Antigenic modulation in vitro. III. Analysis of H-2 antigen modulation on normal and malignant mouse cells. Submitted for publication.

169. Ryan, G. B., Borysenko, J. Z., and Karnovsky, M. J. 1974. Factors affecting the redistribution of surface-bound concanavalin A on human polymorphonuclear leukocytes. J. Cell Biol. 62: 351–365.

170. Sadeghee, S., Hebert, J., Kelley, J., and Abdou, N. I. 1975. Modulation of HL-A antigens by anti-HL-A antiserum: effects on the cytotoxicity assay and mixed leukocyte reaction. J. Immunol. 115: 811–816.

171. Sato, H., Boyse, E. A., Aoki, T., Iritani, C., and Old, L. J. 1973. Leukemia-associated transplantation antigens related to murine leukemia virus. The X.1 system: immune response controlled by a locus linked to H-2. J. Exp. Med. 138: 593–606.

172. Sato, H., Inoué, S., Bryan, J., Barclay, N. E., and Platt, C. 1966. The effect of D_2O on the mitotic spindle. Biol. Bull. 131: 405.

173. Scheid, M. P., Hoffmann, M. K., Komuro, K., Hämmerling, U., Abbott, J., Boyse, E. A., Cohen, G. H., Hooper, J. A., Schulof, R. S., and Goldstein, A. L. 1973. Differentiation of T cells induced by preparations from thymus and by nonthymic agents. J. Exp. Med. 138: 1027–1032.

174. Schlesinger, M. 1970. How cells acquire antigens. Prog. Exp. Tumor Res. 13: 28–83.

175. Schlesinger, M. 1972. Antigens of the thymus. Prog. Allergy 16: 214–299.

176. Schlesinger, M., and Chaouat, M. 1972. Modulation of H-2 antigenicity on the surface of murine peritoneal cells. Tissue Antigens 2: 427–435.

177. Schlesinger, M., and Chaouat, M. 1973. Antibody-induced alteration in the expression of the H-2 antigenicity on murine peritoneal cells: the effect of metabolic inhibitors on antigen modulation and antigen recovery. Transplant. Proc. 5: 105–110.

178. Schlesinger, M., and Golakai, V. K. 1967. Loss of thymus-distinctive serological characteristics in mice under certain conditions. Science 155: 1114–1116.

179. Schlesinger, M., and Hurvitz, D. 1968. Differentiation of the thymus-leukemia (TL) antigen in the thymus of mouse embryos. Israel J. Med. Sci. 4: 1210–1215.

180. Schlesinger, M., Boyse, E. A., and Old, L. J. 1965. Thymus cells of radiation-chimeras: TL phenotype, sensitivity to guinea pig serum, and origin of donor cells. Nature (London) 206: 1119–1121.

181. Schreiner, G. F., and Unanue, E. R. 1976. Membrane and cytoplasmic

changes in B lymphocytes induced by ligand-surface immunoglobulin interaction. *Adv. Immunol.* 24: 37–165.

182. Schwartz, B. D., Kato, K., Cullen, S. E., and Nathenson, S. G. 1973. *H-2* histocompatibility alloantigens. Some biochemical properties of the molecules solubilized by NP-40 detergent. *Biochemistry* 12: 2157–2164.

183. Shimada, A., and Nathenson, S. G. 1971. Removal of neuraminic acid from H-2 alloantigens without effect on antigenic reactivity. *J. Immunol.* 107: 1197–1199.

184. Shipley, W. V. 1971. Immune cytolysis in relation to the growth cycle of Chinese hamster cells. *Cancer Res.* 31: 925–929.

185. Shreffler, D. C., and David, C. S. 1975. The *H-2* major histocompatibility complex and the *I* immune response region: genetic variation, function, and organization. *Adv. Immunol.* 20: 125–195.

186. Siegler, R. 1968. Pathology of murine leukemias. In M. A. Rich (ed.), *Experimental Leukemia,* pp. 51–95. Appleton-Century-Crofts, New York.

187. Silver, J., and Hood, L. 1974. Detergent-solubilized H-2 alloantigen is associated with a small molecular weight polypeptide. *Nature (London)* 249: 764–765.

188. Singer, S. J. 1974. Molecular biology of cellular membranes with applications to immunology. *Adv. Immunol.* 19: 1–66.

189. Singer, S. J., and Nicolson, G. L. 1972. The fluid mosaic model of the structure of cell membranes. *Science* 175: 720–731.

190. Sjögren, H. O., Hellström, I., Bansal, S. C., Warner, G. A., and Hellström, K. E. 1972. Elution of "blocking factors" from human tumors capable of abrogating tumor-cell destruction by specifically immune lymphocytes. *Int. J. Cancer* 9: 274–283.

191. Smith, R. T. 1969. Comment. In M. Landy and W. Braun (eds.), *Immunological Tolerance,* pp. 50–52. Academic Press, New York.

192. Smith, R. T. 1972. Possibilities and problems of immunologic intervention in cancer. *N. Engl. J. Med.* 287: 439–450.

193. Smith, R. T., Klein, G., Klein, E., and Clifford, P. 1968. Studies of the membrane phenomenon in cultured and biopsy cell lines from the Burkitt lymphoma. In J. Dausset, J. Hamburger, and G. Mathé (eds.), *Advances in Transplantation,* pp. 483–493. Williams and Wilkins, Baltimore.

194. Smith, S. R., Lamm, M. E., Powers, M. L., and Boyse, E. A. 1974. Subcellular representation of murine thymus leukemia (TL) antigens in phenotypically TL+ and TL− cells. *J. Immunol.* 113: 1098–1106.

195. Snell, G. D., Graff, R. J., and Cherry, M. 1971. Histocompatibility genes of mice. XI. Evidence establishing a new histocompatibility locus, H-12, and new H-2 allele, H-2^{bc}. *Transplantation* 11: 525–530.

196. Solheim, B. G., and Thorsby, E. 1974. β-2-microglobulin is part of the HL-A molecule in the lymphocyte membrane. *Nature (London)* 249: 36–38.

197. Stackpole, C. W. 1971. Topography of cell surface antigens. *Transplant. Proc.* 3: 1199–1201.

198. Stackpole, C. W. 1977. Topographical differentiation of the cell surface. *Prog. Surf. Membr. Sci.* 12 (in press).

199. Stackpole, C. W., Aoki, T., Boyse, E. A., Old, L. J., Lumley-Frank, J., and

de Harven, E. 1971. Cell surface antigens: serial sectioning of single cells as an approach to topographical analysis. *Science* 172: 472–474.

200. Stackpole, C. W., Jacobson, J. B., and Lardis, M. P. 1974. Two distinct types of capping of surface receptors on mouse lymphoid cells. *Nature (London)* 248: 232–234.

201. Stackpole, C. W., De Milio, L. T., Hämmerling, U., Jacobson, J. B., and Lardis, M. P. 1974. Hybrid antibody-induced topographical redistribution of surface immunoglobulins, alloantigens, and concanavalin A receptors on mouse lymphoid cells. *Proc. Natl. Acad. Sci. U.S.* 71: 932–936.

202. Stackpole, C. W., De Milio, L. T., Jacobson, J. B., Hämmerling, U., and Lardis, M. P. 1974. A comparison of ligand-induced redistribution of surface immunoglobulins, alloantigens, and concanavalin A receptors on mouse lymphoid cells. *J. Cell. Physiol.* 83: 441–448.

203. Stackpole, C. W., Jacobson, J. B., and Lardis, M. P. 1974. Antigenic modulation *in vitro*. I. Fate of thymus-leukemia (TL) antigen-antibody complexes following modulation of TL antigenicity from the surfaces of mouse leukemia cells and thymocytes. *J. Exp. Med.* 140: 939–953.

204. Stackpole, C. W., Jacobson, J. B., and Galuska, S. 1978. Antigenic modulation *in vitro*. II. Modulation of thymus-leukemia (TL) antigenicity requires complement component C3. *J. Immunol.* 120: 188–197.

205. Steinman, R. M., and Cohn, Z. A. 1972. The interaction of soluble horseradish peroxidase with mouse peritoneal macrophages *in vitro*. *J. Cell Biol.* 55: 186–204.

206. Stevens, J. G., and Cook, M. L. 1974. Maintenance of latent herpetic infection: an apparent role for anti-viral IgG. *J. Immunol.* 113: 1685–1693.

207. Stockert, E., Old, L. J., and Boyse, E. A. 1971. The G_{IX} system. A cell surface allo-antigen associated with murine leukemia virus; implications regarding chromosomal integration of the viral genome. *J. Exp. Med.* 133: 1334–1355.

208. Stockert, E., Sato, H., Itakura, K., Boyse, E. A., Old, L. J., and Hutton, J. J. 1972. Location of the second gene required for expression of the leukemia-associated mouse antigen G_{IX}. *Science* 178: 862–863.

209. Stockert, E., Boyse, E. A., Obata, Y., Ikeda, H., Sarkar, N. H., and Hoffman, H. A. 1975. New mutant and congenic mouse stocks expressing the murine leukemia virus-associated thymocyte surface antigen G_{IX}. *J. Exp. Med.* 142: 512–517.

210. Stockert, E., Boyse, E. A., Sato, H., and Itakura, K. 1976. Heredity of the G_{IX} thymocyte antigen associated with murine leukemia virus: segregation data simulating genetic linkage. *Proc. Natl. Acad. Sci. U.S.* 73: 2077–2081.

211. Strom, T. B., Deisseroth, A., Morganroth, J., Carpenter, C. B., and Merrill, J. P. 1974. Modulation of cytotoxic T lymphocyte function by cyclic 3',5'-mononucleotides. *In* W. Braun, L. M. Lichtenstein, and C. W. Parker (eds.), *Cyclic AMP, Cell Growth, and the Immune Response*, Symp. Marco Island, Florida, 1973, pp. 209–222.

212. Stutman, O. 1975. Immunodepression and malignancy. *Adv. Cancer Res.* 22: 261–422.

213. Sundqvist, K. G., Svehag, S. E., and Thorstensson, R. T. 1974. Dynamic aspects of the interaction between antibodies and complement at the cell surface.

Scand. J. Immunol. 3: 237–250.

214. Takahashi, T. 1971. Possible examples of antigenic modulation affecting H-2 antigens and cell surface immunoglobulins. *Transplant. Proc.* 3: 1217–1220.

215. Takahashi, T., Old, L. J., McIntire, K. R., and Boyse, E. A. 1971. Immunoglobulin and other suface antigens of cells of the immune system. *J. Exp. Med.* 134: 815–832.

216. Taylor, R. B., Duffus, W. P. H., Raff, M. C., and de Petris, S. 1971. Redistribution and pinocytosis of lymphocyte surface immunoglobulin molecules induced by anti-immunoglobulin antibody. *Nature (London) New Biol.* 233: 225–229.

217. Thomas, D. B. 1971. Cyclic expression of blood group determinants in murine cells and their relationship to growth control. *Nature (London)* 233: 317–321.

218. Ting, C. C., and Herberman, R. B. 1971. Inverse relationship of polyoma tumour specific cell surface antigen to H-2 histocompatibility antigens. *Nature (London) New Biol.* 232: 118–120.

219. Toyka, K. V., Drachman, D. B., Griffin, D. E., Pestronk, A., Winkelstein, J. A., Fischbeck, K. H., Jr., and Kao, I. 1977. Myasthenia gravis. Study of humoral immune mechanisms by passive transfer to mice. *N. Engl. J. Med.* 296: 125–131.

220. Tung, J.-S., Vitetta, E. S., Fleissner, E., and Boyse, E. A. 1975. Biochemical evidence linking the G_{IX} thymocyte surface antigen to the gp 69/71 envelope glycoprotein of murine leukemia virus. *J. Exp. Med.* 141: 198–205.

221. Unanue, E. R., Perkins, W. D., and Karnovsky, M. J. 1972. Endocytosis by lymphocytes of complexes of anti-Ig with membrane-bound Ig. *J. Immunol.* 108: 569–572.

222. Vitetta, E. S., and Uhr, J. W. 1974. Cell surface immunoglobulin. IX. A new method for the study of synthesis, intracellular transport, and exteriorization in murine splenocytes. *J. Exp. Med.* 139: 1599–1620.

223. Vitetta, E. S., and Uhr, J. W. 1975. Immunoglobulins and alloantigens on the surface of lymphoid cells. *Biochem. Biophys. Acta* 415: 253–271.

224. Vitetta, E., Uhr, J. W., and Boyse, E. A. 1972. Isolation and characterization of H-2 and TL alloantigens from the surface of mouse lymphocytes. *Cell. Immunol.* 4: 187–191.

225. Vitetta, E. S., Uhr, J. W., and Boyse, E. A. 1975. Association of a β_2-microglobulin-like subunit with H-2 and TL alloantigens on murine thymocytes. *J. Immunol.* 114: 252–254.

226. Vitetta, E. S., Artzt, K., Bennett, D., Boyse, E. A., and Jacob, F. 1975. Structural similarities between a product of the *T/t*-locus isolated from sperm and teratoma cells, and H-2 antigens isolated from splenocytes. *Proc. Natl. Acad. Sci. U.S.* 72: 3215–3219.

227. Vitetta, E. S., Poulik, M. D., Klein, J., and Uhr, J. W. 1976. Beta 2-microglobulin is selectively associated with H-2 and TL alloantigens on murine lymphoid cells. *J. Exp. Med.* 144: 179–192.

228. Wang, J. L., McClain, D. A., and Edelman, G. M. 1975. Modulation of lymphocyte mitogenesis. *Proc. Natl. Acad. Sci. U.S.* 72: 1917–1921.

229. Weisenberg, R. C., Borisy, G. G., and Taylor, E. W. 1968. The colchicine-binding protein of mammalian brain and its relation to microtubules. *Biochemistry* 7: 4466–4479.

230. Wessells, N. K., Spooner, B. S., Ash, J. F., Bradley, M. O., Ludueña, M. A., Taylor, E. L., Wrenn, J. T., and Yamada, K. M. 1971. Microfilaments in cellular and developmental processes. *Science* 171: 135–143.

231. Widmer, M. B., Schendel, D. J., Bach, F. J., and Boyse, E. A. 1973. The H(Tla) histocompatibility locus: a study of *in vitro* lymphocyte reactivity. *Transplant. Proc.* 5: 1663–1666.

232. Wilson, J. D., Nossal, G. J. V., and Lewis, H. 1972. Metabolic characteristics of lymphocyte surface immunoglobulin. *Eur. J. Immunol.* 2: 225–232.

233. Winn, H. J. 1960. Immune mechanisms in homotransplantation. I. The role of serum antibody and complement in the neutralization of lymphoma cells. *J. Immunol.* 84: 530–538.

234. Witz, I. P. 1973. The biological significance of tumor-bound immunoglobulins. *Curr. Top. Microbiol. Immunol.* 61: 151–171.

235. Witz, I. P., Kinamon, S., Ran, M., and Klein, G. 1974. Tumour-bound immunoglobulins. The *in vitro* fixation of radioiodine-labelled anti-immunoglobulin reagents by tumour cells. *Clin. Exp. Immunol.* 16: 321–333.

236. Wood, D. C., and Wood, J. 1975. Pharmacologic and biochemical considerations of dimethyl sulfoxide. *Ann. N.Y. Acad. Sci.* 243: 7–19.

237. Yahara, I., and Edelman, G. M. 1972. Restriction of the mobility of lymphocyte immunoglobulin receptors by concanavalin A. *Proc. Natl. Acad. Sci.* 69: 608–612.

238. Yefenof, E., Witz, I. P., and Klein, E. 1976. Interaction of antibody and cell surface localized antigen. *Int. J. Cancer* 17: 633–639.

239. Yu, A., and Cohen, E. P. 1974. Studies on the effect of specific antisera on the metabolism of cellular antigens. I. Isolation of thymus leukemia antigens. *J. Immunol.* 112: 1285–1295.

240. Yu, A., and Cohen, E. P. 1974. Studies on the effect of specific antisera on the metabolism of cellular antigens. II. The synthesis and degradation of TL antigens of mouse cells in the presence of TL antiserum. *J. Immunol.* 112: 1296–1307.

241. Yu, A., Liang, W., and Cohen, E. P. 1975. Detection of a TL(+) murine leukemia cell line that resists the cytotoxic effects of guinea pig complement and specific antiserum. *J. Natl. Cancer Inst.* 55: 299–308.

CHAPTER 3

MEMBRANE ANTIGENS RELATED TO NEOPLASIA AND THEIR POSSIBLE ESCAPE SIGNIFICANCE

Ronald T. Acton,
Kim S. Wise, and
Paul A. Barstad

Diabetes Research and
Training Center and
Department of Microbiology
University of Alabama in Birmingham
Birmingham, Alabama   35294

Despite the fact that neoplastic cells frequently display tumor-specific antigens, the immune system may be ineffective in eliminating aberrant cells. The murine T lymphocyte system provides an excellent model for the study of factors preventing an effective immune response. The thymus leukemic antigen and Gross cell surface antigen often disappear from the cell surface when exposed to antibodies. Other antigens, such as G_{IX}, are found on normal tissues and virions in addition to neoplastic cells. The consequence of oncogenic virion genomes coding for cell surface components related to differentiation events is discussed in regard to recognition by the host immune mechanism and to immunotherapeutic approaches.

INTRODUCTION

In general, neoplastic cells differ from their normal counterparts in their loss of growth control, ability to metastasize, and alterations in membrane structure and function (53, 54, 61, 66, 84). One feature of the neoplastic cell that has attracted the interest of many immunologists is the altered expression of normal cell surface components, as well as the emergence of new components. Since the surface alterations of neoplastic cells are sufficiently aberrant as to be recognized as foreign by the host, causing an immune response, the new components are termed "tumor-specific antigens" (4). In 1943, Gross (34) demonstrated the existence of tumor-specific antigens in inbred animal systems. Other investigators subsequently demonstrated tumor-specific transplantation immunity in several strains of mice and rats (29, 46, 67, 73). Humans have also been found to mount immunologically specific reactions against a variety of neoplastic tissues (5). From these observations, Thomas (79) was led to suggest a normal homeostatic cellular mechanism active in repelling invasion by foreign substances. A basic tenet assumed at this time was that foreign substances induced an immune response whereas "self" components did not. Neoplastic cells were considered to qualify as foreign due to the appearance of tumor specific antigens. Burnet (15) later labeled this homeostatic mechanism "immune surveillance." According to this concept, a major function of the immune system is the detection and elimination of neoplastic cells. Although the concept of immunological surveillance is an attractive hypothesis, it is presently not considered the only factor in tumor rejection. Frequently the immune system either fails to recognize neoplastic cells or neoplastic growth occurs unabated even in the presence of a well-established host response. Why this mechanism is not effective or perhaps not even operative under certain circumstances is one of the major questions in tumor immunology. In this review we will discuss a model system for the study of the mechanism allowing a neoplastic cell to escape detection or elimination by the host immune system.

THE RELATION OF T LYMPHOCYTE DIFFERENTIATION TO LEUKEMOGENESIS

Our approach to understanding malignant transformation of a cell, and its consequence, is to decipher the molecular relationship of normal and malignant cell surface components. Since more is known about the cell surface components of the murine thymocyte than about any other mammalian cell, these cells provide an excellent model for the study of alterations of antigen expression (10, 13, 18, 19). Thymic lymphocytes and leukemia cells derived from them express a number of serologically demonstrable cell surface antigens which reflect normal differentiation events as well as malignant transformation. Some characteristics of these cell surface antigens are summarized in Table 1.

Table 1. Categories of serologically demonstrable murine cell surface antigens

Antigen	Tissue Distribution	Description
H$-$2	Almost all tissue in varying amounts	Alloantigen. Major determinant of graft rejection. Very polymorphic
Thy$-$1	High expression on thymocytes and brain, low expression on T-lymphocytes and epidermal cells	Alloantigen. Marker for T-lymphocytes and nerve endings
Ly$-$1 Ly$-$2 Ly$-$3	Thymocytes and various subsets of T-lymphocytes	Alloantigen. T-helper cells express Ly$-$1, T-cytotoxic killer cells express Ly$-$2, Ly$-$3
TL	Cortical thymocytes of some strains	Alloantigen. TL antigens are often expressed on leukemias of TL$^-$ strain in which case they could be defined as tumor specific antigens
G$_{IX}$	Cortical thymocytes, sperm of some strains	Alloantigen. Antigenic determinant of MuLV[a] gp70. G$_{IX}$ is often expressed on MuLV productively infected leukemias of G$_{IX}-$ strains in which case it could be defined as tumor specific antigen
GCSA[b]	Thymocytes of some strains, leukemic cells, and other cells supporting active MuLV production	MuLV specified. Tumor specific antigen of leukemias induced by Gross-AKR type MuLV

a. MuLV = Murine leukemia virus.
b. GCSA = Gross cell surface antigen.

Cell Surface Antigens Are Markers of T Lymphocyte Differentiation

Figure 1 depicts the quantitative and qualitative variation of these antigens during T lymphocyte maturation. During ontogeny stem cells migrate from yolk sac, primitive blood islands, and/or fetal liver to the thymic epithelial rudiment at about 8–12 days of gestation (49, 51, 64). In the adult these stem cells migrate from bone marrow into the cortex of the thymus, where they differentiate into thymocytes (25, 30, 65). The evidence suggests that maturation is under the influence of the thymic epithelial cells (13, 86). H-2 antigens appear around day 6 of gestation and are fully expressed on thymocytes by 17 days postnatal (26, 71). Simultaneously, a number of other antigens are expressed by cells in an area which will become the thymic cortex (70) (Fig. 1). Responsiveness to phytohemagglutinin (PHA) is acquired during this period. By 18–21 days there are a large number of cells present in the thymus expressing adult levels of cell surface components. These cells also display functional activities characteristic of cells in the adult, such as responsiveness to certain mitogens, ability to respond in a mixed lymphocyte reaction, and cortisone resistance (18, 44, 85). Near the time of birth thymocytes begin to emigrate to peripheral lymphoid tissue, taking up residence first in the lymph nodes. Although the expression of H-2, Thy-1, and TL has been quantified on thymocytes and lymph node cells, the exact density of the other antigens listed is unknown. The composite expression of these cell surface components and functional characteristics reflect the differentiation state of the cells. For example, cells residing in the thymic cortex are relatively immature immunologically, sensitive to cortisone, and express high levels of Thy-1, TL, and G_{IX} and low amounts of H-2 (52, 74). Those cells in the thymic medulla are almost as immunologically mature as peripheral T lymphocytes, cortisone-resistant, and express high levels of H-2, low levels of Thy-1, and no TL or G_{IX}.

Surface Antigens Correlate with Cell Sorting

It would appear that a precise architectural configuration of cell surface components may be essential for T lymphocyte sorting and a reshuffling of these components may occur concomitantly with transition to new differentiation states. There are several lines of evidence which support this hypothesis. First, at least some of the stem cells have an apparent propensity for migrating to the thymus where they receive stimuli in the form of cell–cell contacts and hormones which trigger further differentiation (64). Second, incubation of lymphocytes with glycosidases or neuraminidase impairs their ability to migrate to the

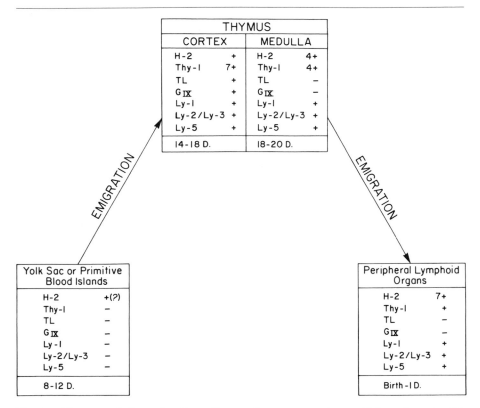

THYMUS	
CORTEX	MEDULLA

H-2	+	H-2	4+
Thy-I	7+	Thy-I	4+
TL	+	TL	−
G IX	+	G IX	−
Ly-I	+	Ly-I	+
Ly-2/Ly-3	+	Ly-2/Ly-3	+
Ly-5	+	Ly-5	+
14-18 D.		18-20 D.	

EMIGRATION

EMIGRATION

Yolk Sac or Primitive Blood Islands	
H-2	+(?)
Thy-I	−
TL	−
G IX	−
Ly -I	−
Ly-2/Ly-3	−
Ly-5	−
8-12 D.	

Peripheral Lymphoid Organs	
H-2	7+
Thy-I	+
TL	−
G IX	−
Ly-I	+
Ly-2/Ly-3	+
Ly-5	+
Birth -I D.	

Fig. 1. The correlation of cell surface antigen expression to T lymphocyte differentiation and migration.

spleen and lymph node, while trypsin appears only to affect migration to lymph nodes (6, 33, 87). Lymphocytes exposed to antilymphocyte serum also have a reduced ability to migrate (78). Finally, the ability of T lymphocytes to migrate to secondary lymphoid tissues is accompanied by a loss of TL and G_{IX} (10, 13, 43).

The Function of Cell Surface Antigens Is Unknown

Although the expression of these alloantigens reflects differentiative changes, their precise function remains obscure. There are recent intriguing observations correlating the presence of certain Ly antigens with T cell subsets having particular functions (16, 17, 19). It has been proposed that the selective loss of Ly antigens parallels the functional maturation of T cells. T cells with killer activity express Ly-2,3 alloantigens on their surface. The maturation of Ly-2,3 cells is amplified by T-cells expressing Ly-1. This is an example of peripheral T lymphocyte subsets being programmed during differentiation to express different immunologic functions in which the Ly alloantigens may play a role. However, it is also possible that the expression of these alloantigens only parallels the differentiation of stem cells into T lymphocytes without actually contributing to the functional differences observed in these cells.

The Thymus Is the Target Organ in Leukemogenesis

It is well known that the thymus is the target organ for overt development of spontaneous or induced murine lymphoid leukemia (35, 36, 48, 50). Since development by Furth (31) years ago, the AKR strain has been particularly useful in studying the malignant process. Most AKR mice develop leukemia within 1 year. Thymectomy greatly reduces the incidence of leukemia (36). The etiological agent for malignancy is the thymotropic Gross-AKR murine leukemia virus (MuLV) imparted by vertical transmission (35, 74). However, other factors most definitely play a role. Genetic background is a major factor in susceptibility to mouse leukemia as are age, thymic humoral factors and exposure to irradiation or carcinogens (47, 50). AKR mice have MuLV genomes integrated at two chromosomal loci which govern the production of virus (20). Other loci that predispose these mice to leukemia have also been defined (48). In AKR mice, virus production is observed shortly after birth and reaches a plateau very early in life (63). At the onset of overt leukemia the output of virus greatly increases. It is of interest that virus infection and production does not qualitatively correlate with malignant transformation. Although AKR mice are producing virus at birth, the highest incidence of leukemia occurs between 6 and 12 months of age. Young mice contain antibodies against various viral antigens and possess killer T cells which can attack leukemic cells from older donors of the same strain (1, 50, 55, 57, 62, 63). Thus, virus production and immunological response to the etiological agent are present in preleukemic mice.

Thymic Cell Populations Are at Risk in Leukemogenesis

One important problem in tumor immunology is to identify the target cell for malignant transformation from the various populations of cells found within the thymus. Analysis of the cell surface of mouse leukemias suggests that these cells are malignant variants of normal thymocytes (10). Using cell surface antigens as markers to define thymocyte subpopulations, investigators have found that different populations of cells are at risk in various strains of mice. Chazan and Haran-Ghera (21) have shown that both spontaneous leukemias in AKR mice and T cell leukemias induced in C57Bl/6 mice have low levels of Thy-1 and high levels of H-2. This pattern is characteristic of the minor (medulla) thymus subpopulation. Kawashima *et al.* (38, 39, 41) demonstrated that thymocytes from 4–6-month-old AKR mice have an altered pattern of cell surface antigens in comparison with 2 month old mice. Thymocytes from 6-month-old mice and thymic leukemia cells frequently have a low Thy-1/high H-2 phenotype (38, 39). Analyzing virus-specific cytoplasmic antigen expression as an index of malignant transformation, Decleve *et al.* (22) observed in C57Bl/Ka that the first detectable sign of MuLV infection was in cells of the outer thymic cortex. They suggest that the immature, large, mitotically active, outer cortical thymocytes are the principal target cells for productive viral infection and subsequent malignant transformation. Our group has analyzed the cell surface phenotype of several murine lymphoblastoid cell lines derived from thymic leukemias of various mouse strains (88). These cell lines express a large amount of TL and Thy-1 and low amounts of H-2, suggesting that they arose from cortical thymocytes. Figure 2 depicts a model consistent with the current data on AKR leukemogenesis. It is our contention that the relative number of cells within each subpopulation changes as a result of a number of contributing factors (e.g., age, irradiation and carcinogens, general health of the animal, and perhaps sex). The end result is that leukemic cells from different AKR mice vary in their cell surface phenotype, reflecting the subpopulation of thymic cortex cells available for transformation. We propose that the transformation event "locks in" the expression of normal cell surface antigens in addition to altering the expression of antigens related to virus production.

TL Is a Normal Differentiation and Leukemia-Specific Antigen

The TL antigen was first discovered by Old *et al.* (59) by immunizing C57Bl/6 mice with mouse leukemia cells. This antiserum would kill C57Bl/6 thymic leukemic cells but not normal C57Bl/6 thymocytes and thus was called the "thymic leukemia" or TL antigen. Subsequent work has shown that this antigen is expressed on normal thymocytes of other strains of mice (7).

The Tla locus is closely linked (1.5 map units) on chromosome 17 with H-2, the major histocompatibility locus (8, 9, 12, 40). The order is Tla:H-2D:H-2K. The Tla locus encodes four antigens, TL.1,2,3, and 4, which have thus far been found only on thymocytes and leukemic cells. Various strains of mice can be divided into three groups with respect to TL expression on their thymocytes. TL$^-$, TL.2, and TL.1,2,3. Many of the

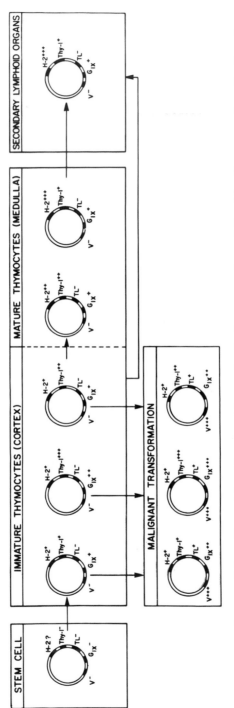
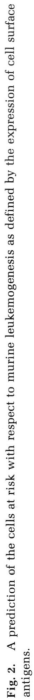

Fig. 2. A prediction of the cells at risk with respect to murine leukemogenesis as defined by the expression of cell surface antigens.

leukemias from TL$^-$ mice are TL$^+$, which suggests that the structural gene for TL synthesis is present in every mouse genome but the gene is only expressed in the leukemic state. All TL$^+$ cells express TL.2. In addition, all TL$^+$ leukemias express TL.1, but TL.1 is not leukemia-specific since it is also found on normal thymocytes in some strains of mice. In contrast, TL.4 is found only in some leukemias. TL.3 is found on both the normal and leukemic cells of various strains. The observation that TL.2 thymocytes express the phenotype TL.1,2 in the leukemic state suggests that TL.1 gene activation has taken place as a result of the transformation process. Since TL.4 is found only in leukemias and TL.3 is found only on leukemias derived from mice expressing TL.3 on thgir thymocytes, it appears that TL.3 represents an antigen reflective of normal differentiation while TL.4 is an antigen of abnormal differentiation. It is possible that TL.4 is an allele of TL.3 as they are never expressed together.

TL$^+$ Leukemic Cells Are Capable of Modulating TL Antigens from Their Cell Surfaces

When it was initially discovered that TL$^+$ leukemias often arise in TL$^-$ animals it was felt that this presented an ideal way to immunize a TL$^-$ animal against their own TL$^+$ leukemias. However, when Boyse et al. (7) injected leukemias into isogeneic recipients which were producing cytotoxic TL antibody, the tumors grew as if the animal had not been previously immunized (7, 11). Further in vitro studies revealed that TL$^+$ thymocytes and leukemic cells exposed to TL antibody in the absence of complement will modulate or stop expressing the TL specificities and become TL$^-$. Fab fragments of TL antibody will also cause antigenic modulation of TL antigens (42). The capacity for TL antibody to effect modulation can be abolished by treating cells with actinomycin D or iodoacetamide, suggesting an active process requiring protein synthesis (7). Modulation is also abolished when the cells are incubated at 0°. Anti-TL.1,3 as well as anti-TL.3 serum will both modulate antigens TL.1,2 and 3 indicating that TL.1,2,3 are closely associated on the cell surface. Modulation cannot be accomplished by anti-TL.2 serum alone although this anti-serum impairs modulation by other TL antibodies. The loss of TL is reversible and is restored by growth for several generations in the absence of TL antisera.

G$_{IX}$ Is a MuLV-Determined Differentiation and Leukemia-Associated Antigen

G$_{IX}$ is an antigen with characteristics of expression somewhat similar to TL (12, 14, 23, 74, 75, 80). It is expressed on normal thymocytes of some mouse strain (G_{IX}^+ strains) but not on the thymocytes of others (G_{IX}^- strains). Thus in G_{IX}^+ strains it is an antigen indicative of thymus-related differentiation. Thymocytes of various mouse strains express quantitatively different amounts of the antigen. G_{IX} induction in a G_{IX}^- strain of mouse appears to be a property of some, but not all, Gross-AKR ecotropic viruses and signals the onset of malignancy in these G_{IX}^- strains. G_{IX} has been shown to be an antigenic specificity associated with the MuLV envelope glycoprotein gp70 (32, 56, 80, 82, 87). This 70,000 mol. wt. glycoprotein of MuLV constitutes the major envelope component of these viruses, and mediates a number of biological events involved in determining interference of viral infection (28), neutralization of virus by antibody (73), and autoimmune reactions in some mouse strain (72). The molecule is antigenically complex, possessing interspecies, group- and type-specific determinants (76).

In addition, extensive polymorphism of gp70 is indicated by multiple antigenic variants found among type-specific antigens associated with this molecule (71), and by peptide maps of variants of the molecule (27). At least three type-specific variants of gp70 have been described. These variants, designated (1) G_{IX}-gp70, (2) X-gp70, and (3) O-gp70 (71), have been defined by serological analysis and are characterized, respectively, by (1) reaction with alloantiserum and standard typing serum recognizing the G_{IX} antigen; (2) reaction with the standard typing serum for the X.1 leukemia-associated alloantigen (69). (This variant is also recognized by the typing serum for the thymus-leukemia antigens, TL.1,2,3. (3) Lack of reaction with these antisera (O-gp70 does precipitate, however, with more broadly reacting determinants of the gp70 molecule, as do the other variants).

Also, the expression of gp70 and some of its associated type specificities is not necessarily dependent upon MuLV production. Thus, 129 mouse thymocytes express G_{IX}-gp70 and B6 mice express O-gp70 without concomitant viral production. Interestingly, the expression of this antigen in 129 mice requires the action of 2 unlinked genes. More than one antigenic form of gp70 may be present on the cell surface. It has been reported (71) that AKR thymocytes and leukemias producing MuLV express the X-gp70 variant. Since AKR thymocytes and leukemias express the G_{IX} antigen (71), both of these type-specific forms of gp70 must be present in AKR thymic tissue and leukemias. Del Villano and Lerner (24, 45) have also shown that the G_{IX}-gp70 component is expressed by a number of different mouse tissues. It is intriguing that this component is a major protein secretion of the mouse genital tract. These investigators suggest that G_{IX} is linked to normal cellular differentiation but that control of its expression is more relaxed than originally recognized. Recently, in a detailed study of gp70 molecules from murine C-type oncoviruses, Elder et *al.* (27) demonstrated by analysis of tryptic peptides that these molecules are polymorphic within a given strain of animal. They can divide gp70 molecules associated with normal tissues into different groups related to gp70 specificities of virus isolates.

Thus, the G_{IX} antigen is a particularly instructive example of the complexity associated with the expression of markers of lymphoid malignancy, and underscores the multiple roles surface components may play as differentiation markers, "tumor-associated" antigens, and structural components of leukemogenic virions.

GCSA Is a Leukemia-Associated Antigen Reflecting MuLV Production

GCSA is a serologically defined cell surface antigen associated with productive infection by Gross-AKR type MuLV (32, 60, 61, 67). Mouse strains like AKR and C58 which are life-long overt carriers of MuLV express GCSA in various organs, whereas other strains such as 129 are GCSA⁻. The spontaneous appearance of overt MuLV infection late in life shows that in some strains there is an age-dependent expression of this MuLV-related antigen. While GCSA appears at the surface of MuLV-producing cells, it has not been shown to be a structural component of the virion. The antigenic determinants composing GCSA may reside on a virus-coded surface molecule containing other virus structural components (77, 83). Also, there are indications that GCSA also may be antigenically polymorphic with more than one specificity involved (2).

It is an interesting situation that both G_{IX} and GCSA appear to be encoded directly by the infecting viral genome, yet reflect distinct events in host differentiation and tumorigenesis (58). It has been speculated that control of the expression of MuLV genome is linked to differentiation, as has been exemplified by the role of G_{IX} in the T lymphocyte system. These structures may play a significant role in the induction or maintenance of morphogenetic patterns. As the molecular nature of these polymorphic cell surface components becomes more defined, these issues should be resolved.

TUMOR-ASSOCIATED ANTIGENS AND THEIR DETECTION BY THE IMMUNE SYSTEM

Thus far, we have examined several cell surface antigens of the murine T lymphoid system which are related to leukemogenesis. Based on these observations, we now discuss their consequence with regard to the immune system. The immune surveillance concept in broad terms states that "tumor antigens" are structures which alert the immune system to the presence of an aberrant cell, resulting in its destruction. The AKR mouse can be shown to mount an immune response against a variety of antigens. This strain can produce high titers of antibodies against the Thy-1.2 antigen and against Friend MuLV gp70 (37, 88). It has also been demonstrated that unimmunized AKR/J mice mount a humoral immune response against gp70 and other MuLV polypeptides (63). Moreover, T lymphocytes from young mice will kill AKR leukemic cells in an in vitro test. However, nearly 100% of young AKR mice succumb even when very small numbers of leukemic cells are injected. Thus, these responses are ineffective in controlling leukemia in this strain. It has been shown that immunization of AKR mice with purified gp70 actually shortens the time prior to the onset of leukemia (37).

Are there observations which might explain how leukemia cells are able to escape the immune system of the AKR host? First, it is of interest that the responding lymphoid cells are probably themselves carriers of MuLV. This may impair the ability of the immune cell to function effectively in eliminating leukemic cells bearing viral surface antigens. Second, MuLV components are shed from infected cells and react with antibodies in the circulation (2). This, coupled with the general viremia present in mice 4–6 months of age, may actually overwhelm any immune response that might be operating against replicating leukemia cells. Third, modulation of TL and GCSA has been observed and may be a means whereby leukemia cells escape detection and/or destruction (3, 7). Moreover, the antigenic determinants on the cell surface may not be readily accessible to antibodies or killer T cells, owing to a combination of the situations just cited. Thus, mechanisms of escape from the immune response are certainly available to the leukemic cell. These examples illustrate the need for reevaluation of the role of the immune system in recognition and elimination of malignant cells.

CONCLUSIONS

Before tumor immunotherapy can become realistic many of the observations derived from mouse models must be confirmed in humans. If the mouse model is indicative of neoplastic cells in general, then immunotherapy in response to "tumor antigens" from cells or virions may be unsuccessful. Immunization with these antigens may initiate autoimmune reactions whose consequences may be as detrimental as the neoplastic disease itself. Much information has been obtained during the last decade on the genetics of cell surface components and virion envelope glycoproteins. As additional knowledge is gained at the molecular level about cell surface components, a clearer understanding of the hosts individuality as compared to a neoplastic cell and a virus should be forthcoming. Then a rational approach to manipulating the immune mechanism to deal with neoplastic cells can be effected.

ACKNOWLEDGMENTS

R. T. Acton's work was done during the tenure of an Established Investigatorship of the American Heart Association.

K. S. Wise was supported by U.S. Public Health Service Institutional National Research Service Award No. T32-GM-07561 from the National Institute of General Medical Science.

P. A. Barstad was supported by U.S. Public Health Service National Research Service Award No. F32A1005423 from the National Institute of Allergy and Infectious Disease.

These investigations were supported by grant no. GB-43575X from the Human Cell Biology section of the National Science Foundation; grant no. IM-33A from the American Cancer Society; U.S. Public Health Service Grants no. CA-15338, no. CA-18609, and no. CA-13148 from the National Cancer Institute, and the Diabetes Trust Fund. The expert technical assistance of Barbara Patterson, Susan Snead and Veda Hayes is gratefully acknowledged.

REFERENCES

1. Aaronoson, S., and Stephensen, J. 1974. Widespread natural occurrence of high titer of neutralizing antibodies to a specific class of endogenous mouse type-C virus. *Proc. Natl. Acad. Sci. U.S.A.* 71: 1957–1961.

2. Aoki, T., Herberman, R. B., Johnson, P. A., Liu, M., and Sturm, M. M. 1972. Wild type Gross leukemia virus: classification of soluble antigens (GSA). *J. Virol.* 10: 1208–1219.

3. Aoki, T., and Johnson, P. A. 1972. Suppression of Gross leukemia cell-surface antigens: A kind of antigenic modulation. *J. Natl. Cancer Inst.* 49: 183–192.

4. Baldwin, R. W., and Price, M. R. 1976. Tumor antigens and tumor-host relationships. *Ann. Rev. Med.* 27: 151–163.

5. Berkelhammer, J. 1974. *In vitro* testing in tumor immunotherapy. *Semin. Oncol.* 1: 397–401.

6. Berney, S. N., and Gesner, B. M. 1970. The circulatory behavior of normal and enzyme altered thymocytes in rats. *Immunology* 18: 681–691.

7. Boyse, E. A., Old, L. J., and Stockert, E. 1965. The TL (thymus leukemia) antigen: a review. In Pierre Graber and Peter A. Miescher (ed.), *Immunopathology: IVth International Symposium*, pp. 23–46. Green and Stratton, New York.

8. Boyse, E. A., Old, L. J., and Stockert, E. 1968. An approach to the mapping of antigens on the cell surface. *Proc. Natl. Acad. Sci. U.S.A.* 60: 886–893.

9. Boyse, E. A., Stockert, E., and Old, L. J. 1968. Isoantigens of the H-2 and TLa loci of the mouse: Interactions affecting their representation on thymocytes. *J. Exp. Med.* 128: 85–95.

10. Boyse, E. A., and Old, L. J. 1969. Some aspects of normal and abnormal cell surface genetics. *Ann. Rev. Genetics.* 3: 269–290.

11. Boyse, E. A., and Old, L. J. 1971. Comment on genetic data relating to expression of TL antigen. *Transplantation.* 11: 561–562.

12. Boyse, E. A., Old, L. J., and Stockert, E. 1972. The relation of linkage group IX to leukemogenesis in the mouse. *In* P. Emmelot and P. Bentuelzen (ed.), *RNA Viruses and Host Genome in Oncogenesis,* pp. 171–185. North-Holland Publishing Co., New York.

13. Boyse, E. A., and Abbott, J. 1975. Surface reorganization as an initial inductive event in the differentiation of prothymocytes to thymocytes. *Fed. Proc.* 34: 24–27.

14. Boyse, E. A. 1977. The G_{IX} system in relation to C-type viruses and heredity. *Immunol. Rev.* 33: 125–145.

15. Burnet, F. M. 1970. *Immunological Surveillance.* Pergamon Press, Sydney, Australia.

16. Cantor, H., and Boyse, E. A. 1975. Functional subclasses of T lymphocytes bearing different Ly antigens. I. The generation of functionally distinct T cell subclasses is a differentiative process independent of antigen. *J. Exp. Med.* 141: 1375–1389.

17. Cantor, H., and Boyse, E. A. 1975. Functional subclasses of T lymphocytes bearing different Ly antigens. II. Cooperation between subclasses of Ly^+ cells in the generation of killer activity. *J. Exp. Med.* 144: 1390–1399.

18. Cantor, H., and Weissman, I. 1976. Development and function of subpopulations of thymocytes and T lymohocytes. *Prog. Allergy* 20: 1–64.

19. Cantor, H., and Boyse, E. A. 1977. Lymphocytes as models for the study of mammalian cellular differentiation. *Immunological Rev.* 33: 105–124.

20. Chattopadhyay, S. K., Rowe, W. P., Teich, N. M., and Lowy, D. R. 1975. Definitive evidence that the murine C-type virus inducing locus AKV-1 is viral genetic material. *Proc. Natl. Acad. Sci. U.S.A.* 72: 906–910.

21. Chazan, R., and Haran-Ghera, N. 1976. The role of thymus subpopulations in "T" leukemia development. *Cell. Immunol.* 23: 356–375.

22. Decleve, A., Travis, M., Weissman, I. L., Lieberman, M., and Kaplan, H. S. 1975. Focal infection and transformation *in situ* of thymus cell subclasses by a thymotropic murine leukemia virus. *Cancer Res.* 35: 3585–3595.

23. Del Villano, B. C., Nave, B., Croker, B. P., Lerner, R. A., and Dixon, F. J. 1975. The oncornavirus glycoprotein gp69/71. A constituent of the surface of normal and malignant thymocytes. *J. Exp. Med.* 141: 172–187.

24. Del Villano, B. C., and Lerner, R. A. 1976. Relationship between the oncornavirus gene product gp70 and the major protein secretion of the mouse genital tract. *Nature* 259: 497–499.

25. Dukor, P., Miller, J. F. A. P., House, W., and Allman, V. 1965. Regulation of thymus grafts I. Histological and cytological aspects. *Transplantation* 3: 639–668.

26. Edidin, M. 1972. Histocompatibility genes, transplantation antigens and pregnancy. In B. D. Kahan and R. Reisfeld (eds.), The Transplantation Antigens, pp. 75–114. Academic Press, New York.

27. Elder, J. H., Jensen, F. C., Bryant, M. C., and Lerner, R. A. 1977. Polymorphism of the major envelope glycoprotein (gp70) of murine C-type viruses: Virion associated and differentiation antigens encoded by a multi-gene family. Nature 267: 23–28.

28. Fischinger, P. J., Nomura, S., and Bolognesi, D. P. 1975. A novel murine oncornavirus with dual ecotrophic and xenotropic properties. Proc. Natl. Acad. Sci. 72: 5150–5155.

29. Foley, E. J. 1953. Antigenic properties of methylcholanthrene-induced tumors in mice of the strain of origin. Cancer Res. 13: 835–837.

30. Ford, C. E., Micklem, H. S., Evans, E. P., Gray, J. G., and Ogden, D. A. 1966. The in-flow of bone marrow cells to the thymus. Ann. N.Y. Acad. Sci. 129: 283–296.

31. Furth, J. 1946. Recent experimental studies on leukemia. Physiol. Rev. 26: 47–64.

32. Geering, G., Old, L. J., and Boyse, E. A. 1966. Antigens of leukemias induced by naturally occurring murine leukemia virus: Their relation to the antigens of gross virus and other murine leukemia viruses. J. Exp. Med. 124: 753–772.

33. Gesner, B. M., and Ginsburg, V. 1964. Effect of glucosides on the fate of transfused lymphocytes. Proc. Natl. Acad. Sci. 52: 750–755.

34. Gross, L. 1943. Intradermal immunization of C_3H mice against sarcoma that originated in animals of the same line. Cancer Res. 3: 326–333.

35. Gross, L. 1951. "Spontaneous" leukemia developing in C_3H mice following inoculation in infancy, with Ak leukemic extracts or Ak embryos. Proc. Soc. Exp. Biol. Med. 76: 27.

36. Gross, L. 1959. Effect of thymectomy on development of leukemia in C_3H mice inoculated with leukemic "passage" virus. Proc. Soc. Exp. Biol. Med. 100: 325–328.

37. Ihle, J. N., Collins, J. J., Lee, J. C., Fischinger, P. J., Pazmino, N., Moenning, U., Shafer, W., Hanna, M. G., Jr., and Bolognesi, D. P. 1976. Characterization of the immune response to the major glycoprotein (gp71) of Friend leukemia virus. III. Influence on endogenous MuLV-mediated pathogenesis. Virology 75: 102–112.

38. Kawashima, K., Ikeda, H., Stockert, E., Takahashi, T., and Old, L. F. 1976. Age related changes in cell surface antigens of preleukemic AKR thymocytes. J. Exp. Med. 144: 193–208.

39. Kawashima, K., Ikeda, H., Hartley, J. W., Stockert, E., Rowe, W. P., and Old, L. J. 1976. Changes in expression of murine leukemia virus antigens and production of xenotropic virus in the late preleukemic period in AKR mice. Proc. Natl. Acad. Sci. U.S.A 73: 4680–4684.

40. Klein, J. 1975. Biology of the mouse histocompatibility-2 complex. Springer Verlag, New York.

41. Krammer, P. H., Citrontauru, R., Read, S. E., Forni, L., and Lang, R. 1976. Murine thymic lymphomas as model tumors for T-cell studies. T-cell markers, immunoglobulin and Fc-receptors on AKR thymomas. Cell. Immunol. 21: 97–111.

42. Lamm, M. E., Boyse, E. A., Old, L. J., Lisowska-Bernstein, B., and Stockert, E. 1963. Modulation of TL (thymus-leukemic) Ag by Fab-fragments of TL ab. J. Immunol. 101: 99–103.

43. Lance, E. M., Cooper, S., and Boyse, E. A. 1970. Antigenic change and cell maturation in murine lymphocytes. Cell. Immunol. 1: 536–544.

44. Leckband, E., and Boyse, E. A. 1971. Immunocompetent cells among mouse thymocytes: A minor population. Science 172: 1258–1260.

45. Lerner, R. A., Wilson, C. B., Del Villano, B. C., McConahey, P. J., and Dixon, F. J. 1976. Endogenous oncornaviral gene expression in adult and fetal mice: Quantitative, histologic and physiologic studies of the major viral glycoprotein, gp70. J. Exp. Med. 143: 151–166.

46. Lewis, M. R., and Aptekman, P. M. 1952. Atrophy of tumors caused by strangulation and accompanied by development of tumor immunity in rats. Cancer 5: 411–413.

47. Lilly, F., and Pincus, T. 1973. Genetic control of murine viral leukemogenesis. In G. Klein, S. Weinhouse, and A. Haddow (eds.), Advances in Cancer Research, pp. 231–277. Academic Press, New York.

48. McEndy, D. P., Boon, M. C., and Furth, J. 1944. On the role of thymus, srleen and gonads in the development of leukemia in a high-leukemic stock of mice. Cancer Res. 4: 377–383.

49. Mandel, T. E., and Russell, P. J. 1971. Differentiation of foetal mouse thymus ultrastructure of organ cultures and of subcapsular grafts. Immunology 21: 659–663.

50. Metcalf, D. 1966. The thymus. In Recent Results in Cancer Research, Vol. 5, Springer-Verlag, New York.

51. Moore, M. A. S., and Owen, J. J. T. 1967. Experimental studies on the development of the thymus. J. Exp. Med. 126: 715–725.

52. Mosier, D. E., and Cohen, P. L. 1975. Ontogeny of mouse T-lymphocytes function. Fed. Proc. 34: 137–140.

53. Nicolson, G. L. 1976. Transmembrane control of the receptors on normal and tumor cells. I. Cytoplasmic influence over cell surface components. Biochem. Biophys. Acta 457: 57–108.

54. Nicolson, G. L. 1976. Transmembrane control of the receptors on normal and tumor cells. II. Surface changes associated with transformation and malignancy. Biochim. Biophys. Acta 458: 1–72.

55. Nowinski, R., and Kaehler, T. 1974. Antibody to leukemia virus: Widespread occurrence in inbred mice. Science 188: 869–871.

56. Obata, Y., Ikeda, H., Stockert, E., and Boyse, E. A. 1975. Relation of G_{IX} antigen of thymocytes to envelope glycoproteins of murine leukemia virus. J. Exp. Med. 141: 188–197.

57. Obata, Y., Stockert, E., Boyse, E. A., Tung, J-S., and Litman, G. W. 1976. Spontaneous autoimmunization to G_{IX} cell surface antigen in hybrid mice. J. Exp. Med. 144: 533–542.

58. O'Donnell, P. V., and Stockert, E. 1976. Induction of G_{IX} antigen and Gross cell surface antigen after infection by ecotropic and xenotropic murine leukemia viruses in vitro. J. Virol. 20: 545–554.

59. Old, L. J., Boyse, E. A., and Stockert, E. 1963. Antigenic properties of

experimental leukemias. I. Serological studies *in vitro* with spontaneous and radiation-induced leukemias. *J. Natl. Cancer Inst.* 31: 977–986.

60. Old, C. J., Boyse, E. A., Stockert, E. 1965. The G (Gross) leukemia antigen. *Cancer Res.* 25: 813–819.

61. Old, L. J., and Boyse, E. A. 1973. Current enigmas in cancer research. The Harvey Lectures, Series 67, pp. 273–315.

62. Oldstone, M. B. A., and Dixon, F. S. 1969. Pathogenesis of chronic disease associated with persistent lymphocytic choriomeningitis viral infection. I. Relationship of antibody production to disease in neonatally infected mice. *J. Exp. Med.* 129: 483–505.

63. Oldstone, M. B. A., Del Villano, B. C., and Dixon, F. J. 1976. Autologous immune responses to the major oncornavirus polypeptides in unmanipulated AKR/J mice. *J. Virol.* 18: 176–181.

64. Owen, J. J. T., and Ritter, M. A. 1969. Tissue interaction in the development of thymus lymphocytes. *J. Exp. Med.* 129: 431–437.

65. Owen, J. J. T., and Raff, M. C. 1970. Studies on the differentiation of thymus-derived lymphocytes. *J. Exp. Med* 132: 1216–1232.

66. Pollack, R. E., and Hough, P. V. C. 1974. The cell surface and malignant transformation. *Ann. Rev. Med.* 25: 431–446.

67. Prehn, R. T., and Main, J. M. 1957. Immunity to methylcholanthrene-induced sarcomas. *J. Natl. Cancer Inst.* 18: 769–778.

68. Rowe, W. P., and Pincus, T. 1972. Quantitative studies of naturally occurring murine leukemia virus infection of AKR mice. *J. Exp. Med.* 135: 429–436.

69. Sato, H., Boyse, E. A., Aoki, T., Iritani, C., and Old, L. J. 1973. Leukemia-associated transplantation antigens related to murine leukemia virus. *J. Exp. Med.* 138: 593.

70. Schlesinger, M., and Hurvitz, D. 1968. Differentiation of the thymus-leukemia (TL) antigen in the thymus of mouse embryos. *Israel J. Med. SciB* 4: 1210–1215.

71. Schlesinger, M. 1972. Antigens of the thymus. *Progress in Allergy 1972,* 16: 214–299.

72. Stephenson, J. R., Peters, R. L., Hino, S., Donahoe, R. M., Long, L. K., Aaronson, S. A., and Kellolf, G. J. 1976. Natural immunity in mice to structural polypeptides of endogenous type C RNA Viruses. *J. Virol.* 19: 890–898.

73. Steves, R. A., Strand, M., and August, J. T. 1974. Structural proteins of mammalian oncogenic RNA virus murine leukemia virus neutralization by antisera prepared against purified envelope glycoprotein. *J. Virol.* 14: 187–189.

74. Stockert, E., Old, L. J., and Boyse, E. A. 1971. The G_{IX} system. A cell surface allo-antigen associated with murine leukemia virus; implications regarding chromosomal integration of the viral genome. *J. Exp. Med.* 133: 1334–1355.

75. Stockert, E., Boyse, E. A., Sato, H., and Itakura, K. 1976. Heredity of the G_{IX} thymocyte antigen associated with murine leukemia virus: Segregation data simulating genetic linkage. *Proc. Natl. Acad. Sci.* 73: 2077–2088.

76. Strand, M., and August, J. T. 1974. Structural proteins of mammalian oncogenic RNA viruses: multiple antigenic determinants of the major internal protein and envelope glycoprotein. *J. Virol.* 13: 171–180.

77. Strand, M., Wilsnack, R., and August, J. T. 1974. Structural proteins of

mammalians oncogenic RNA viruses: immunological characterization of the p15 polypeptide of Rauscher murine virus. *J. Virol.* 14: 1575–1583.

78. Taub, R. N., and Lance, E. M. 1968. Effects of heterologous anti-lymphocyte serum on the distribution of ^{51}Cr-labeled lymph node cells in mice. *Immunology* 15: 633–642.

79. Thomas, L. 1959. Discussion. In H. S. Lawrence (ed.), *Cellular and Humoral Aspects of the Hypersensitive States*, p. 530. Harper and Row, Inc., New York.

80. Tung, J-S., Fleissner, E., Vitetta, E. S., and Boyse, E. A. 1975. Expression of murine leukemia virus envelope glycoprotein gp69/71 on mouse thymocytes. *J. Exp. Med.* 142: 518–523.

81. Tung, J-S., Shen, F-W., Fleissner, E., and Boyse, E. A. 1976. X-gp70 of murine leukemia virus, expressed on mouse lymphoid cells. *J. Exp. Med.* 143: 969–974.

82. Tung, J-S., Vitetta, E. S., Fleissner, E., and Boyse, E. A. 1975. Biochemical evidence linking the G_{IX} thymocyte surface antigen to the gp69/71 envelope glycoprotein of murine leukemia virus. *J. Exp. Med.* 141: 198–205.

83. Tung, J-S., Yoshiki, T., and Fleissner, E. 1976. A core polyprotein of murine leukemia virus on the surface of mouse leukemia cells. *Cell* 9: 573–578.

84. Wallach, D. F. H. 1976. Some biochemical anomalies that can contribute to the malignant behavior of cancer cells. *J. Mol. Med.* 1: 97–107.

85. Weissman, I. L., Baird, S., Gardner, R. L., Papaioannou, V. E., and Raschke, W. 1977. Normal and neoplastic maturation of T-lineage lymphocytes. *Cold Spring Harbor Symposia on Quantitative Biology XLI.* pp. 9–21.

86. Wekerle, H., Cohen, I. R., and Feldman, M. 1973. Thymus reticulum cell cultures confer T cell properties on spleen cells from thymus-deprived animals. *Eur. J. Immunol.* 3: 745–748.

87. Woodruff, J., and Gesner, B. M. 1968. Lymphocytes: Circulation altered by trypsin. *Science* 161: 176–178.

88. Zwerner, R. K., and Acton, R. T. 1975. Growth properties and alloantigenic expression of murine lymphoblastoid cell lines. *J. Exp. Med.* 142: 378–390.

CHAPTER 4

INTRACELLULAR PRESENCE OF THYMUS-LEUKEMIA AND OTHER MURINE CELL SURFACE ANTIGENS

Michael E. Lamm

Department of Pathology
New York University
Medical Center
New York, New York 10016

The question of the intracellular expression of some of the well-studied murine cell surface antigens is considered. Reasons are given why this subject has been relatively neglected, and why it is worth pursuing. Technical problems in the demonstration of antigens in intracellular locations are discussed. The conclusion is drawn that immunoelectron microscopy is potentially a valuable tool. By this means, thymus-leukemia (TL) antigens have been shown to be expressed on internal organelles such as mitochondria. The presence of H-2 antigens within cells is still controversial.

Cell-associated antigens can be classified in various categories (1). For example, alloantigens differ among individual members of a species according to their genetic constitution. Differentiation antigens vary between cells belonging to distinct tissues in the same individual, or between stem cells and mature cells, because of variations in the expression of genes which are uniformly present in all the somatic cells. Tumor-associated antigens are those which appear in neoplasia, not being detectable in the normal counterparts.

For many reasons, these types of antigens have traditionally been considered almost exclusively in terms of the cell surface. First, there is much general interest in how cells interact with and recognize one another. Clearly, the cell surface is involved in such phenomena. Second, in the past the investigator concerned with cell-associated antigens has usually tried both to induce and to measure immune responses with intact cells, rather than subcellular fractions or molecules purified from cells. Such use of intact cells is often a matter of convenience and practicality, and accounts, in part, for the great body of work on lymphocytes and erythrocytes, which occur naturally as suspensions of individual cells, or, in the case of solid lymphoid organs, can easily be placed into suspension. By this means, observation and quantitation are simplified.

The possible existence of some of the well-studied cell surface antigens inside cells has not received a great deal of attention. A priori, it should not be unexpected that particular cell surface elements also occur on internal organelles, since the various membranes of the cell may share constituents, and, furthermore, it is highly likely that the plasma membrane is derived, at least partially, from the intracellular membrane systems (11, 14, 19). Cell surface elements could thus be expressed internally during their synthesis and transit to the exterior. On the other hand, internal expression could also reflect an important functional or structural role within the cell. Moreover, there has not been much effort directed toward finding intracellular tumor-associated antigens which may not be expressed at the cell surface. It is entirely possible that immunological techniques could be highly useful in uncovering significant tumor-related alterations in subcellular constituents. Accordingly, the purpose of the present chapter is to call attention to the relative neglect of this aspect of cellular immunology and tumor immunology, and to discuss, with particular examples of mouse and rat antigens, some of the problems in, and requirements for, demonstrating antigens on intracellular organelles.

Detection of Intracellular Antigens

In the past, most attempts to demonstrate that a particular antigen is associated with an intracellular organelle have employed subcellular fractionation. Classically, a population of cells is disrupted, and the various organelles are separated by differential centrifugation. Purity of a given subcellular fraction is evaluated by the relative specific activities of enzymes associated with particular cell compartments, for instance, 5'-nucleotidase and the plasma membrane, and by the degree of contamination estimated visually by electron microscopy. Unfortunately, these methods are not entirely precise; even so, they generally indicate some degree of impurity. On the other hand, while a particular enzyme may be predominantly associated with a particular organelle, it does not automatically follow, as has often been assumed, that it is specific for that organelle and, therefore, that its presence in preparations of other organelles is necessarily indicative of contamination. In the case of electron microscopy, its value varies according to the organelle being studied. Certain organelles, such as mitochondria, have characteristic features and are readily recognized. In contrast, it may be difficult to decide the origin of a fragment of membrane, perhaps plasma membrane, Golgi apparatus, smooth endoplasmic reticulum, or rough endoplasmic reticulum artifactually stripped of ribosomes.

Although the presence of some degree of contamination may not hinder certain investigations, it can lead to gross errors of interpretation in immunological studies. The occurrence of an antigen in a subcellular fraction has usually been evaluated by two general approaches: (a) injecting the fraction and looking for an immune response such as production of antibodies or sensitization for subsequent accelerated graft rejection in the case of histocompatibility antigens, or (b) testing whether the fraction can inhibit the action of a standard antiserum in an in vitro test system. These methods can be misleading because quantitation is often difficult and a good part of any observed activity could be due to contaminants.

In the author's opinion, the best available approach for firmly demonstrating the presence of an antigen intracellularly is by immunoelectron microscopy. Antibody, or antibody fragments, conjugated to enzymes can be allowed to diffuse into fixed cells, and the antigen subsequently revealed by a reaction product of the enzyme. Or, visual markers such as ferritin and hemocyanin can be used in conjunction with antibody to stain either previously purified subcellular fractions or ultrathin sections of cells embedded in appropriate media. The technology for this last approach is under development (6, 9), and further improvements will undoubtedly be forthcoming. Needless to say, it is crucial in such studies to use highly specific antisera in order to be sure exactly which antigen one is detecting. The ability to use congenic antisera in experimental studies is highly advantageous.

TL Antigens

The TL (thymus-leukemia) antigens, initially described by Boyse, Old and colleagues, have several important properties (1). They are normally expressed by the thymocytes of some, but not all, strains of mice (TL+ strains), but in the strains which are normally TL−, TL antigens may be expressed by leukemias, in which case they are tumor-associated antigens. Much of the interest in these antigens has centered around the phenomenon of "antigenic modulation," a term used to describe a change (mechanism not clear) in which cells bearing TL antigens become resistant to lysis by antibody and complement if there is a sufficient interval before the addition of the complement, either alone or with fresh antibody (3, 7, 13, 17, 20). The in vivo counterpart is the apparent change to a TL− phenotype, rather than killing, undergone by TL+ leukemia cells after injection into mice previously immunized against TL (2). The modulation phenomenon has been cited as an example of a possible means by which tumor cells evade immunological defense mechanisms.

Reasons for interest in cell surface TL antigens are evident. Since nothing was known regarding their possible expression internally, Smith et al. (15, 16) studied this question in the traditional way, namely by separating various subcellular fractions by centrifugation and testing for the presence of TL antigens in various organelles by inhibition of cytotoxicity. Indeed, appreciable TL antigen activity, which could not be explained on the basis of contamination by plasma membrane, was found in mitochondrial and microsomal fractions prepared from phenotypically TL+ cells, but not from phenotypically TL− cells. Because the plasma membrane comprises only a small portion of the total cell, it appeared that most of the TL antigen activity actually lies intracellularly.

In order to confirm the tentative conclusion that TL antigens are in fact expressed internally, as well as on the cell surface, direct visual confirmation was sought by immunoelectron microscopy in more recent

---

Fig. 1.   Mitochondria, prepared by differential centrifugation of homogenates of mouse lymphoid cells, were incubated successively with congenic anti-TL antiserum and a covalent conjugate of rabbit antimouse immunoglobulin and hemocyanin. Thin sections were stained with uranyl acetate and lead citrate. Hemocyanin particles are distributed along the margins of several mitochondria that were isolated from phenotypically TL+ cells, indicative of the presence of TL antigen. A variety of control preparations always showed less staining. Magnification × 47,500. (Preparation by Drs. M. Jeng and M. Feingold.)

studies (M. Jeng, M. Finegold, R. Basch, and M. Lamm, in press). Mitochondria were used because of their characteristic morphology in electron micrographs, unlike fragments of membrane whose origin may be uncertain. The presence of visual marker overlying the surface of typical mitochondria afforded such confirmation (Fig. 1).

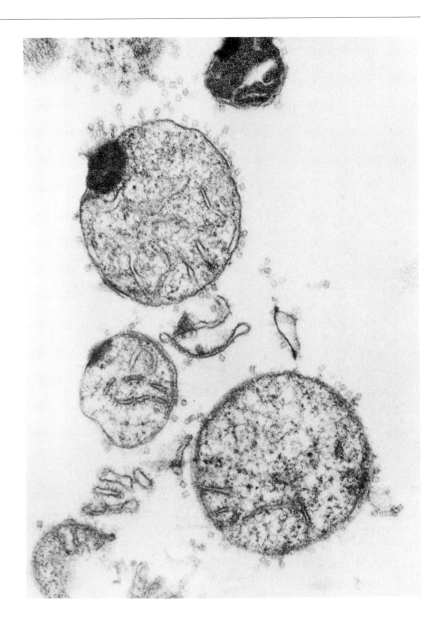

H-2 Antigens

Although the H-2 system of antigens has been studied mostly from the viewpoint of the cell surface, there have been a number of investigations dealing with their presence elsewhere. Nearly every organelle has been reported by one or more laboratories to contain H-2 antigens (reviewed in Refs. 5 and 12). However, when taken as a whole, the literature on this subject is highly controversial. Some authors claim high intracellular contents, and others none at all.

In addition to those already discussed, there have been several other approaches to the expression of H-2 on the various cellular membranes. The contents of histocompatibility antigens (mouse H-2 and rat Ag-B) on whole cells and in cell lysates have been compared to see whether rupture exposes new, that is, formerly intracellular, antigenic determinants. Haughton (4) and Letarte-Muirhead et al. (8) found most of the activity at the surface. Molnar et al. (10) looked for H-2 activity in various subcellular fractions after the lactoperoxidase-catalysed radioiodination of intact cells. They used the radioactivity of each fraction as a measure of plasma membrane content and inhibition of cytotoxicity as the measure of antigen content, and concluded that H-2 is confined to the cell surface. Vitetta and Uhr (18) studied the migration of newly synthesized, radiolabeled H-2 antigen by a method in which anti-H-2 antibody is bound to surface H-2 of intact cells, following which the cells are lysed. Complexes of H-2 antigen and its antibody, containing only H-2 that had been on the surface, were then removed from non-complexed, that is, formerly internal H-2. The data were interpreted as indicating that newly synthesized H-2 antigen enters a small, membrane-bound, intracellular pool. It would certainly be useful to reinvestigate the intracellular representation of H-2 antigens via immunoelectron microscopy.

Thy-1 Antigen

The activity of the rat Thy-1 (θ) antigen was found to be mostly at the surface when whole cells and their detergent lysates were compared (8).

Conclusions

By a number of criteria, including immunoelectron microscopy, TL antigens have been shown to be present intracellularly, as well as on the plasma membrane. Although several laboratories have examined H-2 antigens in this regard, no firm conclusions can be drawn at present because of the conflicting evidence. It would not be surprising if some H-2 antigens were present on intracellular membranes if current views on the interrelationship of the various cellular membranes are correct. Other murine cell surface antigens have not been well studied from the viewpoint of intracellular expression.

ACKNOWLEDGMENT

Studies performed in the author's laboratory were supported by NIH grant CA-08627.

REFERENCES

1. Boyse, E. A., and Old, L. J. 1969. Some aspects of normal and abnormal cell surface genetics. *Ann. Rev. Genet.* 3: 269–290.

2. Boyse, E. A., Old, L. J., and Luell, S. 1963. Antigenic properties of experimental leukemias. II. Immunological studies *in vivo* with C57B1/6 radiation-induced leukemias. *J. Natl. Cancer Inst.* 31: 987–995.

3. Esmon, N. L., and Little, J. R. 1976. Different mechanisms for the modulation of TL antigens on murine lymphoid cells. *J. Immunol.* 117: 919–926.

4. Haughton, G. 1966. Transplantation antigen of mice: Cellular localization of antigen determined by the H-2 locus. *Transplantation* 4: 238–244.

5. Klein, J. 1975. *Biology of the Mouse Histocompatibility-2 Complex*, pp. 337–339. Springer-Verlag, New York.

6. Kraehenbuhl, J. P., and Jamieson, J. D. 1972. Solid-phase conjugation of ferritin to Fab-fragments of immunoglobulin G for use in antigen localization on thin sections. *Proc. Natl. Acad. Sci. USA* 69: 1771–1775.

7. Lamm, M. E., Boyse, E. A., Old, L. J., Lisowska-Bernstein, B., and Stockert, E. 1968. Modulation of TL (thymus-leukemia) antigens by Fab-fragments of TL antibody *J. Immunol.* 101: 99–103.

8. Letarte-Muirhead, M., Acton, R. T., and Williams, A. F. 1974. Preliminary characterization of Thy-1.1 and Ag-B antigens from rat tissues solubilized in detergents. *Biochem. J.* 143: 51–61.

9. McLean, J. D., and Singer, S. J. 1970. A general method for the specific staining of intracellular antigens with ferritin-antibody conjugates. *Proc. Natl. Acad. Sci. USA* 65: 122–128.

10. Molnar, J., Klein, G., and Friberg, Jr., S. 1973. Subcellular localization of murine histocompatibility antigens in tumor cells. *Transplantation* 16: 93–102.

11. Morré, D. J., Keenan, T. W., and Huang, C. M. 1974. Membrane flow and differentiation: Origin of Golgi apparatus membranes from endoplasmic reticulum. *Adv. Cytopharmacol.* 2: 107–125.

12. Nathenson, S. G. 1970. Biochemical properties of histocompatibility antigens. *Ann. Rev. Genetics* 4: 69–90.

13. Old, L. J., Stockert, E., Boyse, E. A., and Kim, J. H. 1968. Antigenic modulation. Loss of TL antigen from cells exposed to TL antibody. Study of the phenomenon *in vitro. J. Exp. Med.* 127: 523–539.

14. Schnaitman, C. A. 1969. Comparison of rat liver mitochondrial and microsomal membrane proteins. *Proc. Natl. Acad. Sci. USA* 63: 412–419.

15. Smith, S. R., Lamm, M. E., and Powers, M. L. 1975. Spleen cells of phenotypically TL+ mice do not contain intracellular TL antigens. *Immunogenetics* 1: 591–594.

16. Smith, S. R., Lamm, M. E., Powers, M. L., and Boyse, E. A. 1974. Subcellular representation of murine thymus-leukemia (TL) antigens in phenotypically TL+ and TL− cells. *J. Immunol.* 113: 1098–1106.

17. Stackpole, C. W., Jacobson, J. B., and Lardis, M. P. 1974. Antigenic modulation *in vitro*. I. Fate of thymus-leukemia (TL) antigen-antibody complexes following modulation of TL antigenicity from the surfaces of mouse leukemia cells and thymocytes. *J. Exp. Med.* 140: 939–953.

18. Vitetta, E. S., and Uhr, J. W. 1975. Synthesis of surface H-2 alloantigens in murine splenocytes. *J. Immunol.* 115: 374–381.

19. Whaley, W. G., Dauwalder, M., and Kephart, J. E. 1972. Golgi apparatus: Influence on cell surfaces. *Science* 175: 596–599.

20. Yu, A., and Cohen, E. P. 1974. Studies on the effect of specific antisera on the metabolism of cellular antigens. II. The synthesis and degradation of TL antigens of mouse cells in the presence of TL antiserum *J. Immunol.* 112: 1296–1307.

CHAPTER 5

ANTITUMOR DEFENSE MECHANISMS AND THEIR SUBVERSION

Robert J. North,
George L. Spitalny, and
David P. Kirstein

Trudeau Institute, Inc.
Saranac Lake, New York 12983

Evidence is introduced to support the proposition that it is macrophages, and not lymphocytes, that most likely have the potential to function in native surveillance against incipient neoplasms. Progressive tumor growth, however, eventually results in the generation of a state of concomitant antitumor immunity, which is mediated by cytotoxic T cells and can call forth activated macrophages. To survive concomitant immunity, therefore, a primary tumor must possess mechanisms that can locally subvert the function of both types of host effector cells. This may well be caused by the tumor cell secretion of pharmacologically active molecules that either suppress the function of host effector cells, or discourage their accumulation at the site of neoplastic growth.

INTRODUCTION

The changes that send a cell and its progeny on the path to malignant behavior depend ultimately on a sequence of stable changes in its genome. There is no doubt that these genetic changes can either occur "spontaneously," or they can be caused, or their onset hastened by the action of carcinogenic agents or oncogenic viruses. The recent arguments by Cairns (21) for a major role for environmental carcinogens in the cause of the more common cancers in humans is compelling. The suggestion by this author (22) that the increased frequency of cancers in older people indicates the need for a long incubation period because of the requirement for an accumulated sequence of genetic mutations, and does not necessarily indicate increased susceptibility to cancer with age, is supported by recent experimental evidence.

It has been shown (121) for instance, that the reason why there is an increased incidence of chemically induced experimental tumors in older mice is because of the long period of time required for the carcinogen to cause malignant conversion. Since most mutations are caused by replication errors that occur during cell division (29), it is not surprising that tumors arise more frequently in older age in those tissues with large populations of constantly dividing cells. The need for an accumulation of mutations over a long period of time for conversion to malignancy is evidenced by the descriptions (63) of a definite sequence of phenotypic changes in epithelial cells over an 18-year period preceding the onset of carcinoma of the vagina, and of similar sequences of morphological changes in epithelial cells which precede the emergence of cervical and bronchial carcinomas (9, 148).

Additional evidence for a sequence of changes leading to malignancy is demonstrated by distinct initiator and promoter stages in the induction of neoplasms with chemical carcinogens (159).

With a view to a more refined analytical approach to the study of the changes that result in malignancy, a great deal of effort is currently being devoted to discovering the causes of malignant transformation of cells in culture. In support of in vivo evidence, it is well established that the physiological and morphological changes that characterize cellular transformation in vitro can either occur "spontaneously," or can be induced with carcinogenic agents or oncogenic viruses. The characteristic ability of transformed cells to multiply continuously and "uncontrollably" and to overgrow normal cells in culture obviously is a characteristic without which they could not form tumors in vivo. The trouble with these studies, however, is that despite the sophisticated knowledge that is being discovered about the acquisition of the capacity for unrestricted growth in vitro, very few spontaneous or chemically transformed cells in vitro prove to be truly malignant when injected into animals of the strain of origin. Instead, they either fail to grow, or are destroyed. In many cases, therefore, transformation is being studied for its own sake, except by those who hypothesize that in vitro transformation, as currently defined, represents the phenotypic expression of only some of the necessary steps that lead to malignancy.

Thus, while many in vitro studies, on the one hand, provide evidence that "spontaneous" mutation and transformation of somatic cells can occur with a high frequency, they show, on the other hand, that most of these transformations may not have survived if they had occurred in the host animal. The additional knowledge that many in vitro transformed cells that do not form tumors when implanted in a syngeneic host do so when implanted in a host that is immunologically immature or that has been immunologically depressed, suggests the possibility that an essential additional requirement for a cell to be defined as malignant is a capacity for avoiding destruction by a mechanism(s) of host resistance that would otherwise act to destroy it. Indeed, there is now ample evidence for hypothesizing that metazoan animals possess mechanisms that have evolved to protect them against colonization of their tissues by neoplastic cells. A corollary of this statement, therefore, is that those neoplastic cells that are seen as frank tumors have been naturally selected to avoid destruction by antitumor defense mechanisms.

The purpose of this chapter is to briefly examine the evidence for the existence of host mechanisms that might naturally defend against tumors, and to discuss the ways that tumor cells might employ to avoid being destroyed by them.

MAJOR DEFENSE MECHANISMS THAT TUMORS NEED TO SUBVERT

Immunosurveillance

The concept that the immune apparatus of mammals, in particular that component that rejects tissue allografts, evolved primarily for defense against colonization by neoplastic cells was first put forward by Thomas (153). The concept was later popularized and expanded into a hypothesis by Burnet (20), who documented the evidence to support it, and predicted a number of findings that would prove to be consistent with it. Most of the evidence on which the hypothesis is based, however, is circumstantial, and is subject to alternative interpretations. For this and other reasons, the hypothesis of immunosurveillance has recently been severely and justifiably criticized (103, 127, 137).

Obviously, the formulation of a hypothesis of immunosurveillance must rest on a knowledge that most neoplastic cells that arise possess tumor-specific antigens that enable the immune apparatus of the host to recognize and eliminate them before they have a chance to form progressive malignancies. It is paradoxical, therefore, that most of the evidence for the immunogenicity of malignant tumors comes from studies with the cells obtained from frank progressive tumors: tumors that should not have arisen in the presence of an immunosurveillance mechanism. It must be assumed, therefore, that for these particular tumors either immunosurveillance was genetically defective, or that they were somehow selected to avoid destruction by immunosurveillance. The second possibility is the more acceptable one because the genetic intactness of the immune system in the hosts of origin is indicated by the demonstration of immunogenicity of these tumors in syngeneic animals. In fact, most solid experimental tumors so far examined have been shown to be immunogenic to varying degrees in syngeneic hosts. This means that they evoke, when implanted in subtumorigenic doses or after lethal irradiation, the generation of a state of specific immunity to growth of a subsequent tumor challenge. When adequately investigated (59, 115) moreover, it has been found that the immunity generated is cell-mediated, meaning that like immunity to strong transplantation antigens, it is a function of thymus-dependent or T lymphocytes. This subject of "immunization immunity" has been reviewed by Herberman and Oldham (61) and will not be discussed here.

While there is no doubt, therefore, that an adaptive immune response can be artificially evoked by the appropriate presentation of tumor cells, the view has nevertheless been expressed that the immune system is incapable under natural conditions of recognizing the early emergence of a malignant tumor in the form of a small nascent nest of tumor cells because of the relative "weakness" of tumor specific antigens. It could be argued, however, that this does not at present invalidate the hypothesis of immunosurveillance because it does not take into account the possibility that these so-called weakly antigenic tumors represent only a small fraction of the total number of tumors that actually arise and which are antigenically strong enough to be recognized and destroyed before they become visible. This defense of the theory is cancelled, however, by experiments which show (128) that those tumors that arise in the absence of an immune mechanism are no more immunogenic than those that arise in normal animals. Thus, it is apparent that there is no selection pressure in normal animals which favors the emergence and escape of only those tumors that are weakly immunogenic. It should be realized, nevertheless, that the meaning of the terms antigenic strength and immunogenic strength are not fully understood. This is particularly so when the terms are applied to autochthonous and syngeneic tumors where a variety of techniques, some relatively crude, have been employed to test and to grade the immunizing properties of tumors. Indeed, most workers appear to be unaware of the distinct possibility that the failure of an immunizing regimen with a transplantable tumor to give an appreciable level of immunity to a subsequent tumor challenge may depend on factors in addition to the tumor's immunogenicity. It could also depend, for instance, on a selected capacity of tumor cells to actively resist destruction by what by other criteria might have been viewed as a potentially strong immunity.

Among other things, some tumor cells may avoid immune destruction because of a capacity for rapid growth, or by possessing a plasma membrane, that despite its content of antigen, may be adapted to resist immune lysis. After all, it is the *expression* of immunity that is always measured, and this involves measuring the suppression of growth of a challenge of live tumor cells that undoubtedly possess adaptive capabilities (39, 114).

The fact is that most *in vitro* transformed cells are also antigenic, but there is as yet no convincing evidence (83) that those few that can form tumors *in vivo* are any less antigenic than those that cannot. On the contrary, there is some paradoxical evidence (83) that the acquisition of the ability of *in vitro* spontaneously transformed cells to form tumors *in vivo* is coincident with the acquisition of immunogenicity: evidence that would support a concept of immunostimulation of tumor growth (127). It seems clear, therefore, that more experimental refinement needs to be introduced into the study of tumor immunogenicity, and deeper thought given to its meaning. Based on the present state of the art, however, there is little doubt that many workers favor the view that most immunogenic malignant cells in the form of a small incipient tumor represent too small an antigenic mass to be recognized by the immune apparatus.

The hypothesis of immunosurveillance can be even more strongly criticized on the grounds that one of its key predictions, that there should be an increased frequency of *all* types of tumors in mammals that have been immunologically comprised, is not supported by fact. Instead, the general finding is that although immunodeficient individuals show an above normal frequency of spontaneous neoplasms, a very large portion of these neoplasms are represented by a single type of tumor, the lymphoreticulum cell sarcoma. An increased incidence of this tumor has been documented in humans with immunodeficiency diseases (99), as well as in humans maintained on immunosuppressive therapy following organ transplants (69). Congenitally athymic nude mice, that are devoid of a mechanism of T-cell-mediated immunity, also show an increased incidence of only this one particular tumor (119). Schwartz (137) has justifiably argued, therefore, that these findings do not support the hypothesis of immunosurveillance, and rightly points out that this type of tumor could well result from a severe disturbance, because of T cell deficiency, in immunologic control mechanisms: a suggestion that is supported by the evidence (94, 152) that lymphoreticulum sarcomas are in reality lymphomas of B cell origin.

Additional evidence against the concept of immunosurveillance is represented by the finding (51, 119) that athymic nude mice do not show an above normal incidence of tumors in response to the application of chemical carcinogens. Neither do mice (51) and rats (2) that have been made T cell deficient as adults by thymectomy and X-irradiation. In fact, T-cell-deficient mice can show an increased capacity for retarding the growth of implanted syngeneic tumor cells (51). In the same vein, it was demonstrated by Martinez (98) that neonatally thymectomized mice show a lower than normal incidence of mammary carcinoma. In view of this evidence, then, there seem to be no sound reasons for believing that the immune apparatus generally functions to detect and destroy neoplastic cells before they form visible tumors. It is safe to assume, moreover, that additional evidence that is inconsistent with the hypothesis of immunosurveillance will be forthcoming.

Immunity Against Established Tumors

While there is no direct evidence that the immune apparatus has the capacity to detect and eliminate small incipient autochthonous neoplasms, there is a substantial amount of evidence to show that it nevertheless is capable of responding to such neoplasms after they become visibly established as frank progressive tumors. This is convincingly shown by the numerous descriptions of the generation of a state of concomitant antitumor immunity which enables a host with a large progressive tumor burden to paradoxically destroy a challenge of cells of the same tumor implanted at a distant site. There are enough published examples to suggest that concomitant immunity may represent a fairly common response to growing solid tumors. It is known to be generated both against autochthonous as well as syngeneic transplantable tumors (reviewed in Ref. 158), and in most cases to be strikingly effective in terms of the size of the tumor cell challenge that it is capable of rejecting. Its existence in humans is suggested by the report (145) that many cancer patients are capable of rejecting autografts of their own tumors.

It is surprising that, compared to "immunization immunity," this natural example of antitumor immunity has received so little attention. This may be due to the belief that concomitant immunity serves little or no purpose because the host is doomed to die in spite of it. There is convincing evidence, however, to contradict this belief. Indeed, there is now reason for believing that although concomitant immunity cannot reject the primary tumor burden, it can nevertheless function to retard the disease process by suppressing the spread and growth of metastases. It has seemed a puzzle to many investigators (42, 105, 130, 161), why so relatively very few secondary tumors emerge in spite of the very large numbers of viable tumor cells that are constantly shed from the primary tumors into blood and lymph. Indeed, it was considered a foregone conclusion that the large majority of these cells are rapidly and efficiently destroyed (39, 40) before they settle in the tissues.

Gershon and his colleagues (48) suggested a role for concomitant immunity in this process on the basis of the finding that a nonmetastasizing fibrosarcoma that evokes a strong concomitant immunity in hamsters, underwent rapid metastasis when the hamsters were treated with an immunosuppressive regimen of antilymphocyte globulin. Likewise, it has been shown that (71) treatment of mice carrying subcutaneous implants of the lewis lung carcinoma with antilymphocyte globulin results in a much more rapid emergence and a larger number of lung metastases. Again, Crile and Deodhar (26), who appreciate the distinction between true concomitant immunity, and immunity that develops after removal of a primary tumor, showed that the rapid decay of concomitant immunity that followed tumor excision was associated with an increased rate of development of pulmonary metastases. It should also be mentioned that there is convincing evidence (102, 129, 166) that a state of concomitant immunity reduces the number of artificial metastases caused by the infusion of tumor cells intravenously.

Concomitant immunity, then, deserves a lot more experimental attention than it has received, particularly when one considers that in many experimental cases it has been shown to rapidly decay after surgical removal of a primary tumor. An additional possibility that should be kept in mind is that concomitant immunity may contribute significantly to the successful chemotherapy of tumors, so that care should be taken not to completely suppress it.

There is good evidence that concomitant immunity, like immunity generated in response to an experimental immunizing regimen, is cell-mediated rather than antibody-mediated. This appears to have been convincingly shown first by the work of Gershon et al. (48), who demonstrated with the Winn neutralization assay that concomitant immunity to a syngeneic hamster fibrosarcoma can be transferred to normal recipients with lymphoid cells, but not with serum, from tumor-immune donors. Direct evidence that concomitant immunity is mediated by sensitized T cells was supplied by the demonstration (77, 111) that it is not generated in T-cell-deficient mice, and that tumor growth can be specifically neu-tralized in normal test recipients by θ-positive T cells from the draining lymph nodes of concomitantly immune donors (111). An additional im-portant finding was that the generation of concomitant immunity requires the presence of a large tumor mass, and is independent of the length of the latency period that follows the implantation of tumor cells (111). The position on the scale of immunogenicity of those tumors that are not immunogenic in terms of the classical accepted definition, but which give strong concomitant immunity to a growing tumor, has yet to be consid-ered.

Additional evidence for the proposition that concomitant immunity may represent a common response to most progressive neoplasms is pro-vided by the numerous demonstrations of the presence in the circulation of tumor-bearing humans and animals (4, 59) of lymphocytes that are specifically cytotoxic for tumor cells in vitro. For obvious reasons, this in vitro cytotoxicity of tumor-bearers' lymphocytes has been the subject of a very large number of publications, particularly with regard to the way in which its inhibition in vitro by antigen, antibody, or antigen-antibody complexes in serum can help explain the paradox of concomitant immun-ity in vivo. In spite of its possible importance, however, doubts have been expressed (3, 14, 62, 97) about the validity of the microcytotoxicity assay that has been almost exclusively employed to demonstrate it. This assay involves a comparison between the ability of normal and immune lym-phoid cells to detach adherent tumor cells from the bottom of microtest plates after a long (up to 3 days) incubation period in vitro. Not only is this incubation period long enough to allow the initiation and expression of an in vitro immune response, but the results obtained with the assay are at variance with those obtained with another well established in vitro assay (92, 93, 138), as well as with in vivo assays (70). There is enough evidence to show that unlike the ^{51}Cr-release assay, where there is no doubt that the cytotoxic activity of sensitized T cells is measured, a posi-tive microcytotoxicity test does not require the presence of T cells. The kinetics of production of the cell type involved, moreover, is unlike that of cytotoxic T cells. Doubt remains, therefore, about the type of in vivo host immunity that the microcytotoxicity assay is supposed to reveal. There are certainly enough different types of in vitro defined effector cells to choose from. There is little doubt at the moment, however, that the most important of these is the macrophage.

Macrophages as Participants in Antitumor Surveillance and Immunity

There are three main lines of evidence that support the belief that macrophages possess the potential for playing an important role in natural defense against neoplastic disease: (a) The response to an established progressive tumor can include an activation of the host's macrophage system as evidenced by a significant increase in its capacity for phagocytosing intravenously injected colloids; (b) animals whose macrophage systems have been activated by infectious and other agents display an enhanced capacity for resisting the growth of tumor cell implants; and (c) macrophages harvested from mice with an activated macrophage system display a striking capacity for destroying or inhibiting the growth of tumor cells in vitro.

Beginning with the natural response to the tumor itself, there are numerous examples in animals and humans to show that the response to progressive tumor growth can involve a systemic activation of macrophages. The earlier literature on the possible importance of this activation in defense against cancer has been discussed by Old and colleagues (116). The general conclusion was that macrophages possess mechanisms with at least a potential for defending against neoplastic cells. More recent evidence for a macrophage response against malignant growth is supplied by descriptions (13, 75, 76) of a large increase in the capacity of the reticuloendothelial system of tumor-bearing animals for phagocytosing intravenously infused inert colloids. It is significant that, as is the case with concomitant immunity, increased phagocytic activity of the RES was not seen until the tumors reached a large size. Similar findings have been described in humans. It was shown by Magarey and Baum (95), for example, that the majority of the large number of cancer patients they examined displayed a much greater capacity than controls for clearing radiolabeled aggregated albumin from their blood. Here again, it was found that the highest levels of RES phagocytic activity were expressed by those patients with the larger tumor burdens. So much so, that surgical removal of tumors resulted in a return to normal clearance levels. These findings in humans essentially confirmed those of others (135).

Increased phagocytic activity of the RES is not the only sign of a macrophage response to tumor growth. A response by these cells may also be indicated by a systemic increase in the rate of their division. It was shown by Nelson and Kearney (106) that subcutaneous growth of murine sarcomas can result in a significant increase in the proportion of peritoneal macrophages synthesizing DNA. This finding fits with that of others (11) who revealed that the bone marrow of tumor-bearing animals can show the presence of an increased number of macrophage precursor cells capable of forming macrophage colonies in vitro. None of these findings, however, provide direct evidence that activated macrophages play a role in antitumor resistance. Evidence for a direct role for activated macrophages is supplied, instead, by numerous reports that animals whose macrophage systems have been activated by microbial infection display an increased nonspecific capacity for destroying challenge implants of tumor cells, and that macrophages harvested from these animals display potent antitwmor acvivity *in vitro*.

Before describing this evidence, however, it is desirable to first bridge it with a discussion of the significance of systemic macrophage activation as it may be a consequence of, and participate in, the expression of concomitant immunity. There is enough evidence to suggest that the above discussed increase in macrophage function that occurs in response to tumor growth may serve as an indication of the possession of a state of concomitant immunity. In other words, that macrophage activation is a consequence of the generation of T-cell-mediated concomitant immunity, as is the case for macrophage activation in T-cell-mediated antimicrobial immunity (110). Thus, concomitant immunity and systemic macrophage activation both require the presence of a large progressive tumor, they both develop in parallel (111), and decline after removal of the tumor burden. Moreover, neither macrophage activation nor concomitant immunity develop in response to tumor growth in T-cell-deficient animals (111).

A significant additional finding (111, 113) about macrophage activation in response to the growth of certain murine tumors was that macrophages so activated gave the host a strikingly enhanced capacity for resisting infection with microbial parasites. This represents, therefore, the reciprocal of the general finding (see below) that a macrophage system activated by microbial infection can nonspecifically express antitumor resistance. There can be little doubt that activated macrophages acquired by concomitantly immune animals are responsible for nonspecific resistance expressed against antigenically unrelated tumor cells (77, 78, 111).

Yet a different type of evidence for the participation of macrophages in the natural response against established tumors is seen in the stromal reaction that is characteristic of many tumors. The evidence for lymphoreticular cell infiltration into tumors, and its correlation with more favorable prognoses has been discussed by Underwood (157). Direct evidence that many of these infiltrating cells are macrophages has been supplied by workers in several laboratories (35, 36, 57, 133) who identified them as macrophages on morphological and physiological grounds. A surprisingly large number of macrophages have been recovered from cell suspensions obtained from a variety of solid tumors. In fact, on the basis of a comparative study of the content of macrophages in different tumors, it has been suggested (31) that an inverse relationship exists between the degree of macrophage infiltration and the rate of metastatic spread. Direct evidence that the macrophages that infiltrate solid tumors possess antitumor activity was supplied by the demonstration (57) that macrophages isolated from rat sarcomas suppress colony formation of tumor cells *in vivo*.

The remaining and by far the most convincing direct evidence that supports a role for macrophages in antitumor defense is that which shows that animals whose macrophage systems have been activated by microbial infection and certain other agents display nonspecific resistance to the growth of tumor cell implants, and that macrophages harvested from such animals display a capacity for destroying tumor cells *in vitro*. This subject has recently undergone a vigorous revival, to a large extent, because of the work of Hibbs and colleagues (64, 65, 66, 67), who showed that activation of the macrophage system of mice by infection with *Toxoplasma* or *Besnoitia*, or by treatment with Freund's complete adjuvant, results in a lower incidence of certain types of spontaneous tumors, as well as in the acquisition of a powerful capacity to resist the growth of syngeneic tumor implants. Direct evidence that activated macrophages were responsible for the acquired antitumor resistance displayed by these animals was soon supplied by these as wgll as a number of other workers who demonstrated that macrophages harvested from such animals display the capacity for either destroying or inhibiting the growth of tumor cells *in vitro* (10, 25, 30, 47, 65, 66, 67, 79, 80, 81, 82, 85, 89, 90, 108, 123). Similar convincing *in vitro* findings were described for human blood monocytes activated by lymphokines *in vitro* (68). Since it is generally agreed, moreover, that the expression of this antitumor activity requires contact between macrophages and target tumor cells, it is unlikely that inhibition of tumor growth as mostly measured by inhibition of ^{3}H-thymidine into DNA is the result of an artifact caused by the release of cold thymidine from macrophages (118). There has been at least one report, however, (23) that cytostatic activity can be achieved by way of a soluble macrophage mediator.

An important general point to emphasize about this antitumor activity of macrophages is that it is nonspecifically mediated. It is apparent, therefore, that activated macrophages, and to a lesser extent normal macrophages, can discriminate between neoplastic and normal cells in the absence of specific antitumor immunity (66). The distinct possibility must be considered, therefore, that this discriminative ability may give these cells the capacity for functioning as key agents in native antitumor surveillance.

Indeed, a hypothesis of antitumor surveillance based on the discriminative and tumoricidal powers of macrophages would help to explain some apparently puzzling findings. It could explain, for instance, why there is a lower than normal incidence of spontaneous as well as chemically-induced tumors in T-cell-deficient mice, and why these mice also show increased resistance to the growth of tumor implants. These findings need not support a theory of immunostimulation as interpreted by Prehn (128). Instead, they can be explained more easily on the basis of

the recent revelation (24) that T-cell-deficient mice possess a highly activated macrophage system that compensates them for their immunodeficiency. Indeed, their macrophage systems must be considered similar to
those of mice whose macrophages have been activated by microbial infection, and which also show (116, 154) a lower incidence of spontaneous
and chemically induced tumors, and display resistance to the growth of
tumor implants. Simply stated, the compensatory activation of the macrophage system of T-cell-deficient mice would be expected to give them
a greatly enhanced macrophage-mediated mechanism of native antitumor
surveillance. This proposition is nicely supported by the recent interesting discoveries that conventionally raised athymic nude mice possess a
greater capacity than normal mice for destroying intravenously injected
tumor cells (142), and that macrophages harvested from conventionally
reared nude mice, in contrast to germ-free nudes, display enhanced
tumoricidal activity in vitro (100).

It should also be realized that any increase in tumor incidence in
animals and humans treated with immunosuppressive drugs need not
represent evidence that the increased tumor incidence is the result of
suppressed immunity. In fact, these drugs are equally capable of suppressing macrophage surveillance because of their toxicity for replicating
macrophage precursors in bone marrow.

It is predicted, in view of the foregoing discussion, therefore, that
more experimental emphasis will eventually be given to testing a
hypothesis of antitumor surveillance based on the discriminative activity
of macrophages, rather than on one based on the recognition powers of
lymphocytes. Indeed, it is well to realize that a surveillance hypothesis
based on the immune apparatus alone is extremely limited in that it cov-
ers only one phylum of the animal kingdom. The fact is, that invertebrate
species do not possess a lymphocyte-based immune mechanism, but must
somehow protect themselves against neoplastic colonization (27). To survive as species, therefore, they need an antitumor surveillance
mechanism just as much as vertebrates. It is perhaps significant that the
only major cellular defense mechanism they are known to possess in
common is one based on the discriminative powers of their phagocytic
cells; cells that show many properties and functions in common with the
vertebrate macrophages.

MECHANISMS OF SUBVERSION

The foregoing discussion dealt with evidence that supports the
proposition that the mammalian host possesses, and is capable of generating, mechanisms with at least the potential for combating colonization of

its tissues by neoplastic cells. Aside from certain purely *in vitro* defined mechanisms of defense such as the antitumor activity of null killer cells and antibody-dependent cellular cytotoxicity, the host has two major defense mechanisms against solid tumors at its disposal: T cell-mediated immunity, and the antitumor activity of macrophages.

There is still doubt, however, about the capacity of the immune apparatus to recognize and respond to the small antigenic mass presented by incipient tumors. There is no doubt, on the other hand, that a state of adaptive cell-mediated immunity can be generated, in many cases, against established progressive tumors, and that this immunity can call forth activated macrophages. Despite the eventual generation of antitumor immunity, however, autochthonous and syngeneic tumors continue to grow to kill their hosts. Malignant tumors, therefore, must be selected to avoid the host's defenses at two levels: at the level of native surveillance and at the level of acquired surveillance.

Subversion of Immune Surveillance

Some explanation is required, therefore, to explain why a malignant tumor with proven immunogenicity is not detected and destroyed in its incipiency by the immune apparatus and the macrophage system. One such mechanism is suggested by the discovery (18, 117) of antigenic modulation by certain leukemia cells exposed to the action of lytic antibodies and complement *in vitro*. This ability of tumor cells to hide their antigenicity would obviously enable them to avoid immune destruction. It has yet to be discovered, however, how common this capacity is. There is more recent evidence to suggest, moreover, that both the phenomenon of antigenic modulation and its interpretation are more complicated than originally thought (34).

The most popular and most often quoted explanation for escape from immune surveillance is based on the concept of "sneak through" (115), which simply proposes that a weakly immunogenic tumor cannot be recognized until it reaches a size that is too large for the subsequent adaptive immune response to reject it. This concept originated from the finding (sometimes erroneously quoted in reverse) that whereas a small inoculum of tumor cells takes and grows in a syngeneic host, a large inoculum, in contrast, is often rejected. It is obvious from only a brief review of the literature, however, that this does not apply to all tumors. In fact, the concept is contradicted by the reverse finding inherent in a well established procedure for immunizing against a large tumor implant, and which involves repeated inoculation with very small subtumorigenic numbers of viable tumor cells. There can be little doubt, therefore, that the means whereby antigenic tumors escape from mechanisms of surveillance are more complicated than that proposed by "sneak through," particularly when one considers the evidence for the reverse proposal by Prehn (127) that an immune response may actually be necessary to stimulate the growth of incipient neoplasms.

In fact, there could be no better indication that an explanation of tumor escape is more complicated than one based on the weakness of tumor antigens than the recent fascinating findings by Bonmasser and colleagues (16, 17). These workers have revealed the possibility that tumor cells can exert an active subversive influence on the immune apparatus. They have shown that lethal "dilution escape" of certain murine lymphomas employed as allografts depends on the capacity of tumor cells when implanted in very small numbers to actively inhibit the initiation of a T-cell-mediated immune response to strong H-2 antigens. A host injected with 10^4 or less tumor cells was shown to be incapable, after 24 hours, of mounting the strong immune rejection mechanism that it normally generates in response to a much larger implant. This tumor-induced state of immunologic refractoriness is long-lived and apparently nonspecific. Moreover, it is not caused by antibody enhancement, and is not due to contaminating viruses. It appears to be caused, instead, by a soluble factor(s) secreted by the tumor cells. Similar findings were reported by Mengersen and colleagues (88, 101) who described "dilution escape" with a syngeneic murine mastocytoma, and interpreted their findings as indicating that a small dose of tumor cells induces a state of low dose tolerance. In this system, for instance, there was some evidence that the tumor-induced state of immunologic refractoriness was specific for the tumor that induced it.

There are a number of other descriptions of immunosuppressive activity associated with soluble extracts from tumor cells. Tumor ascites fluids, as well as sera from tumor-bearing animals, have also been shown to possess immunosuppressive properties. It has been shown, for instance, (162) that infusions of serum from tumor bearing mice can greatly delay the rejection of skin allografts, as can infusions of cell free extracts of ascites tumors (55). Again, ascites tumor fluid has been demonstrated (104) to contain factors that interfere with the trapping of lymphocytes in lymphoid organs responding to antigenic stimulation. All of these examples, then, point to the possibility that the cells of many tumors secrete molecules that might function pharmacologically to actively inhibit the initiation of the immune response. The selective advantage of such molecules to neoplastic cells growing in an immunocompetent host must surely be considered in any hypothesis that attempts to explain the ability of antigenic tumors to avoid early destruction by the immune apparatus. It has yet to be discovered, however, how universal such molecules might be, and whether different tumors produce different molecules.

Most of the examples quoted, and in particular the "dilution escape factor" of Bonmasser et al. (16), give a potent suppressive effect systemically. However, failure to find similar systemic effects with certain tumors would not necessarily mean that they do not produce antisurveillance factors. On the contrary, the secretion of small quantities of such factors might limit their sphere of influence to the vicinity of the tumor. The possibility also arises from this discussion that the systemic liberation of immunosuppressor molecules at later stages of tumor growth might well facilitate the emergence of metastases by actively subverting or reducing the effectiveness of concomitant immunity.

Before discussing the ways in which established tumors might subvert mechanisms of acquired surveillance, however, it is first necessary to discuss how incipient tumors might avoid destruction by the other major component of native surveillance, the macrophage system.

Subversion of Macrophage Surveillance

It was recently demonstrated (112) that subcutaneous implantation of 10^5 or 10^6 cells from any one of 5 syngeneic murine tumors resulted within 24 hours in a severe systemic suppression of the capacity of mice to express native resistance to infection with the bacterial parasites, Listeria monocytogenes and Yersinia enterocolitica. Because it is well established that the initial destruction of these bacteria is achieved by way of the phagocytic and bactericidal activity of macrophages, it was concluded that the implanted tumor cells caused a systemic suppression of macrophage function. It was next shown, in support of this conclusion, that the greatly enhanced nonspecific antibacterial activity of a macrophage system activated either by infection with BCG or by treatment with Corynebacterium parvum was also severely suppressed by the implantation of tumor cells. As expected, the suppressive effect was caused by a factor liberated into the circulation, in that macrophage-mediated antibacterial resistance was suppressed in normal recipients by an infusion of a small volume of serum from tumor-treated donors. It is significant, moreover, that the half-life of suppressed antimicrobial resistance in the recipients was about 24 hours, and that the suppressor factor was small enough to pass through a dialysis membrane.

The relevance of these findings to tumor escape mechanisms was indicated by the additional finding that the state of suppressed macrophage-mediated antimicrobial resistance was associated with a state of decreased native resistance to growth of a tumor cell inoculum. This was evidenced by a substantial decrease in the period of latency before a subcutaneous challenge implant began to grow progressively, and also by a substantial delay before an intraperitoneal tumor cell inoculum began to multiply as measured by ^{3}H-thymidine incorporation into DNA (112). Since there is enough information (87) to show that the length of the latency period is inversely proportional to the number of tumor cells implanted, it was concluded that the decreased latency period observed in tumor-suppressed mice was caused by suppression of a native defense mechanism that normally acts to destroy a large part of a syngeneic tumor cell implant. It was further concluded that this mechanism of native surveillance was based on the antitumor capacity of macrophages.

There is additional evidence for the existence of a macrophage-mediated mechanism of native resistance to implanted tumor cells. It has been reported, for example, that a large proportion of an inoculum of radiolabelled tumor cells injected intravenously into normal animals is rapidly destroyed (38), as is a large proportion of similarly labeled cells injected subcutaneously (120) and intraperitoneally (41, 43). The destruction of implanted tumor cells occurs much too rapidly, moreover, to be caused by an immune response. It seems highly more likely, instead, that this antitumor activity represents a mechanism of native surveillance based on the antitumor activity of macrophages, particulary since it seems almost a foregone conclusion that a more rapid destruction of tumor cells would occur in animals with a BCG- or C. parvum-activated macrophage system.

It is also important to discuss in this context the possible meaning of the well-known Révész effect (131) which refers to the significant "enhancement" of growth (decreased period of latency) of implanted tumor cells when they are admixed with a large number of lethally X-irradiated tumor cells. There have been a number of attempts to explain this puzzling phenomenon including one based on the "feeder" effects of the irradiated cells. Another explanation proposes (120) that the presence of irradiated cells results in a larger deposit of fibrin that functions to retain a larger number of viable tumor cells at the site of implantation. Neither of these explanations, however, is satisfactory in the light of recent unpublished experiments in this laboratory (147) which indicate that the Révész effect is caused by the suppression of a preexisting macrophage-mediated mechanism of tumor cell destruction. This was deduced from the simple finding that the greatly increased antitumor activity expressed against a tumor cell implant by mice with a BCG-activated macrophage system is significantly suppressed by the inclusion of a large number of X-irradiated tumor cells with the viable inoculum. Or, stated in reverse, the presence of an activated macrophage system can greatly decrease the magnitude of the Révész effect. Additional experiments have revealed that a Révész effect can be obtained either by the local or systemic injection of bacterial lipopolysaccharide, which in the first instance is known to be a suppressor of macrophage function. It is highly significant, more-over, that animals so treated, besides showing enhanced growth of a tumor inoculum implanted in their hind footpad, also allowed a striking enhancement of growth of an inoculum of *Listeria monocytogenes* in-jected in the same site. Since the initial destruction of a large proportion of an inoculum of this bacterium is known to be achieved by macro-phages, the possibility must be considered that the observed endotoxin-induced enhancement of tumor growth was likewise caused by suppres-sion of macrophage function.

There is yet an additional means that incipient tumors might employ to escape from native macrophage surveillance. They could secrete molecules that function pharmacologically to prevent macrophages from migrating to their vicinity and confronting them. In fact, a recent publica-tion has shown (124) that subcutaneous injection of small numbers of cells from certain murine tumors results in a greatly reduced capacity of the host for directing macrophages into a site of peritoneal inflammation. It was further shown that the same suppressive effect could be obtained by injecting the host with a small molecular weight dialysable factor released from disrupted tumor cells. More to the point, this factor was shown to suppress the chemotactic response of macrophages *in vitro*. This factor then might be the same as the one which suppresses macrophage-mediated resistance to bacterial infection, particularly since they both were shown to cause enhanced growth of a tumor cell inoculum. Additional evidence that the same factor is involved is supplied by recent unpublished experiments in this laboratory which show that dialysates of sera from tumor-treated mice which cause suppression of antibacterial resistance also cause a 60% reduction in the number of leukocytes that emigrate into peritoneal inflammation. The possibility must be consid-ered, therefore, that incipient tumors are able to subvert macrophage-mediated surveillance by secreting molecules that prevent macrophages (and perhaps other cells) from migrating to sites of tumor cell multiplica-tion. Considering the possibility that antigen processing by macrophages is an essential step in the initiation of an immune response, the local influence of an antiinflammatory factor might also result in failure to mount an immune response, and thus cause escape from immune surveil-lance.

The foregoing discussion, then, has dealt with mechanisms that might give incipient tumors the capacity to break through mechanisms of native antitumor surveillance and emerge as progressive malignancies. It was suggested that the ability of tumors to do this, in spite of their posses-sion of antigens that might trigger an immune response, and of surface characteristics that make them vulnerable to destruction by macrophages, might rest with their possession of mechanisms that allow them to directly or indirectly subvert surveillance mechanisms by pharmacological means. There is certainly enough information for at least the proposal that there is probably a lot more to an explanation for the escape of immunogenic tumors than an explanation based simply on the inability of the immune system to detect weak tumor specific antigens. The knowledge that the immune response to tumors with strong transplantation antigens, can be nonspecifically subverted by prior exposure to numbers of tumor cells small enough to stimulate natural tumor emergence suggests the need to reexaming what is meant by the term, weak immunogenicity. The problem at the moment, however, is that there is no way of guessing how universal these types of tumor subversive mechanisms might prove to be. As mentioned above, some could be relatively weak in that their subversive action is limited to the tumor site, while others may be potent enough to suppress surveillance systemically. Indeed, the latter possibility could be responsible for the frequent emergence of multiple primary tumors.

The high incidence of multiple primary tumors in human cancer patients is well illustrated by the fact that there is a special section devoted to the subject in Index Medicus. In view of the commonness of multiple primaries, the distinct possibility must be considered that one established tumor can subvert surveillance against others.

Subversion of Acquired Mechanisms of Resistance

There are many published examples of the paradox of progressive tumor growth in the face of an acquired mechanism of antitumor immunity. As stated in a preceding section, a major segment of the evidence for this statement is based on the numerous reports of the presence in humans and animals with progressive tumors of lymphocytes that are specifically cytotoxic for tumor cells in vitro, and also on numerous descriptions in animals of concomitant immunity to a tumor cell challenge. In many cases, therefore, an acquired immunologic effector mechanism with the potential for ridding the host of its tumor burden exists. The problem is thus to explain why this immunity fails to carry out its function.

Before discussing the possible reasons for the paradox of concomitant immunity, however, it is important to point out that in contrast to tumor syngrafts, most tumor allografts after a period of growth, are vigorously rejected by a powerful mechanism of T cell-mediated immunity that is generated against their strong histocompatibility antigens. Thus, the fact that an allograft is presented in the form of a malignant tumor, in most cases, makes little difference to the capacity of an immune effector mechanism to reject it, although there appear to have been no definitive studies that have compared the rejection times of grafts of normal and malignant tissues. It might be assumed on the basis of this knowledge, therefore, that the paradox of concomitant immunity can be explained on the basis that the immunity generated against a tumor syngraft is comparatively weak.

Whether the term "weak immunity" refers to the presence of fewer cytotoxic T cells, or whether, instead, the cytotoxic T cells generated against syngeneic tumors are less cytotoxic than those generated against allografts, appears not to be known. It is timely to suggest, however, that caution should be exercised when comparing antisyngraft and antiallograft immunity. This is indicated by the recent important demonstration (139) that the T cells that are cytotoxic for syngeneic tumor cells are of a different cell lineage than those that are cytotoxic for allogeneic tumor cells, and may therefore possess different properties. Add this knowledge to that (136) which suggests that the lysis of syngeneic tumor cells requires that the cytotoxic T cells and the tumor cells share the same H-2 antigens, and one is forced to consider the likelihood that allogeneic tumors may represent invalid models for analyzing immunity to malignant neoplasms.

It is entirely possible that a mechanism that subverts the action of T cells cytotoxic for tumor syngrafts may have no effect on the T cells that are cytotoxic for tumor allografts, and vice versa. It is for this reason that this chapter, except for special circumstances, has not included in its discussion examples of immunity to allogeneic tumors.

The Role of Serum Blocking Factors in Subversion of Acquired Immunity

The paradox of the presence in humans and animals with progressive tumors of circulating lymphocytes that are specifically cytotoxic for tumor cells in vitro has received a great deal of experimental investigation. Since the presence of these lymphocytes indicates the successful generation of a state of acquired cell-mediated immunity, it seems obvious that these cells represent the effectors of concomitant immunity. The paradox of concomitant immunity demonstrates, therefore, that it is the efferent or effector arm of the immune response, and not the afferent and central arms, that is being subverted.

The most popular explanation of why acquired cytotoxic lymphocytes in apparently large numbers fail to reject the tumor that evoked their generation is based on the demonstration that their cytotoxicity in vitro can be blocked by prior exposure of the tumor target cells to the tumor bearer's serum. The large amount of evidence for the existence of factors in serum that specifically block in vitro cytotoxicity of tumor-sensitized lymphocytes has been adequately reviewed (4, 60). There is evidence (6,

141) that blocking factors are complexes of antibody with tumor specific antigens. Furthermore, because such antigens almost certainly are shed into the circulation in large quantities from large progressive tumors, a good case was made by Baldwin et al. (7) for implicating them directly in blocking activity. These authors conceptualize that the expected presence of large quantities of antigen, and antigen-antibody complexes within a large tumor mass, would serve to severely paralyze the local expression of cytotoxicity by swamping sensitized lymphocytes with the tumor antigens to which they have been sensitized.

Indeed, there is a need to emphasize that the action of blocking factors may not be expressed systemically, but limited to the site of the tumor itself. Otherwise, it would be difficult to explain why the presence of these factors in serum does not inhibit the expression in tumor-bearers of high levels of concomitant immunity. For this reason it is difficult to reconcile the evidence (8) for the expression of concomitant immunity with the blocking effects of infusions of comparatively small amounts of blocking serum. Aside from the fact that the in vivo blocking effects were observed as enhanced growth of an inoculum of implanted tumor cells which bears little resemblance to conditions within vascularized established tumors, there is also the possibility that antigen-dependent blocking factors are not responsible for the observed enhancement of growth. It is possible, instead, that the blocking serum employed may also have contained molecules like those discussed above, which subvert macrophages or lymphocyte function pharmacologically. Another finding that throws some doubt on the in vivo significance of serum blocking factors is that strong in vitro blocking activity can be demonstrated with serum taken from animals that have been made highly immune to a tumor cell challenge (5).

In fact, most of the correlations between tumor growth and regressions and the corresponding presence and absence of serum blocking activity have been demonstrated with Moloney-virus-induced sarcomas in mice. Because these tumors, more often than not, progress and then regress, it is doubtful whether they should be considered as malignant and representative of tumors in general. It should also be realized that the viremia that results from implantation of this type of tumor may be immunosuppressive in its own right (44). The complexity of this and of similar systems that are used as models for demonstrating the in vivo significance of serum blocking factors was well illustrated by Pierce (122). This author made the interesting observation that even though there was no blocking activity in serum taken from mice whose Moloney tumors were regressing under the influence of acquired immunity, infusions of this same regressor serum nevertheless caused a greater enhancement of growth of a tumor implant than a progressor serum with high in vitro blocking activity.

A recent finding published from this laboratory (156) also throws some doubt on an explanation of the paradox of concomitant immunity based on blocking factors. This finding stemmed from a study which showed that Corynebacterium parvum-potentiated cell-mediated immunity to a murine fibrosarcoma could be transferred to normal recipients with short-lived replicating T cells from immune donors. Not only did an infusion of immune T cells prevent the growth of a tumor cell challenge, it also dramatically halted the growth for 6 or 7 days of relatively large established tumors. This hardly supports the notion that established tumors contain blocking factors that act locally to neutralize the antitumor activity of sensitized lymphocytes. Even so, it could well be suggested that the sensitized tumor-specific T cells generated under the immunopotentiation action of C. parvum, like those that mediate antiallograft immunity, are different from the effector T cells that arise naturally by the generation of concomitant immunity. There is no doubt from an overall consideration of the foregoing discussion, however, that it requires more than a consideration of the action of in vitro defined blocking factors to explain why a host with a population of effector lymphocytes is unable to make use of these cells to rid itself of its tumor burden.

Nonspecific Antagonism of Host Defenses in Established Tumors

A possible alternative or additional explanation for failure of a tumor to be rejected by an acquired mechanism of immunity is that the environ of an established tumor may be pharmacologically antagonistic not only to the expression of antitumor defenses, but to host defenses in general. This concept was recently investigated in this laboratory (146) by testing the prediction that a tumor-bearing host that acquires a mechanism of T-cell-mediated immunity to the bacterial parasite, Listeria monocytogenes, is incapable of expressing this immunity against a bacterial challenge inoculated into the bed of its primary tumor. The general finding with 4 different murine tumors either growing subcutaneously, or intraperitoneally in ascites form, is illustrated in Figure 1. It shows that whereas bacteria inoculated into a normal footpad first grew for 2 days and were then progressively and efficiently eliminated, the same numbers of bacteria inoculated into the contralateral footpad carrying a 6-day fibrosarcoma were not eliminated, but remained in high numbers in the tumor until the mice died. Bacteria were not eliminated from the tumor, furthermore, in spite of an acquired mechanism of T cell-mediated im-

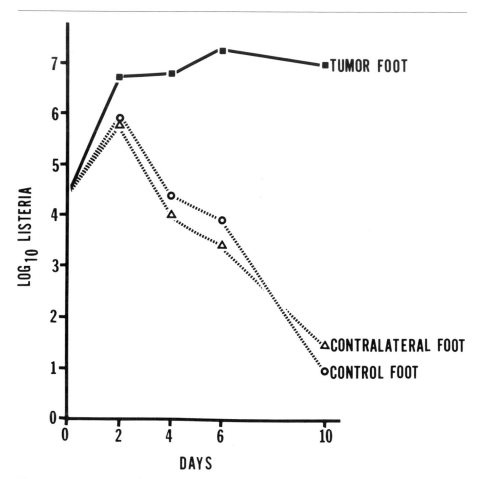

Fig. 1. Comparison between the growth of the bacterial parasite *Listeria monocytogenes* in a tumor-bearing footpad and its growth in the normal contralateral footpad. While the host was quite capable after 2 days of progressively and efficiently eliminating the organism from its tumor-free footpad, it was incapable of eliminating the organism from its tumor footpad. Included is the growth curve of bacteria in the footpads of tumor-free control mice.

munity that gave the tumor-bearing mice the capacity to eliminate lethal challenges of *Listeria* injected either subcutaneously or intravenously.

The similarities between this situation and concomitant antitumor immunity are obvious. While both types of immunity can be efficiently expressed systemically, neither can be fully expressed inside the tumor. A preliminary histological study revealed, moreover, that most of the bacteria in solid and ascites tumors were located inside macrophages, many of which were heavily parasitized. That this observation is more than of academic interest is shown by recent descriptions (140, 144) of human cancer patients with tumors heavily parasitized with L. monocytogenes. It is apparent from these results, therefore, that conditions within a primary tumor may be antagonistic to host defense mechanisms in general, either because they inhibit the entry of effector cells, or suppress their function after they enter.

Anti-Inflammation Factors in Subversion of Acquired Immunity

Mahoney and Leighton (96) described an interesting difference between the cellular reaction that occurred in response to a cotton thread implanted inside an established tumor and a thread implanted in normal tissues. Whereas the presence of the thread in normal tissues resulted in 7 days in a considerable influx of inflammatory cells, the response to its presence within a primary tumor mass was minimal. A similar observation was later made by other workers (28) who showed that the number of leukocytes that emigrated into areas of injured skin was much lower in cancer patients than in normal people or in patients with other diseases. It was mainly because of a greatly decreased number of emigrant macrophages, moreover, that a lower number of inflammatory cells was observed. Additional evidence for a suppressed capacity by tumor bearers for mounting inflammatory responses was supplied by a study with guinea pigs carrying intramuscular hepatomas (12). It was revealed that guinea pigs with established tumors possessed a greatly reduced capacity for directing blood leukocytes into turpentine-induced inflammation in the skin and peritoneal cavity, and this was associated with a reduced capacity for mounting delayed sensitivity reactions. Less leukocyte emigration occurred, moreover, even though the tumor bearers contained larger than normal numbers of leukocytes in their circulation.

These results have been essentially confirmed with tumor-bearing mice in this laboratory. Very similar results have also been reported by Johnson et al. (72, 73, 74) for human cancer patients. Indeed, these authors have shown that failure to elicit delayed responses to chemical sensitizers in humans with cancer is more likely the result of an inability to mount inflammatory responses in general, rather than the result of suppressed cell-mediated immunity. They rightly quote examples of situations in which animals with negative skin tests can nevertheless be shown to possess sensitized lymphocytes that respond to test antigens in vitro.

There is now a substantial amount of evidence which suggests that the reduced responses to inflammatory stimuli observed in tumor-bearing animals are at least partly caused by tumor-induced suppression of macrophage function. A series of papers from Snyderman and colleagues (124, 143) have revealed that mice carrying subcutaneous implants of syngeneic tumors show a greatly decreased influx of mobile macrophages into peritoneal inflammation. They have also shown that the inhibitor of macrophage migration in vivo is a small molecular weight (10,000 MW) factor released by cells of the tumors, and that this factor can inhibit macrophage chemotaxis in vitro. These observations support the notion of Fauve et al. (37), who showed that injection of a small molecular weight factor from tumor cell extracts was capable of locally inhibiting the emigration of leukocytes into sites of subcutaneous inflammation.

More recently, additional reports (37, 109, 149) have shown that the greatly reduced emigration of leukocytes into inflammation in tumor-bearing animals is associated with a greatly reduced capacity of their macrophages to respond chemotactically in vitro. Human cancer patients also have been shown to possess macrophages with an impaired ability to respond to chemotactic stimuli in vitro (15, 58, 132, 134). Given the possibility that the assay for measuring in vitro chemotaxis may also measure differences in the rate of random locomotion, there seems little doubt that these findings show that macrophage function is strikingly defective. Considering the convincing evidence for a role for macrophages in defense against neoplasia, it is obvious that tumor-induced suppression of macrophage function must figure in any hypothesis that attempts to explain the escape of tumors from mechanisms of native and acquired surveillance.

Tumor-Induced Immunosuppression

The subject of impaired immunoresponsiveness in cancer patients has been reviewed by Harris and Copeland (56) who interpret the evidence as showing that the phenomenon is quite common, and mainly involves patients with advanced disseminated disease. The evidence consists of demonstrations of a depressed ability of tumor-bearers to mount delayed skin reactions to recall antigens that more likely than not they became sensitized to at some stage of life, and to mount an immune response to a chemical sensitizing agent to which they have not been previously exposed. The importance of immune responsiveness to a favorable prognosis has been discussed by Eilber and Morton (33).

Additional evidence for generalized immunodepression in tumor bearers is that their lymphocytes can show a significantly reduced capacity for responding to mitogenic substances in vitro: an apparent indication of suppressed immunocompetence. This has been shown with lymphocytes harvested from tumor-bearing animals (1, 49, 50) and from tumor-bearing humans (19, 46, 53, 164). It is significant that in many cases both *in vivo* and *kn vitro* responsiveness return to normal after removal of the primary tumor burden. It is well to point out, however, that many of the results obtained with mitogens *in vitro* employed an assay that compares the response of a standard number of control lymphocytes with the response of the same number of experimental lymphocytes. This experimental design, therefore, does not cover the likely possibility that a reduced response to mitogens by tumor bearers' lymphocytes could simply be a reflection of a decrease in the proportion of those lymphocytes capable of responding. This would occur, for instance, if blood and lymphoid organs acquired a large proportion of either sensitized cytotoxic lymphocytes or antibody-forming cells in response to the tumor. Indeed, it seems a little contradictory (160) to interpret a reduced PHA response of lymphocytes from lymphoid organs from tumor-bearing animals as indicating the presence of a state of depressed immunoresponsiveness, when these same lymphoid organs were shown to have acquired committed T cells capable of lysing tumor cells *in vitro*.

This type of criticism is partly answered, however, by the additional evidence that the serum of immunodepressed tumor-bearers can contain soluble factors that inhibit lymphocyte responses *in vivo* and *in vitro* (19, 52, 107, 125, 151, 163, 165). In some cases these factors are of relatively large molecular weight, while in others they are the size of small peptides. It must be assumed, therefore, that in many cases tumors are capable of systemically suppressing immune responsiveness by secreting pharmacologically active suppressor molecules. There is evidence (126), moreover, that tumor-synthesized prostoglandins may function in this capacity.

The impaired immunoresponsiveness of tumor-bearers has also been explained in terms of the immunoregulatory function of suppressor T cells (86). The general literature on suppressor T cells is rapidly expanding, and it currently shows that there are both antigen-specific and non-specific suppressor cells. Antigen-specific suppressor T cell systems have been described which can inhibit the generation of primary immune responses, while others have been shown to be capable of inhibiting the expression of an already established immunity. It was recently shown (45) that tumor-bearing mice generate T cells that are capable of partially suppressing the expression of an already established immunity in tumor-immunized mice. This evidence supports that published by others (155) who have demonstrated in tumor-bearing mice the presence of T cells capable of enhancing the growth of a tumor cell implant in normal recipients. These *in vivo* results give credence to those which show (54, 84) that T cells from tumor-bearing mice can suppress lymphocyte responses to mitogens in vitro, although this type of in vitro result supports a nonspecific role for suppressor T cells.

Perhaps the most meaningful evidence for a role for suppressor T cells comes from sequential studies of the properties of T cells produced at different stages of tumor growth. According to the results from two different laboratories (91, 150), early growth of syngeneic tumors evokes the generation of T cells that are cytotoxic for tumor cells in vitro, while T cells generated at later stages of tumor growth can inhibit the cytotoxic activity of early phase cells. An interesting interpretation of such results was offered by Kuperman et al. (91), who suggest that suppressor T cells prevent the rejection of immunogenic tumors by inhibiting the continuous generation of short-lived cytotoxic effector T cells from acquired-memory precursor T cells.

None of this evidence about suppressor T cells supports a role for antigen- and antibody-dependent serum blocking factors in the suppression of acquired antitumor immunity. In fact, it supports an alternative explanation. It cannot, however, fully explain the paradox of concomitant antitumor immunity which by definition is expressed in spite of the presence of suppressor T cells. Again, according to some authors, suppressor cells are apparently absent during the early growth of tumors at a time when functional numbers of cytotoxic T cells are present. There must be some other reason, therefore, why these early cytotoxic effector cells fail to reject the tumor.

CONCLUSIONS

This chapter has attempted to show that since most malignant neoplastic cells are immunogenic to a larger or lesser degree, and possess surface characteristics that can be recognized by macrophages, they must be naturally selected to avoid being destroyed at some stage of tumor growth by the immune apparatus and the macrophage system. While most of the evidence indicates that an incipient neoplasm in the form of a small nest of malignant cells represents too small an antigenic mass to trigger an immune response, there is some evidence that macrophages possess at least the potential for detecting and destroying such cells.

The possibility was discussed that the apparent inability of the immune apparatus and the macrophage system to recognize and respond against an incipient immunogenic neoplasm might be caused by the release of molecules from tumor cells that pharmacologically subvert the function of host effector cells. If these molecules functioned locally or systemically to subvert native surveillance against incipient tumors, they would also be capable of subverting acquired surveillance in the form of concomitant immunity that is eventually generated against large established tumors. It has been demonstrated, for instance, that tumor cells secrete factors capable of inducing a state of immunological refractoriness and of suppressing macrophage function.

Perhaps the most important recent finding, however, was that tumor cells secrete a small molecular weight factor that can inhibit macrophage chemotaxis in vitro, and prevent the emigration of leukocytes from blood into sites of inflammation. If an antiinflammatory molecule is indeed found to be secreted by most types of tumors, then there would be no need to consider incomplete explanations of the paradox of concomitant antitumor immunity based on the action of serum blocking factors and suppressor T cells. The local action of a molecule that prevents the transit of host effector cells from small blood vessels into the tumor mass, obviously, would in itself represent an adequate explanation for the failure of native and acquired mechanisms of antitumor surveillance to eliminate a malignant neoplasm. It would also explain why a large malignant tumor represents an environment that is antagonistic to the expression of host defenses in general.

The problem, however, is that it is not yet possible to judge how common the possession of these types of pharmacologically active molecules by tumor cells might prove to be. There is not enough information currently available to formulate a general hypothesis based on the action of such molecules to explain how tumors avoid destruction by native and acquired surveillance. It is anticipated, however, that evidence for the association of similar suppressor molecules with many types of tumors will form the subject matter of a large number of publications in the future.

ACKNOWLEDGMENT

This work was supported by grants No. CA16642 from the National Cancer Institute and No. 5501-RR05705 from the Division of Research Resources.

REFERENCES

1. Adler, W. H., Takiguchi, T., and Smith, R. T. 1971. Phytohemagglutinin unresponsiveness in mouse spleen cells induced by methylcholanthrene sarcoma. Cancer Res. 31: 864–867.

2. Allison, A. C., and Taylor, R. B. 1967. Observations on thymectomy and carcinogenesis. Cancer Res. 27: 703–707

3. Baldwin, R. W. 1975. *In vitro* assays of cell-mediated immunity to human solid tumors: Problems of quantitation, specificity and interpretation. *J. Natl. Cancer Inst.* 55: 745–748.

4. Baldwin, R. W., Embleton, M. J., and Robins, R. A. 1973. Humoral factors influencing cell-mediated immune responses to tumor-associated antigens. *Proc. Roy. Soc. Med.* 66: 466–468.

5. Baldwin, R. W., Embleton, M. J., and Robins, R. A. 1973. Cellular and humoral immunity to rat hepatoma specific antigens correlated with tumor status. *Int. J. Cancer.* 11: 310–319.

6. Baldwin, R. W., Price, M. R., and Robins, R. A. 1972. Blocking of lymphocyte-mediated cytotoxicity for rat hepatoma cells by tumor-specific antigen-antibody complexes. *Nature New Biol.* 238: 185–187.

7. Baldwin, R. W., Price, M. R., and Robins, R. A. 1973. Inhibition of hepatoma-immune lymph-node cell cytotoxicity by tumor-bearer serum, and solubilized hepatoma antigen. *Int. J. Cancer* 11: 527–535.

8. Bansal, S. C., Hargreaves, R., and Sjogren, H. O. 1972. Facilitation of polyoma tumor growth in rats by blocking sera and tumor eluate. *Int. J. Cancer.* 9: 97–108.

9. Barron, B. A., and Richart, R. M. 1968. A statistical model of the natural history of cervical carcinoma based on a prospective study of 557 cases. *J. Natl. Cancer Inst.* 41: 1343–1353.

10. Basic, I., Milas, L., Grdina, D. J., and Withers, H. R. 1975. *In vitro* destruction of tumor cells by macrophages from mice treated with *Corynebacterium granulosum. J. Natl. Cancer Inst.* 55: 589–595.

11. Baum, M., and Fisher, B. 1972. Macrophage production by the bone marrow of tumor-bearing mice. *Cancer Res.* 32: 2813–2817.

12. Bernstein, I. D., Zbar, B., and Rapp, H. J. 1972. Impaired inflammatory responses in tumor-bearing guinea pigs. *J. Natl. Cancer Inst.* 49: 1641–1647.

13. Blamey, R. W., Crosby, D. L., and Baker, J. M. 1969. Reticuloendothelial activity during growth of rat sarcomas. *Cancer Res.* 29: 335–337.

14. Bloom, B. R., Cepellini, R., Cerottini, J-C., *et al.* 1973. *In vitro* methods in cell-mediated immunity: A progress report. *Cell. Immunol.* 6: 331–347.

15. Boetcher, D. A., and Leonard, E. J. 1974. Abnormal monocyte chemotactic response in cancer patients. *J. Natl. Cancer Inst.* 52: 1091–1099.

16. Bonmasser, E., Bonmasser, A., Goldin, A., and Cudkowicz, G. 1973. Depression of antilymphoma allograft reactivity by tumor associated factors. *Cancer Res.* 33: 1054–1061.

17. Bonmasser, E., Menconi, E., Goldin, A., and Cudkowicz, G. 1974. Escape of small numbers of allogeneic lymphoma cells from immune surveillance. *J. Natl. Cancer Inst.* 53: 475–479.

18. Boyse, E. A., and Old, L. J. 1963. Antigenic properties of experimental leukemias. II. Immunological studies *in vivo* with C57Bl/6 radiation induced leukemias. *J. Natl. Cancer Inst.* 31: 987–1108.

19. Brooks, W. H., Netsky, M. G., Normansell, D. E., and Horwitz, D. A. 1972. Depressed cell-mediated immunity in patients with primary intracranial tumors: Characterization of a humoral immunosuppressive factor. *J. Exp. Med.* 136: 1631–1647.

20. Burnet, F. M. 1970. The concept of immunological surveillance. *Prog. Exp. Tumor Res.* 13: 1–27.

21. Cairns, J. 1975. The cancer problem. *Scientific American* 233: 64–78.

22. Cairns, J. 1975. Mutation selection and the natural history of cancer. *Nature (Lond.)* 255: 197–200.

23. Calderon, J., Williams, R. T., and Unanue, E. R. 1974. An inhibition of cell proliferation released by cultures of macrophages. *Proc. Natl. Acad. Sci. U.S.A.* 71: 4273–4277.

24. Cheers, C., and Waller, R. 1975. Activated macrophages in congenitally athymic nude mice and thymectomized lethally-irradiated mice. *J. Immunol.* 115: 844–847.

25. Cleveland, R. P., Meltzer, M. S., and Zbar, B. 1974. Tumor cytotoxicity *in vitro* by macrophages from mice infected with *Mycobacterium bovis* strain BCG. *J. Natl. Cancer Inst.* 52: 1887–1895.

26. Crile, G., and Deodhar, S. D. 1971. Role of preoperative irradiation in prolonging concomitant immunity and preventing metastasis in mice. *Cancer* 27: 629–634.

27. Dawe, C. J., and Harshbarger, J. C. 1969. Neoplasms and related disorders of invertebrate and lower vertebrate animals. *Natl. Cancer Inst. Monogr.* 31: 1–769.

28. Dizon, Q. S., and Southam, C. M. 1963. Abnormal cellular response to skin abrasions in cancer patients. *Cancer* 14: 1288–1292.

29. Drake, J. W. 1970. *The Molecular Basis of Mutation*, Holden-Day, San Francisco.

30. Droller, M. J., and Remington, D. S. 1975. A role for the macrophage in *in vivo* and *in vitro* resistance to murine bladder tumor cell growth. *Cancer Res.* 35: 49–53.

31. Eccles, S. A., and Alexander, P. 1974. Macrophage content of tumors in relation to metastatic spread and host immune reaction. *Nature.* 250: 667–669.

32. Eccles, S. A., Bandlow, G., and Alexander, P. 1976. Monocytosis associated with the growth of transplanted syngeneic rat sarcomata differing in immunogenicity. *Brit. J. Cancer.* 34: 20–27.

33. Eilber, F. R., and Morton, D. L. 1970. Impaired reactivity and recurrence following cancer surgery. *Cancer* 25: 362–367.

34. Esmon, N. L., and Little, J. R. 1976. An indirect radioimmunoassay for thymus leukemia (TL) antigens. *J. Immunol.* 117: 911–918.

35. Evans, R. 1972. Macrophages in syngeneic animal tumors. *Transplantation.* 14: 468–473.

36. Evans, R. 1973. Macrophages and the tumor bearing host. *Brit. J. Cancer.* 28: (Suppl. 1) 19–25.

37. Fauve, R. M., Hevin, B., Jacobs, H., Gaillard, J. A., and Jacob, F. 1974. Antiinflammatory effects of murine malignant cells. *Proc. Natl. Acad. Sci. U.S.A.* 71: 4052–4056.

38. Fidler, I. 1970. Metastasis: Quantitative analysis of distribution and fate of tumor emboli labeled with ^{125}I-5-Iodo-2'-deoxyuridine. *J. Natl. Cancer Inst.* 45: 773–782.

39. Fidler, I. J. 1973. Selection of successive tumor lines for metastasis. *Nature New Biol.* 242: 148–149.

40. Fidler, I. J., and Zeidman, I. 1972. Enhancement of experimental metastasis by X-ray: A possible mechanism. *J. Med. (Basel)* 3: 172–177.

41. Fioretti, M. C., Liberati, M., Bonmasser, E., and Cudkowicz, G. 1975. Immune inhibition of lymphoma cells in the peritoneal cavity of mice. *Cancer Res.* 35: 30–36.

42. Fisher, E. R., and Turnbull, R. B. 1955. Cytological demonstration and significance of tumor cells in mesenteric venous blood in patients with colorectal carcinoma. *Surg. Gynec. Obst.* 100: 102–108.

43. Forman, J., Ketchel, M. M., and Hofer, K. G. 1972. Tumor immunity *in vivo*. Use of the [125]IUdR prelabeling technique to monitor cell death in immune animals. *Transplant.* 14: 166–174.

44. Friedman, H., and Walter, S. G. 1975. Immunosuppression in the etiology of cancer. In *Immunological Aspects of Neoplasia*, pp. 253–292. Williams and Wilkins Co., Baltimore.

45. Fujimoto, S., Green, M. I., and Sehon, A. H. 1976. Regulation of the immune response to tumor antigens. I. Immunosuppressor cells in tumor-bearing host. *J. Immunol.* 116: 791–799.

46. Gatti, R. A., Garrioch, D. B., and Good, R. A. 1970. Depressed PHA responses in patients with non-lymphoid malignancies. In Proceedings Fifth Leukocyte Culture Conference , 1970, pp. 339–358. Academic Press, New York.

47. Germain, R. N., Williams, R. M., and Benacerraf, B. 1975. Specific and nonspecific antitumor immunity. II. Macrophage-mediated nonspecific effector activity induced by BCG and similar agents. *J. Natl. Cancer Inst.* 54: 709–720.

48. Gershon, R. K., Carter, R. L., and Kondo, K. 1967. On concomitant immunity in tumor-bearing hamsters. *Nature* 213: 674–676.

49. Gillette, R. W., and Boone, C. W. 1973. Changes in phytohemagglutinin response due to presence of tumors. *J. Natl. Cancer Inst.* 50: 1391–1393.

50. Gillette, R. W., and Boone, C. W. 1975. Changes in mitogen response of lymphoid cells with progressive tumor growth. *Cancer Res.* 35: 3774–3779.

51. Gillette, R. W., and Fox, A. 1975. The effect of T lymphocyte deficiency on tumor induction and growth. *Cell. Immunol.* 19: 328–335.

52. Glasgow, A. H., Nimberg, R. B., Menzoian, J. O., Saporoschetz, I., Cooperband, S. R., Schmid, K., and Mannick, J. A. 1974. Association of anergy with immunosuppressive peptide fraction in the serum of patients with cancer. *N. Engl. J. Med.* 291: 1263–1267.

53. Golub, S. H., O'Connell, T. X., and Morton, D. L. 1974. Correlation of *in vivo* and *in vitro* assays of immunocompetence in cancer patients. *Cancer Res.* 34: 1834–1837.

54. Gorczynski, R. M. 1974. Immunity to murine sarcoma virus-induced tumors. II. Suppression of T-cell-mediated immunity by cells from progressor animals. *J. Immunol.* 112: 1826–1838.

55. Gresser, I., Vignaux, I., Maury, C., and Lindahl, P. 1975. Factor(s) from Ehrlich ascites cells responsible for delayed rejection of skin allografts in mice and its assay on lymphocytes *in vitro*. *Proc. Soc. Exp. Biol. Med.* 149: 83–88.

56. Harris, J., and Copeland, D. 1974. Impaired immunoresponsiveness in tumor patients. *Ann. N.Y. Acad. Sci.* 230: 56–85.

57. Haskill, J. S., Proctor, J. W., and Yamamura, Y. 1975. Host responses

within solid tumors. I. Monocytic effector cells within rat sarcomas. *J. Natl. Cancer Inst.* 54: 387–393.

58. Hausman, M. S., Brosman, S., Synderman, R., Mickey, M. R., and Fahey, J. 1975. Defective monocyte function in patients with genitourinary carcinoma. *J. Natl. Cancer Inst.* 55: 1047–1054.

59. Hellström, K. E., and Hellström, I. 1969. Cellular immunity against tumor antigens. *Adv. Cancer Res.* 12: 167–223.

60. Hellström, I., Sjögren, H. O., Warner, G., and Hellström, K. E. 1971. Blocking of cell-mediated tumor immunity by sera from patients with growing neoplasms. *Int. J. Cancer.* 7: 226–273.

61. Herberman, R. B. 1974. Cell-mediated immunity to tumor cells. *Adv. Cancer Res.* 19: 207–253.

62. Herbermann, R. B., and Oldham, R. K. 1975. Problems associated with study of cell-mediated immunity to human tumors by microcytotoxicity assays. *J. Natl. Cancer Inst.* 55: 749–753.

63. Herbst, A. L., Ulfelder, H., and Poskanzer, D. C. 1971. Association of maternal stilbestrol therapy with tumor appearance in young women. *N. Engl. J. Med.* 284: 878–881.

64. Hibbs, J. B., Lambert, L. H., and Remington, J. S. 1971. Resistance to murine tumors conferred by chronic infection with intracellular protozoa, *Toxoplasma gondii* and *Besnoitia jellisoni*. *J. Infec. Dis.* 124: 587–592.

65. Hibbs, J. B., Lambert, L. H., and Remington, J. 1972. Adjuvant induced resistance to tumor development in mice. *Proc. Soc. Exp. Biol. Med.* 139: 1053–1056.

66. Hibbs, J. H., Lambert, L. H., and Remington, J. S. 1972. Possible role of macrophage mediated nonspecific cytotoxicity in tumor resistance. *Nature New Biol.* 235: 48–50.

67. Hibbs, J. B., Lambert, L. H., and Remington, D. S. 1972. Control of carcinogenesis: A possible role for the activated macrophage. *Science.* 177: 998–1000.

68. Holtermann, O. A., Djerassi, I., Lisafeld, B. A., Elias, E. G., Papermaster, B. W., and Klein, E. 1974. *In vitro* destruction of tumor cells by human monocytes. *Proc. Soc. Exp. Biol. Med.* 147: 456–459.

69. Hoover, R., and Fraumeni, J. F. 1973. Risk of cancer in renal-transplant recipients. *Lancet* 2: 55–57.

70. Howell, S. B., Esber, E. C., and Law, L. W. 1974. Cellular immunity in mice with simian virus 40-induced mKSA tumors: Comparison of three assays of tumor immunity. *J. Natl. Cancer Inst.* 52: 1361–1363.

71. James, S. E., and Salsbury, A. J. 1973. Facilitation of metastasis by antithymocyte globulin. *Cancer Res.* 34: 367–370.

72. Johnson, M. W., Maibach, H. I., and Salmon, S. E. 1971. Impaired delayed sensitivity or faulty inflammatory response. *N. Engl. J. Med.* 284: 1255–1257.

73. Johnson, M. W., Maibach, H. I., and Salmon, S. E. 1972. Dinitrochlorobenzene: Inflammatory response and delayed cutaneous hypersensitivity. *N. Engl. J. Med.* 286: 1162–1165.

74. Johnson, M. W., Maibach, H. I., and Salmon, S. E. 1973. Quantitative impairment of primary inflammatory responses in patients with cancer. *J. Natl.*

Cancer Inst. 51: 1075–1076.

75. Kampschmidt, R. F., and Pulliam, L. A. 1972. Changes in the opsonin and cellular influences on phagocytosis during the growth of transplantable tumors. J. Reticuloendothel. Soc. 11: 1–10.

76. Kampschmidt, R. F., and Upchurch, H. F. 1968. Stimulation of the reticuloendothelial system in tumor-bearing rats. J. Reticuloendothel. Soc. 5: 510–519.

77. Kearney, R., Basten, A., and Nelson, D. S. 1975. Cellular basis for the immune response to methylcholanthrene-induced tumors in mice. Heterogeneity of effector cells. Int. J. Cancer. 15: 438–450.

78. Kearney, R., and Nelson, D. S. 1973. Concomitant immunity to syngeneic methylcholanthrene-induced tumors in mice: Occurrence and specificity of concomitant immunity. Aust. J. Exp. Biol. Med. Sci. 51: 723–735.

79. Keller, R. 1973. Cytostatic elimination of syngeneic rat tumor cells in vitro by nonspecifically activated macrophages. J. Exp. Med. 138: 625–644.

80. Keller, R. 1974. Modulation of cell proliferation by macrophages: A possible function apart from cytotoxic tumor rejection. Brit. J. Cancer. 30: 401–415.

81. Keller, R. 1974. Mechanisms by which activated normal macrophages destroy syngeneic rat tumor cells in vitro. Cytokinetics, noninvolvement of T lymphocytes, and effect of metabolic inhibitors. Immunology 27: 285–298.

82. Keller, R., Keist, R., and Ivatt, R. J. 1974. Functional and biochemical parameters of activation related to macrophage cytostatic effects on tumor cells. Int. J. Cancer. 14: 675–683.

83. Kieler, J. 1972. Antigenic modification of mammalian cells undergoing "spontaneous" malignant conversion. Series Haematol. 5: no. 4, 93–122.

84. Kirchner, H., Chused, T. M., Herberman, R. B., Holden, H. T., and Lavrin, D. H. 1974. Evidence of suppressor cell activity in spleens of mice bearing primary tumors induced by Moloney sarcoma virus. J. Exp. Med. 139: 1473–1487.

85. Kirchner, H., Holden, H. T., and Herberman, R. B. 1975. Inhibition of in vitro growth of lymphoma cells by macrophages from tumor-bearing mice. J. Natl. Cancer Inst. 55: 971–975.

86. Kirkwood, J. M., and Gershon, R. K. 1974. A role for suppressor T cells in immunological enhancement of tumor growth. Prog. Exp. Tumor Res. 19: 157–179.

87. Klein, G., and Révész, L. 1953. Quantitative studies on the multiplication of neoplastic cells in vivo. I. Growth curves of the Ehrlich and MCIM ascites tumors. J. Natl. Cancer Inst. 14: 229–277.

88. Kölsch, E., Mengersen, R., and Diller, E. 1973. Low dose tolerance preventing tumor immunity. Eur. J. Cancer. 9: 879–882.

89. Krahenbuhl, J. L., and Lambert, L. H. 1975. Cytokinetic studies of the effects of activated macrophages on tumor target cells. J. Natl. Cancer Inst. 55: 1433–1437.

90. Krahenbuhl, J. L., and Remington, J. S. 1974. The role of activated macrophages in specific and nonspecific cytostasis of tumor cells. J. Immunol. 113: 507–516.

91. Kuperman, O., Fortner, G. W., and Lucus, Z. J. 1975. Immune response to syngeneic mammary adenocarcinoma. II. Development of memory and suppressor

functions modulating cellular cytotoxicity. *J. Immunol.* 115: 1282–1287.

92. Lamon, E. W., Wigzell, H., Klein, E., Andersson, B., and Skurzak, H. M. 1973. The lymphocyte response to primary Moloney sarcoma virus tumors in Balb/c mice. *J. Exp. Med.* 137: 1472–1493.

93. Leclerc, J. C., Senik, A., Gomard, E., Plata, F., and Levy, J. P. 1973. Cell-mediated antitumor immune reactions under syngeneic conditions. *Transplantation.* 5: 1431–1434.

94. Lukes, R. J., and Collins, R. D. 1974. Immunologic characterization of human malignant lymphomas. *Cancer.* 34: 1488–1503.

95. Magarey, C. J., and Baum, M. 1970. Reticuloendothelial activity in humans with cancer. *Brit. J. Surg.* 57: 748–752.

96. Mahoney, M. J., and Leighton, J. 1962. The inflammatory response to a foreign body within transplantable tumors. *Cancer Res.* 22: 334–339.

97. Martin, J. W., Esber, E., and Wunderlich, J. R. 1973. Evidence for the suppression of the development of cytotoxic lymphoid cells in tumor-immunized mice. *Fed. Proc.* 32: 173–179.

98. Martinez, C. 1964. Effect of early thymectomy on development of mammary tumors in mice. *Nature.* 203: 1188.

99. Melief, C. J. M., and Schwartz, R. S. 1975. *In* F. F. Becker (ed.), *Immunocompetence and Malignancy: A Comprehensive Treatise.* Vol. 1, pp. 121–160. Plenum Press, New York.

100. Meltzer, M. S. 1976. Tumoricidal response *in vitro* of peritoneal macrophages from conventionally housed and germ-free nude mice. *Cell. Immunol.* 22: 176–182.

101. Mengersen, R., Schick, R., and Kölsch, E. 1975. Correlation of "sneaking through" of tumor cells with specific immunological impairment of the host. *Eur. J. Immunol.* 5: 532–537.

102. Milas, L., Hunter, N., Mason, K., and Withers, H. R. 1974. Immunological resistance to pulmonary metastases in C3Hf/BU mice bearing syngeneic fibrosarcoma of different sizes. *Cancer Res.* 34: 61–71.

103. Möller, G., and Möller, E. 1975. Considerations of some current concepts of cancer research. *J. Natl. Cancer Inst.* 55: 755–759.

104. Mongini, P. K. A., and Rosenberg, L. T. 1975. Inhibition of lymphocyte trapping by cell-free ascitic fluids cultivated in syngeneic mice. *J. Immunol.* 114: 650–654.

105. Moore, G. E., Sandberg, A., and Schubarg, J. R. 1957. Clinical and experimental observations of occurrence and fate of tumor cells in the blood stream. *Ann. Surg.* 146: 580–587.

106. Nelson, D. S., and Kearney, R. 1976. Macrophages and lymphoid tissues in mice with concomitant immunity. *Br. J. Cancer* 34: 221–226.

107. Nimberg, R. B., Glasgow, A. H., Menzoian, J. O., Constantain, M. B., Cooperband, S. R., Mannick, J. A., and Schid, K. 1975. Isolation of immunosuppressive peptide fraction from the serum of cancer patients. *Cancer Res.* 35: 1489–1494.

108. Norbury, K. C., and Fidler, I. J. 1975. *In vitro* tumor cell destruction by syngeneic mouse macrophages: Methods for assaying cytotoxicity. *J. Immunol. Methods.* 7: 109–121.

109. Normann, S. J., and Sorkin, E. 1976. Cell-specific defect in monocyte function during tumor growth. *J. Natl. Cancer Inst.* 57: 135–140.

110. North, R. J. 1974. Cell-mediated immunity and the response to infection. In R. T. McCluskey and S. Cohen (eds.), *Mechanisms of Cell-Mediated Immunity*, pp. 185–220. John Wiley, New York and London.

111. North, R. J., and Kirstein, D. P. 1977. T cell-mediated concomitant immunity to syngeneic tumors. I. Activated macrophages as expressors of nonspecific immunity to unrelated tumors and bacterial parasites. *J. Exp. Med.* 145: 275–292.

112. North, R. J., Kirstein, D. P., and Tuttle, R. L. 1976. Subversion of host defense mechanisms by murine tumors. I. A circulating factor that suppresses macrophage-mediated resistance to infection. *J. Exp. Med.* 143: 559–573.

113. North, R. J., Kirstein, D. P., and Tuttle, R. L. 1976. Subversion of host defense mechanisms by murine tumors. II. Counter-influence of concomitant antitumor immunity. *J. Exp. Med.* 143: 574–584.

114. Nowell, P. C. 1976. The clonal evolution of tumor cell populations. *Science.* 194: 23–28.

115. Old, L. J., Boyse, E. A., Clarke, D. A., and Carswell, E. 1962. Antigenic properties of chemically induced tumors. *Ann. N.Y. Acad. Sci.* 101: 80–106.

116. Old, L. J., Clarke, D. A., Benacerraf, B., and Goldsmith, M. 1960. The reticuloendothelial system and the neoplastic process. *Ann. N.Y. Acad. Sci.* 88: 264–280.

117. Old, L. J., Stockert, E., Boyse, E. A., and Kim, J. H. 1968. Antigenic modulation. *J. Exp. Med.* 127: 523–536.

118. Opitz, H-G., Neithammer, D., Jackson, R. C., Lemke, H., Huget, R., and Flad, H-D. 1975. Biochemical characterization of a factor released by macrophages. *Cell. Immunol.* 18: 70–75.

119. Outzen, H. C., Custer, R. P., Eaton, G. J., and Prehn, R. T. 1975. Spontaneous and induced tumor incidence in germ-free "nude" mice. *J. Reticuloendothel. Soc.* 17: 1–9.

120. Peters, L. J., and Hewitt, H. B. 1974. The influence of fibrin formation on the transplantability of murine tumor cells: Implications for the mechanism of the Révész effect. *Brit. J. Cancer.* 29: 279–291.

121. Peto, R., Roe, F. J. C., Lee, P. N., Levy, L., and Clack, J. 1975. Cancer and ageing in mice and men. *Brit. J. Cancer.* 32: 411–426.

122. Pierce, G. E. 1971. Enhanced growth of primary Moloney virus-induced sarcomas in mice. *Int. J. Cancer.* 8: 22–31.

123. Piessens, W. F., Churchill, W. H., and David, J. R. 1975. Macrophages activated *in vitro* with lymphocyte mediators kill neoplastic but not normal cells. *J. Immunol.* 114: 293–299.

124. Pike, M. C., and Snyderman, R. 1976. Depression of macrophage function by a factor produced by neoplasms: A mechanism for abrogation of immune surveillance. *J. Immunol.* 117: 1243–1249.

125. Pwosky, M. A., Ziffroni-Gallon, Y., and Witz, I. P. 1975. Suppression of immune response to sheep red blood cells in mice treated with preparations of tumor cell components and in tumor-bearing mice. *Eur. J. Immunol.* 5: 444–450.

126. Plescia, O. J., Smith, A. H., and Grinwich, K. 1975. Subversion of im-

mune system by tumor cells and role of prostoglandins. *Proc. Natl. Acad. Sci. U.S.A.* 72: 1848–1851.

127. Prehn, R. T. 1971. Perspectives on oncogenesis: Does immunity stimulate or inhibit neoplasia. *J. Reticuloendothelial Soc.* 10: 1–16.

128. Prehn, R. T. 1976. Tumor progression and homeostasis. *Adv. Cancer Res.* 23: 203–233.

129. Proctor, J. W., Rudenstam, C-M., and Alexander, P. 1974. A preliminary investigation into the role of immunity in modifying the blood-borne spread of chemically induced rat sarcomas. *J. Natl. Cancer Inst.* 53: 1671–1676.

130. Pruitt, J. C., Hilberg, A. W., and Kaiser, R. F. 1958. Malignant cells in blood. *N. Engl. J. Med.* 259: 1161.

131. Révész, L. 1958. Effect of lethally damaged tumor cells upon the development of admixed viable cells. *J. Natl. Cancer Inst.* 20: 1157–1186.

132. Rubin, R. H., Cosimi, A. B., and Goetzl, E. 1976. Defective human mononuclear leukocyte chemotaxis as an index of host resistance to malignant melanoma. *Clin. Immunol. Immunopath.* 6: 376–388.

133. Russell, S. W., Doe, W. F., Hoskins, R. G., and Cochrane, C. G. 1976. Inflammatory cells in solid murine neoplasms. I. Tumor disaggregation and identification of constituent inflammatory cells. *Int. J. Cancer.* 18: 322–330.

134. Ruutu, T., Ruutu, P., Vuopio, P., Franssila, K., and Linden, E. 1975. An inhibitor of chemotaxis and phagocytosis in reticulum cell sarcoma. *Scand. J. Haematol.* 15: 27–34.

135. Salby, N. K., DiLuzio, N. R., Levin, A. G., and Goldsmith, H. S. 1967. Phagocytic activity of the reticuloendothelial system in neoplastic disease. *J. Lab. Clin. Med.* 70: 393–403.

136. Schrader, J. W., and Edelman, G. M. 1976. The participation of the H-2 antigens of tumor cells in their lysis by syngeneic T cells. *J. Exp. Med.* 143: 601–614.

137. Schwartz, R. S. 1975. Another look at immunologic surveillance. *N. Eng. J. Med.* 293: 181–184.

138. Scollard, D. 1975. Cellular cytotoxicity assays detect different effector cell types *in vitro. Transplantation.* 19: 87–93.

139. Shiku, H., Takahashi, T., Bean, M. A., Old, L. J., and Oettgen, H. F. 1976. Ly phenotype of cytotoxic T cells for syngeneic tumor. *J. Exp. Med.* 144: 1116–1120.

140. Simon, H. B. 1974. Case record of the Mass. General Hospital. *N. Engl. J. Med.* 291: 516–524.

141. Sjögren, H. O., Hellström, I., Bansal, S. C., and Hellström, K. E. 1971. Suggestive evidence that "blocking antibodies" of tumor-bearing individuals may be antigen-antibody complexes. *Proc. Natl. Acad. Sci. U.S.A.* 68: 1372–1375.

142. Skov, C. B., Holland, J. M., and Perkins, E. H. 1976. Development of fewer tumor colonies in lungs of athymic nude mice after intravenous injection of tumor cells. *J. Natl. Cancer Inst.* 56: 193–196.

143. Snyderman, R., Pike, M. C., Blaylock, B. L., and Weinstein, P. 1976. Effects of neoplasms on inflammation: Depression of macrophage accumulation after tumor implantation. *J. Immunol.* 116: 585–589.

144. Sohier, W. 1976. Case record of the Mass. General Hospital. *N. Engl. J.*

Med. 295: 828–834.

145. Southam, C. M., and Brunschwig, A. 1961. Quantitative studies of auto-transplantation of human cancer. Cancer 14: 971–978.

146. Spitalny, G. L., and North, R. J. 1977. Subversion of host defense mechanisms by malignant tumors: An established tumor as a privileged site for bacterial growth. J. Exp. Med. 145: 1264–1277.

147. Spitalny, G. L., and North, R. J. 1977. Evidence that the Révész effect is caused by suppression of macrophage function. J. Exp. Med. (in press).

148. Spriggs, A. I. 1971. Follow-up of untreated carcinoma-in-situ of cervix uteri. Lancet ii: 599–600.

149. Stevenson, M. M., and Meltzer, M. S. 1976. Depressed chemotactic response in vitro of peritoneal macrophages from tumor-bearing mice. J. Natl. Cancer Inst. 57: 847–852.

150. Takei, F., Levy, J. G., and Kilburn, D. G. 1976. In vitro induction of cytotoxicity against syngeneic mastocytoma and its suppression by spleen and thymus cells from tumor-bearing mice. J. Immunol. 116: 288–293.

151. Tanapatchaiyapong, P., and Zolla, S. 1974. Humoral immunosuppressive substances in mice bearing plasmacytomas. Science 185: 748–750.

152. Taylor, C. R. 1976. Immuno-histological observations on the development of reticulum cell sarcoma in the mouse. J. Pathol. 118: 201–219.

153. Thomas, L. 1959. Reactions to homologous tissue antigens in relation to hypersensitivity. In H. S. Lawrence (ed.), Cellular and Humoral Aspects of the Hypersensitive States, 1959, pp. 529–532. Hoeber, New York.

154. Tokunaga, T., Yamamoto, S., Nakamura, R. M., and Kataska, T. 1974. Immunotherapeutic and immunoprophylactic effects of BCG on 3-methylcholanthrene-induced autochthonous tumors in Swiss mice. J. Natl. Cancer Inst. 53: 459–466.

155. Treves, A. J., Treinin, C. C., Feldman, M., and Cohen, I. R. 1974. Enhancing T lymphocytes from tumor-bearing mice suppress host resistance to a syngeneic tumor. Eur. J. Immunol. 4: 727–731.

156. Tuttle, R. L., and North, R. J. 1976. Mechanisms of the antitumor action of Corynebacterium parvum: The generation of cell-mediated tumor specific immunity. J. Reticuloendothel. Soc. 20: 197–208.

157. Underwood, J. C. E. 1974. Lymphoreticular infiltration in humor tumors: Prognostic and biological implications: A review. Br. J. Cancer. 30: 538–547.

158. Vaage, J. 1971. Concomitant immunity and specific depression of immunity by residual or reinfected syngeneic tumor tissue. Cancer Res. 31: 1655–1662.

159. Van Duuren, B. L. 1969. Tumor-promoting agents in two stage carcinogenesis. Proc. Exp. Tumor Res. 11: 31–68.

160. Veit, B. C., and Feldman, J. D. 1976. Altered lymphocyte functions in rats bearing syngeneic Moloney sarcoma tumors. I. Mitogen responses, mixed lymphocyte reactions (MLR) and mixed lymphocyte tumor reactions (MLTR). J. Immunol. 117: 646–654.

161. Watre, A. L., Moore, G. E., and Hatiboglu, I. 1960. Cancer cells in thoracic duct lymph. Proc. Amer. Cancer Res. 3: 72.

162. Wexler, M. R., Kripke, M., and Weiss, D. W. 1971. Prolonged survival of male to female skin isografts and of allografts from normal mice following treatment of recipient or graft with sera from tumor-bearing mice. Cancer Res. 31: 122–126.

163. Whitney, R. B., and Levy, J. G. 1975. Mode of action of immunosuppressive substances in sera of tumor-bearing mice. J. Natl. Cancer Inst. 55: 1447–1452.

164. Whittaker, M. G., Rees, K., and Clark, C. G. 1971. Reduced lymphocyte transformation in breast cancer. Lancet 1: 892–893.

165. Wong, A., Mankovitz, R., and Kennedy, J. 1974. Immunosuppressive and immunostimulatory factors produced by malignant cells in vitro. Int. J. Cancer. 13: 530–542.

166. Yuhas, J. M., Pazimino, H. G., and Wagner, E. 1971. Development of concomitant immunity in mice bearing the weakly immunogenic line 1 lung carcinoma. Cancer Res. 35: 237–241.

CHAPTER 6

REGULATION OF THE IMMUNE RESPONSE BY TUMORS

Susan Zolla-Pazner,
Shelley Fleit and
Jean-Pierre Kolb

Departments of Pathology
Manhattan VA Hospital and
New York University
Medical Center
New York, New York   10010

Some tumors are capable of affecting immune impairment directly by producing suppressive substances. Others appear to carry viruses which are immunosuppressive to the tumor hosts. Still other tumors are indirectly suppressive, generating non-malignant regulatory cells. Plasma cell tumors in men and mice cause a unique pattern of immunodeficiency. Hosts of these tumors are defective in their capacity to produce antibodies to newly encountered antigens. In all other respects they appear to be immunologically normal. This tumor, therefore, allows us to analyse the immunoregulation of B cells and provides a model for the study of a unique tumor-induced regulatory phenomenon.

Work from many laboratories has shown that most tumors affect the immune response of their hosts whether by providing an immunologic stimulus to which the host responds or by causing an impairment in immune functions. When tumor-induced immunologic defects have been studied in tumor hosts, it has usually been the T lymphocytes or both the T and B lymphocytes that have been found to be functionally depressed. In most instances, for example, both antibody production and cell-mediated immunity are depressed in mice with viral-induced leukemias (17, 34, 37). However, normal antibody production with concurrent depression of cell-mediated immunity, and of in vitro T lymphocyte activity, is the most characteristic immunologic pattern in patients and animals bearing solid tumors (1, 28, 39).

Several mechanisms have been proposed to explain the suppressive effects of tumors on the immune system. These generally can be grouped into three categories: (a) suppressor cells are induced and/or activated by malignant cells in tumor-bearing hosts; (b) tumors produce immunosuppressive factors; and (c) viruses carried by tumors (and/or tumor-inducing viruses) may induce immunosuppression.

Suppressor cells of several different types have been described in tumor-bearing mice. Cerny and Stiller (7), for instance, have characterized a suppressor cell in the T-cell-enriched fraction of spleens and lymph nodes from mice bearing Moloney-leukemia-virus-induced lymphomas. Kuperman et al. (31) have demonstrated, but not yet characterized, a cell in the spleens of mice bearing mammary carcinoma which prevents the differentiation of cytotoxic spleen cells. And several papers have been published on the properties of a cell with suppressive activity found in mice bearing Moloney-virus-induced tumors; this latter cell was characterized as a macrophage by Kirchner et al. (29), and as a B cell by Gorczynski (20). As studied by these two groups, this cell exerts its negative regulatory effect selectively on T lymphocyte functions. In order to be effective, however, the suppressor cell-enriched spleen populations must be co-cultured with normal spleen cells at ratios no higher than 1:4. Eggers and Wunderlich (12) have also found evidence for a suppressor cell, in this case, a non-T cell, in the spleens of mice with progressively growing methylcholanthrene-induced tumors. The mechanism by which these different cell populations exert their suppressive effects is unknown.

Immunosuppression in tumor-bearing hosts has also been ascribed to soluble factors produced by tumor cells. These factors have been extracted from tumors (25, 32) or found in ascites fluid and serum of tumor-bearing animals (8, 23, 25), or found in the supernatant of cultured tumor cells (41). With few exceptions, however (35), the chemical nature of these soluble factors has not been elucidated and the target cell(s) affected by these factors has not been defined.

In the case of viral-induced neoplasms, immunosuppression has been related to the effects of the etiologic agent or passenger viruses. In vitro studies have shown suppressed immunologic responses of normal spleen cells when they were mixed with spleen cells from mice carrying Friend leukemia virus tumors (26), or with culture fluids of EL-4 (G⁻) ascites cells which contain minute virus of mice (2). The suppression was alleviated if antivirus antiserum was included in the culture medium.

A unique tumor-induced immunodeficiency syndrome is manifested by patients with multiple myeloma and by mice bearing plasmacytomas (PC). Because the pattern of immune impairment in these tumor hosts is so unusual, we undertook a study of the mechanism by which malignant plasma cells affect their hosts' immune response. The use of the murine model of this disease was utilized because it caused an immunodeficiency syndrome that appeared to be closely analogous to that found in patients with multiple myeloma. Published clinical studies provided a firm basis on which to build an experimental program.

Many patients with multiple myeloma were found to have frequent and fatal bacterial infections (14), to be deficient with respect to their ability to mount a primary antibody response, but to be capable of responding normally to antigens like diphtheria and tetanus toxoids, if they had been immunized with these agents prior to the onset of their disease (10). Peripheral blood leukocytes (PBL) from these patients, stimulated with pokeweek mitogen, could not synthesize immunoglobulins as did PBL from normal individuals (3). These patients were able to respond normally to a battery of skin test antigens and PBL from these patients gave as vigorous a response to T-cell mitogens as did PBL from normal individuals (11). These data suggest that B cell function in patients with multiple myeloma is defective, while T cell activity appears to be normal or only minimally affected.

An analogous picture has emerged as the immune system of PC-bearing mice has been studied. It was first noted that there was a decreased titer of antibodies after primary immunization in PC-bearing mice (PC mice) (6, 13); the secondary antibody response, however, appeared to be normal. These findings were later confirmed by Hirano et al. (22) and in our laboratory (42, 43), using the Jerne plaque technique (24). Recently, Fenton and Havas (15) have documented that serum immunoglobulin levels (of classes other than that of the myeloma protein) are reduced in unimmunized PC mice. These studies in mice, and others in humans (38), established that low antibody levels were not due to an increase in the catabolic rate of immunoglobulins but rather to a decrease in the amount of antibodies being produced.

On the basis of the work by others, summarized above, and our own work, summarized below, it seems evident that PC, like many other malignancies, are capable of exerting negative regulatory effects on their hosts' immune systems. Unlike other tumors, however, PC apparently affect only a specific function of the immune response, i.e., the capacity to produce antibodies in response to antigenic challenge. This inhibition of the humoral immune response is mediated by a cell with suppressive activity and by a soluble factor.

Parameters of the Immunodeficiency in PC-Bearing Mice

In studying the characteristics of PC-induced immunosuppression we have found that the depression of the primary immune response in PC mice is (a) proportional to tumor size. (This relationship is depicted in Figure 1a.) The immune impairment was also shown to be (b) independent of paraprotein synthesis and (c) demonstrable whether the animals had been stimulated with thymus-dependent or -independent antigens. (d) All PC we have studied depress the primary antibody response of their hosts though some do it to a greater degree than do others; (e) the demonstration of this immunodepression often depends on the use of a suboptimal dose of antigen. (f) In most cases, the secondary antibody response is normal although it is depressed in those mice bearing PC which maximally depress the primary response. (g) The precursors of antibody-forming cells are present in PC mice but are apparently unable to proliferate and/or differentiate normally. These experiments documenting the parameters of PC-induced immunosuppression have been carried out in mice bearing several PC; the phenomenon described seems to be unique to PC mice since our studies of mice bearing other solid tumors (a thymic lymphoma, a pigmented melanoma and a non-T cell lymphoblastic lymphoma) have not shown a similar pattern of immune impairment (42, 43, 44).

T Cell Activity in PC Mice

Having previously determined that B cell function was depressed in the process of antibody production, we undertook studies of T lymphocyte function in PC mice. For this we used mice bearing three PC previously found to cause a severe reduction in the number of antibody-forming cells per spleen after i.v. injection of antigen (MPC-11, TEPC-183, and SPQC-11). Since several of the T cell studies involved the use of

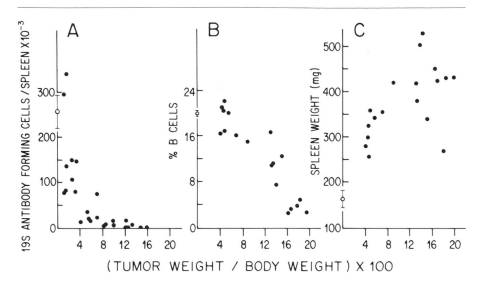

Fig. 1. (a) Depression of the primary immune response in mice bearing SPQC-11 plasmacytomas as a function of tumor size. The response of tumor-bearing mice (●) measured by the Jerne plaque technique was compared to the response of normal mice (○). The data are expressed as the numbers of 19S antibody forming cells per spleen. Ten normal mice were used as controls and their mean response ± S.E. is shown. Mice with SPQC-11 were immunized i.v. with 4×10^7 SRC on the 25th day after tumor implantation; control mice were immunized on the same day and with the same dose. Determination of the immune response was made four days after immunization.   (b)   Determination of the percentage of complement receptor positive lymphocytes (B cells) in the spleens of normal (○) and SPQC-11-bearing mice (●). The number of B cells was determined by the method of Nussenzweig et al. (33). The per cent of B cells in spleens of normal mice was determined by studying six normal spleen; the mean ± S.E. is shown.   (c)   The relationship between spleen size and tumor size. The spleens and/or tumors from normal (○) and tumor-bearing (●) mice were dissected and weighed. The mean weight of six normal spleens ± S.E. is shown.

lymph node cells (LNC) from PC mice, we first had to determine if there was a depression of the antibody response of lymph nodes draining the site of antigen injection in mice bearing these tumors. Because we had previously determined that suboptimal stimulation with antigens was most effective for demonstrating PC-induced immune deficiency in the spleens of PC-bearing mice, we used a suboptimal dose of 1×10^6 sheep red blood cells (SRC) injected into the left front foot pad of mice bearing PC on their right flanks. The antigen-draining nodes of SRC-immunized PC mice gave a markedly poorer anti-SRC response than did the draining nodes of similarly immunized normal mice (44). Histologic examination of nodes from unimmunized PC mice showed a diffuse hyperplasia and retention of follicular architecture even when metastatic tumor was found at the periphery of the nodes. Some PC were found regularly to metastasize to the nodes (MPC-11) while others appeared not to do so (SPQC-11). The depression of the response was therefore not due to the destruction of lymph node architecture by the tumor.

Having established that lymph nodes of PC mice exhibited a decreased ability to respond to antigen with antibody production, we tested the axillary and inguinal nodes (contralateral to the tumor) for their ability to respond to phytohemagglutinin (PHA) and to allogeneic cells. The results indicated that LNC from PC mice gave as vigorous a response as did LNC from normal mice to PHA and to irradiated allogeneic cells. Neither the kinetics nor the height of the response of LNC from PC mice was altered (44).

We also used an in vivo measure of delayed hypersensitivity to determine T cell function in PC mice. In this model, mice were sensitized by cutaneous application of dinitrofluorobenzene; three days after the last sensitizing dose the animals were challenged on the ear with the sensitizing antigen. Ear swelling was measured 24 hours after challenge and found to be comparable in magnitude whether the test mice bore PC or were tumor-free. After measurement of ear swelling, the non-tumor-draining axillary and inguinal lymph nodes of the mice in the experimental and control groups were tested for their reactivity in vitro to the hapten, dinitrobenzene sulfonate (DNBS). Again there was no difference in response to DNBS between sensitized PC-mice and sensitized nontumor-bearing mice. By both in vivo and in vitro criteria, therefore, PC-mice were found to be normally reactive to an agent which elicits delayed hypersensitivity and antigen-specific T cell proliferation (44).

A Soluble Immunosuppressive Factor Demonstrable in PC-Bearing Mice

To determine if a soluble factor mediated PC-induced immunosuppression, we implanted in normal and tumor-bearing mice, diffusion chambers containing normal syngeneic spleen cells and SRC. The diffusion chambers were constructed of lucite rings and Millipore membranes with 0.1 μ pores. The contents of the chambers were assayed six days after chamber implantation by the Jerne plaque technique. We found that the number of plaque-forming cells per chamber was reduced in chambers implanted in PC mice compared to the number of plaque forming cells per chamber recovered from chambers in normal mice. Mice bearing one of three different PC were used for these experiments. These findings suggested that a humoral substance, capable of passing through a Millipore membrane, mediates PC-induced immunosuppression. We extended these studies to mice bearing non-PC tumors. The response of cells enclosed in chambers implanted in mice bearing a thymic lymphoma, a non-T cell lymphoblastic lymphoma, or a melanoma was comparable to the response of chamber-enclosed cells in normal mice. Therefore, the immunosuppressive substance demonstrated in PC mice was not found in mice with other lymphoid and non-lymphoid tumors, and so appears to be specifically associated with plasma cell malignancies (40).

We did find that the number of cells recovered from the chambers in PC mice was slightly but significantly reduced compared to the recovery of cells from chambers in normal mice. This appeared to be due to the failure of cells in chambers in PC mice to proliferate after the initial period in the chamber when a large proportion of cells die. The presence of a humoral, nonspecific cytotoxic factor seemed unlikely since such a factor would be expected to affect equally all types of cells; this would result in the ratio of antibody-forming cells to chamber-enclosed cells to be equal in normal and PC mice. This ratio does differ, however, supporting the concept that the immunocompetent cells within the chambers are failing to proliferate and reaffirming our previous conclusions (43) that a block in proliferation of antibody forming cells was a probable cause of this tumor-induced immune impairment.

The phenomenon of PC-induced immunodeficiency has also been studied by Heller et al. (21), Giacomoni et al. (19), and Katzman et al. (27). This group believes that RNA molecules released from PC are capable of causing the circulating B lymphocytes of mice bearing these tumors to acquire and express surface immunoglobulins with the idiotype of the immunoglobulin secreted by the PC. They suggest also that this conversion from the expression of normal immunoglobulin to paraprotein on the surface of lymphocytes disables these lymphocytes as antigen-binding cells, thus producing the immunologic deficiency seen in PC mice. While the RNA described by these workers could be the soluble factor that causes the immunosuppression of the chamber-enclosed cells in our experiments, we would refrain from drawing such a speculative conclusion until a clearer and firmer correlation can be drawn between these two sets of data.

In attempting to define further the biological and chemical nature of the soluble factor demonstrated in the diffusion chamber experiments, we have extensively studied supernatants from cultured PC tumor cells and homogenates of PC tumors grown in vivo. In none of these studies, conducted both in vivo and in vitro, have we been able to demonstrate a factor that is immunosuppressive. In addition, we have examined the serum from PC-bearing mice for the putative immunosuppressive factor. These latter studies have been complicated by the fact that mouse serum is toxic to mouse spleen cells in Mishell-Dutton cultures; however, mouse serum can be added to Mishell-Dutton cultures without adverse effects if the spleen cells have been primed with antigen *in vivo*. We therefore added fresh serum from PC-mice to Mishell-Dutton cultures of spleen cells from mice which had been primed with SRC six hours prior to sacrifice. Final culture concentrations of 1–10% serum from normal or PC mice showed comparable effects (Fig. 2): a final concentration of 1.0% mouse serum was somewhat depressive but this never reached significant levels; nor did a 5% concentration of normal or PC-serum give a significant depressive or enhancing effect; a 10% concentration of serum was stimulatory in all cases. Clearly, no immunosuppressive factor was demonstrable in the serum of PC mice.

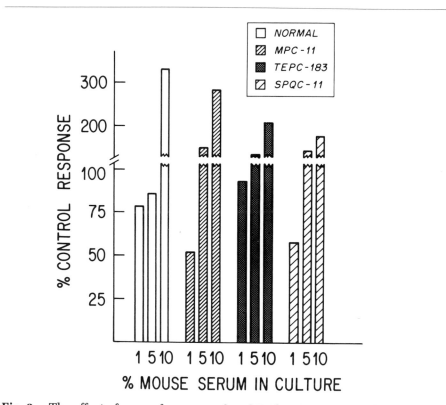

Fig. 2. The effect of serum from normal and PC-bearing mice on the response of 6 hour-primed spleen cells in Mishell-Dutton cultures. Serum from normal mice (□) or mice bearing MPC-11, TEPC-18, or SPQC-11 was added to Mishell-Dutton cultures in varying amounts. The results are expressed as a percentage of the response of similar cultures containing no mouse serum.

Lymphoid Cells from PC-Bearing Mice Exhibit a Suppressive Effect on the Immune System

Spleen cells from PC-bearing mice are unresponsive in Mishell-Dutton cultures; however, we had previously noted in our in vivo experiments that the immunosuppression in PC mice could be overcome in vivo by increasing the dose of antigen used for immunization. Therefore, we tried to overcome the unresponsiveness in culture by increasing the number of SRC added to the culture. Three million SRC are normally added per Mishell-Dutton culture. Increasing this to 60 million SRC per culture did not cause a significant increase in the response of spleen cells from PC mice. The solution to the problem of unresponsiveness was therefore not simply a matter of antigen dose.

In attempting to understand this phenomenon, we postulated that perhaps the population of cells in the spleens of PC-bearing mice was so altered as to prevent these cells from responding. In particular, we were concerned with the possible depletion of splenic B cells. We therefore studied the proportion of B cells in the spleens of PC-bearing mice to determine if there was a significant decrease as the size of the PC increased. For this project, we identified splenic B cells by the EAC rosette technique of Nussenzweig et al. (33). By this method, we showed that the percentage of B cells in the spleens of PC mice did not begin to show a substantial drop until the tumor had reached 10% of the hosts' body weight (Fig. 1b). By this point, the primary immune response had already dropped to less than 10% of normal (Fig. 1a). The fact that the spleens of PC mice were significantly enlarged when tumor sizes were still small (Fig. 1c) and before the percent of B cells began to drop, suggests that the drop in the percent of splenic B cells was not simply a reflection of the dilution of B cells due to infiltration or replication of other cellular elements during the course of splenic enlargement.

We next questioned whether the lack of response could be attributed to a negative regulatory cell (a "suppressor cell") in the spleens of PC mice. Therefore, we tested the effect of splenocytes from PC mice on the ability of normal splenocytes to respond to antigen in Mishell-Dutton cultures; twelve to 20 million normal spleen cells and 3 million SRC were mixed with varying numbers of spleen cells from PC mice (hereafter called PC spleen cells). We found that increasing the number of PC spleen cells in these mixed cultures decreased the response of the normal spleen cells. The cell recovery in all cultures was comparable, indicating that the immunosuppression was not the result of a cytotoxic effect of the PC spleen cells (30). These experiments have been repeated using spleen cells from mice bearing three different PC; we have also done control experiments with mice bearing the thymic lymphoma RL♂1, the mammary adenocarcinoma TA3-Ha, and the malignant melanoma HP. Spleen cells from mice with these latter tumors show no consistent pattern of suppression in these mixing experiments.

Mixing experiments were also done in which lymph node cells or thymus cells from PC mice were added to Mishell-Dutton cultures. Addition of 10^3–10^6 of these cells caused no diminution in the response of normal spleen cells in Mishell-Dutton cultures. Therefore, the suppressor cell in PC mice is concentrated in the spleens of these animals.

Since PC spleen cells were able to suppress antibody formation *in vitro*, we tested the ability of cells from PC mice to affect the *in vitro* proliferative response of normal lymph node and spleen cells to Br-cyclic GMP and PHA (B and T cell mitogens, respectively). We therefore mixed PC-spleen and normal spleen cells or PC lymph node and normal LNC in ratios from 1:2 to 1:50 and cultured them in the presence of either mitogen. The level of incorporation of ^{3}H-thymidine by these mixed stimulated cultures did not differ from the level of stimulated cultures containing the identical number of normal cells but no cells from PC mice. Therefore, although the ratio of PC spleen to normal spleen cells was comparable or even lower than the ratio that gives suppression of Mishell-Dutton cultures, no suppression of this mitogen-stimulated proliferative response was noted (30).

An extensive series of experiments have been performed to identify the nature of the suppressor cell found in PC-bearing mice. As mentioned above, suppressor cells are found in the spleens but not in the lymph nodes or thymuses of PC-bearing mice. Suppressor cells have also been demonstrated in cells washed from the peritoneum of mice bearing these tumors. The suppressor cells are radiation-resistant since irradiation with 3000 R does not inhibit their suppressive activity in mixed Mishell-Dutton cultures (30).

The suppressor cells were not affected by treatment with anti-Thy 1.2 and complement or with anti-Ig and complement indicating that they lack the two markers that distinguish the surfaces of T and B cells, respectively. Suppressor cells are, however, sensitive to treatment with silica. These latter experiments, were performed *in vivo*, and the results are shown in Figure 3. Normal or PC-bearing mice were injected with 4 mg of 5 μ silica particles, i.v. Twenty-four hours later they and previously untreated normal and PC mice were immunized with 4×10^7 SRC, iv. Four days later, the number of plaque-forming cells per spleen in each mouse was determined. The data show that tumor-bearing mice that were not treated with silica had a severely depressed immune response compared to non-tumor bearing controls. However, PC mice which had been treated with silica prior to immunization had an immune response that was 12-fold higher than that of immunized PC mice which had not been treated with silica. Although silica is known to have nonspecific effects, these

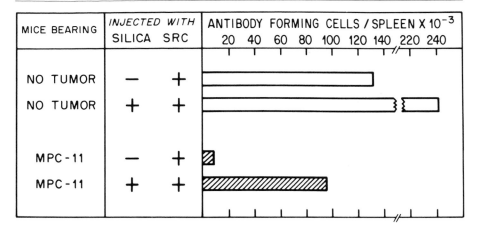

Fig. 3. Effect of silica on the immune response of normal and PC-bearing mice. Normal mice (□) and mice bearing subcutaneous MPC-11 tumors (hatched box) were immunized i.v. with 4×10^7 SRC. One day prior to immunization, normal and tumor-bearing mice in the experimental groups received 4 mg of silica particles, i.v. All mice were sacrificed four days after immunization and the number of antibody forming cells per spleen was determined by the Jerne plaque technique.

data suggest that, like macrophages, the activity of PC suppressor cells is abrogated by silica treatment.

We have also shown that PC suppressor cells can be enriched by several techniques. Suppressor cells from the spleens of PC mice were found to adhere to nylon wool and Sephadex G10 columns. After washing off the non-adherent cells with medium containing EDTA, the adherent cell fraction containing suppressor cells was recovered. Morphologic examination of the cells eluted from nylon wool showed them to contain 92–97% mononuclear cells. This technique reduced the percent of polymorphonuclear cells to 1/2 or 1/3 that found in the original, unfractionated population.

Suppressor cells were also found to adhere to plastic culture dishes; thus, incubating PC spleen cells in culture dishes for 2 hours at 37° in an atmosphere of 5% CO_2 resulted in a monolayer of cells that was able to suppress the antibody response of macrophage-depleted normal spleen cells that were incubated on these PC spleen monolayers.

If we remove adherent cells from PC spleen cells we can partially restore the response of these cells in Mishell-Dutton cultures. For example in one experiment, spleen cells from normal mice gave 1,586 PFC/culture and spleen cells from MPC-11 bearing mice gave 618 PFC/culture. Cultures of these latter PC spleen cells after removal of adherent cells, by passage through Sephadex G-10, allowed a response of 1,058 PFC/culture. Thus, a significant increase in the in vitro responsiveness was obtained by removing cells which we have shown to have suppressive activity.

These experiments lead to the conclusion that the cells from the PC mice with suppressive activity share the characteristics of macrophages.

Our findings that a soluble factor and a suppressor cell mediate PC-induced immunodeficiency have led us to postulate that plasma cell tumors elicit the immune impairment indirectly, i.e., that malignant plasma cells are able to induce the appearance or the expression of regulatory activity by macrophages. It is these suppressor macrophages, not the tumor cells, that are responsible for the negative regulation of the primary (and, less frequently, of the secondary) antibody response; neither the tumor cells nor the macrophages seem to affect the function of T cells. Thus the phenomenon of PC-induced immunosuppression is at least a two-step process. In the first phase, the generation, or stimulation, of suppressor macrophages may be induced by a soluble factor produced by the tumor; alternatively, a population of circulating monocytes may be converted to supppessor cells as they pass through the tumor bed. In the second step, suppressor macrophages may affect the cells involved in antibody production either by means of a soluble factor or through direct cell-to-cell contact. Having previously shown that a soluble factor does play a role in the mediation of PC-induced immunosuppression, we believe that at least one of these steps is mediated by a soluble substance.

The involvement of a suppressor macrophage in this system indicates that the immunosuppression observed in PC mice belongs to the growing list of normal and malignant conditions in which immune responses are regulated, at least in part, by macrophages (5, 9, 16, 29, 36). Immunodepressed mice bearing PC, therefore, probably reflect an exaggerated case of one form of macrophage-mediated immune responses—in this case, a situation that is, apparently, generated by the presence of an uncommonly large number of plasma cells.

ACKNOWLEDGMENT

This work was supported in part by United States Public Health Service Grants CA15585 and CA16247 and by a grant from the Veterans Administration.

REFERENCES

1. Adler, W. H., Smith, R. T., and Takiguchi, T. 1971. Phytohemagglutinin unresponsiveness in mouse spleens induced by methylcholanthrene sarcomas. Cancer Res. 31: 864.

2. Bonnard, G. D., Campbell, D. A., Jr., Mandeis, E. K., Herberman, P. B., and Collins, M. J., Jr. 1976. Immunosuppressive activity of a subline of the mouse EL-4 lymphoma. Evidence for minute virus of mice causing the inhibition. *J. Exp. Med.* 143: 187.

3. Broder, S., Humphrey, R., Durm, M., Blackman, M., Meade, B., Goldman, C., Strober, W., and Waldmann, T. 1975. Impaired synthesis of polyclonal (non-paraprotein) immunoglobulin by circulating lymphocytes from patients with multiple myeloma. *N. Engl. J. Med.* 293: 887.

4. Brooks, W. H., Netsky, M. G., Normansell, D. E., and Horwitz, D. A. 1972. Depressed cell-mediated immunity in patients with primary intracranial tumors. Characterization of a humoral immunosuppressive factor. *J. Exp. Med.* 136: 1631.

5. Calderone, J., Kiely, J. M., Lefko, J. L., and Unanue, E. R. 1975. The modulation of lymphocyte functions by molecules secreted by macrophages. I. Description and partial biochemical analysis. *J. Exp. Med.* 142: 151.

6. Carlson, P. J., and Smith, F. 1968. Effect of plasma cell tumor on antibody production by mouse spleen cells. *Proc. Soc. Exp. Biol.* 127: 212.

7. Cerny, J., and Stiller, R. A. 1975. Immunosuppression by spleen cells from Moloney leukemia. Comparison of the suppressive effect on antibody response and on mitogen-induced response. *J. Immunol.* 115: 943.

8. Chan, P. L., and Sinclair, N. 1972. Immunologic and virologic properties of chemical and γ-irradiation-induced thymic lymphoma in mice. *J. Natl. Cancer Inst.* 48: 1629.

9. Chen, C., and Hirsch, J. G. 1972. Effects of mercaptoethanol and of peritoneal macrophages on the antibody-forming capacity of non-adherent mouse spleen cells. *J. Exp. Med.* 136: 604.

10. Cone, L., and Uhr, J. W. 1964. Immunologic deficiency disorders associated with chronic lymphocytic leukemia and multiple myeloma. *J. Clin. Inv.* 43: 2241.

11. Douglas, S. D., Kamin, R. M., and Fudenberg, H. H. 1969. Human lymphocytic response to phytomitogens *in vitro*: normal agammaglobulinemic and paraproteinemic individuals. *J. Immunol.* 103: 1185.

12. Eggers, A. E., and Wunderlich, J. R. 1975. Suppressor cells in tumor-bearing mice capable of non-specific blocking of *in vitro* immunization against transplant antigens. *J. Immunol.* 114: 1554.

13. Fahey, J. L., and Humphrey, J. H. 1962. Effect of transplantable plasma cell tumors on antibody response in mice. *Immunology.* 5: 110.

14. Fahey, J. L., Scoggins, R., Utz, J. P., and Szwed, C. F. 1963. Infection, antibody response and gamma-globulin components in multiple myeloma and macroglobulinemia. *Amer. J. Med.* 35: 698.

15. Fenton, M. R., and Havas, F. 1975. The effect of plasmacytomas on serum immunoglobulin levels of BALB/c mice. *J. Immunol.* 114: 793.

16. Folch, H., Yoshinaga, M., and Waksman, B. Y. Regulation of lymphocytic response *in vitro*. III. Inhibition by adherent cells of the T-lymphocytic responses to PHA. *J. Immunol.* 110: 835.

17. Friedman, H., and Ceglowski, W. S. 1968. Cellular basis for the immunosuppressive properties of a leukamogenic virus. *Nature* 218: 1232.

18. Gatti, R. A., Garrioch, D. B., and Good, R. A. 1970. Depressed PHA re-

sponses in patients with non-lymphoid malignancies. *In Proceedings Fifth Leukocyte Culture Conference.* Academic Press, New York, p. 339.

19. Giacomoni, D., Yakulis, V., Wong, S. R., Cooke, A., Dray, S., and Heller, P. 1974. *In vitro* conversion of normal mouse lymphocytes by plasmacytoma RNA to express idiotypic specificities on their surface characteristic of the plasmacytoma Ig. *Cell. Immunol.* 11: 389.

20. Gorczynski, R. W. 1974. Immunity to murine sarcoma-virus-induced tumors. II. Suppression of T cell-mediated immunity by cells from progressor animals. *J. Immunol.* 112: 1826.

21. Heller, P., Bhoopalam, N., Cabana, V., Costea, N., and Yakulis, V. 1973. The role of RNA in the immunological deficiency of plasmacytoma. *Ann. N.Y. Acad. Sci.* 207: 468.

22. Hirano, S., Immamura, Y., Takaku, F., and Nakao, K. 1972. Immune response in mice with plasma cell tumor assayed by agar plaque technique. *Blood* 31: 252.

23. Hrsak, I., and Marotti, T. 1975. Mechanism of the immunosuppressive effect of Ehrlich ascitic tumor. *Eur. J. Cancer.* 11: 181.

24. Jerne, N. K., and Nordin, A. A. Plaque formation in agar by single antibody producing cells. *Science* 140: 405.

25. Kamo, F., Patel, C., Kateley, J., and Friedman, H. 1975. Immunosuppressive and immunostimulatory factors produced by malignant cells *in vitro. Int. J. Cancer* 13: 530.

26. Kateley, J. R., Kamo, I., Kaplan, G., and Friedman, H. 1974. Effect of leukemia virus-infected lymphoid cells on *in vitro* immunization of normal splenocytes. *J. Natl. Canc. Inst.* 53: 1371.

27. Katzman, J., Giacomoni, D., Yakulis, V., and Heller, P. 1975. Characterization of two plasmacytoma fractions and their RNA capable of changing surface immunoglobulin. *Cell. Immunol.* 18: 98.

28. Kirchner, H., Herberman, R. B., Glaser, M., and Larvin, D. H. 1974. Suppression of *in vitro* lymphocyte stimulation in mice bearing primary Moloney sarcoma virus-induced tumors. *Cell. Immunol.* 13: 32.

29. Kirchner, H., Chused, T. M., Herberman, R. B., Holden, H. T., and Larvin, D. H. 1974. Evidence of suppressor cell activity in spleens of mice bearing primary tumors induced by Moloney sarcoma virus. *J. Exp. Med.* 139: 1473.

30. Kolb, J. P., Arrian, S., and Zolla-Pazner, S. 1977. Suppression of the humoral immune response by plasmacytomas: mediation by an adherent mononuclear cell. *J. Immunol.* 118: 702.

31. Kuperman, O., Fortner, G. W., and Lucas, Z. J. 1975. Immune response to a syngeneic mammary adenocarcinoma. III. Development of memory and suppressor functions modulating cellular cytotoxicity. *J. Immunol.* 115: 1282.

32. Masaki, M., Takatsu, K., Hamaoka, T., and Kitagawa, M. 1972. Immunosuppressive activity of chromatin fraction derived from nuclei of Ehrlich ascites tumor cells. *Gann* 63: 633.

33. Nussenzweig, V., Bianco, C., Dukor, P., and Eden, A. 1971. Receptors for C3 on B lymphocytes: possible role in the immune response. *In* B. Amos (ed.), *Progress in Immunology,* Vol. 1, p. 73. Academic Press, New York.

34. Notkins, A. L., Mergenhagen, S. E., and Howard, R. J. 1970. Effect of virus

infections on the function of the immune system. *Annu. Rev. Microbiol.* 24: 525.

35. Plescia, O. J., Smith, A. H., and Grinwich, K. 1975. Subversion of immune system by tumor cells and role of prostaglandins. *P.N.A.S.* 72: 1848.

36. Ptak, W., and Gershon, R. K. 1975. Immunosuppression effected by macrophage surfaces. *J. Immunol.* 115: 1346.

37. Siegel, B. V., and Morton, J. I. 1966. Depressed antibody response in the mouse infected with Rauscher leukemia virus. *Immunology* 10: 559.

38. Solomon, A., Waldmann, T. A., and Fahey, J. L. 1963. Metabolism of normal 6.6S γ-globulin in normal subjects and in patients with macroglobulinemia and multiple myeloma. *J. Lab. Clin. Med.* 62: 1.

39. Solowey, A. C., and Rapaport, F. T. 1965. Immunologic responses in cancer patients. *Surg. Gynecol. Obst.* 121: 756.

40. Tanapatchaiyapong, P., and Zolla, S. 1974. Humoral immunosuppressive substance in mice bearing plasmacytomas. *Science* 186: 748.

41. Wong, A., Markovitz, R., and Kennedy, J. C. 1974. Immunosuppressive and immunostimulatory factors produced by malignant cells *in vitro*. *Int. J. Cancer* 13: 530.

42. Zolla, S. 1972. The effect of plasmacytomas on the immune response of mice. *J. Immunol.* 108: 1039.

43. Zolla, S., Naor, D., and Tanapatchaiyapong, P. 1974. Cellular basis of immunodepression in mice with plasmacytomas. *J. Immunol.* 112: 2068.

44. Zolla-Pazner, S., Sullivan, B., and Richardson, D. 1976. Cellular specificity of plasmacytoma-induced immunosuppression. *J. Immunol.* 117: 563.

CHAPTER 7

ANTI-INFLAMMATORY EFFECTS OF CANCER: A MACROPHAGE-MODULATING FACTOR PRODUCED BY CANCER CELLS

G. Sundharadas,
H. T. Cheung, and
W. D. Cantarow

Immunobiology Research Center
and the Department
of Medical Microbiology
University of Wisconsin
Madison, Wisconsin   53706

Growth and spread of cancer in spite of the surveillance mechanisms of the host may in part be due to the ability of the cancer cells to subvert host immune mechanisms. Studies presented here show that mouse neoplasms possess a factor of molecular weight less than 3500 Daltons capable of affecting macrophages in vitro, resulting in a modulation of their properties. This tumor factor also inhibits in vitro immune responses. These effects could be an indication that this factor has a role in the subversion of in vivo macrophage function by cancer cells.

The tumor-host relationship is paradoxical, as the spread of cancer occurs in spite of host surveillance mechanisms. It is quite reasonable to hypothesize that cancer cells have the capacity to subvert immune surveillance mechanisms of the host and escape destruction. Recent findings suggest a surveillance role for macrophages against cancer and inflammatory reactions involving the influx of these cells may be important in destroying neoplasms (1, 4, 8, 9, 11, 15, 16). Several studies indicate that the presence of neoplasm results in an impairment of the inflammatory response of the host and this may be mediated by factor(s) produced by the neoplasm and released into the circulation (12, 20, 21, 22, 27, 28). Mouse neoplasms have been shown to possess a factor capable of inhibiting macrophage chemotaxis *in vitro* (22, 27); a factor with anti-inflammatory activity has also been detected in culture supernatants of different mouse tumor cell lines (12). Here we present data showing that several murine neoplasms possess a low molecular weight factor(s) capable of affecting peritoneal macrophages *in vitro* resulting in the modulation of their properties. The tumor factor causes an enhancement in their random migration and inhibits their ability to attach to substratum and spread. These effects observed *in vitro* could be an indication that this macrophage-modulating tumor factor (MMTF) has a role in the subversion of macrophage function *in vivo* by tumor cells.

Macrophages and Surveillance Against Cancer

Recent findings strongly suggest that macrophages mediate surveillance against cancer and the importance of this macrophage-mediated surveillance has been receiving increasing support. The evidence supporting this concept will not be described here as this topic has been reviewed elsewhere (8, 16). It appears that macrophages in the activated state have the ability to recognize neoplastic cells and destroy them in a nonspecific manner. The activated macrophages have the ability to differentiate between normal cells and cells that have undergone neoplastic transformation. This probably depends upon cell surface changes associated with neoplastic transformation. Activated macrophages capable of killing neoplastic cells can be generated by exposure to lymphokines, as a result of chronic infections with agents such as *Toxoplasma gondii*, Bacillus Calmette-Guerin (BCG), etc., or by treatment with adjuvants such as double-stranded RNA, bacterial lipopolysaccharide, etc. (7, 8).

Anti-inflammatory Effects of Cancer

Inflammatory reactions involving the influx of macrophages and other cell types appear to mediate destruction of tumors. Berg, in a study of breast cancer patients, observed an association between increased inflammation about the cancers and increased survival and better prognosis. In the group of patients who had survived postoperatively, 73% showed infiltration by inflammatory cells at the junction of tumor and normal tissue (4). This infiltration was correlated with degenerative changes in the cancer cells. In the control lethal series, significant inflammation was rare. Similar findings were made in a study of patients with gastric carcinoma (5). Studies in rat also show an impressive inverse correlation between the capacity to metastasize and the macrophage content of the different tumors studied (1). These findings suggest that those tumors that have the ability to metastasize and spread also have a mechanism to subvert macrophages and prevent them from infiltrating and destroying the tumors. In fact, some studies strongly suggest that malignant tumors have the ability to exert an anti-inflammatory effect in vivo.

Rats bearing transplanted syngeneic sarcomas have a reduced capacity to mount an inflammatory reaction and delayed hypersensitivity response to unrelated antigens (1). The impairment increases progressively as the tumor grows. It is possible that in the presence of the tumor, the properties of the circulating macrophages are modified in such a way that they do not respond to chemotactic stimuli and enter into inflammatory sites. This possibility is substantiated by the following findings.

Tumor-bearing mice have a depressed ability to mobilize macrophages to an inflammatory site in vivo; also the in vitro chemotactic responsiveness of peritoneal macrophages recovered from such animals is markedly depressed (27, 28). Macrophages derived from cancer patients exhibit a depressed chemotactic response in vitro, whereas surgical removal of the neoplasm results in a reversal to a normal response (6, 26). The impairment of the inflammatory response of macrophages in vivo and their chemotactic response in vitro may be mediated by factor(s) produced by the tumors and released into the circulation. In fact, Fauve et al. demonstrated the ability of different mouse tumor cell lines to produce in vitro and release into the culture medium, a low-molecular-weight factor or factors (between 1000 and 10,000 Daltons) having anti-inflammatory activity when injected in vivo (12). Snyderman and Pike were able to extract from different in vivo–grown tumors a low-molecular-weight fraction (between 6000 and 10,000 Daltons) capable of having anti-inflammatory effect in vivo and inhibiting the chemotactic response of normal peritoneal macrophages in vitro (27).

In our laboratory we have made the observation that several mouse neoplasms possess a low molecular weight (less than 3,500 Daltons) factor or factors capable of modulating different properties of macrophages *in vitro*. Our findings suggest that this factor has the capacity to affect macrophages in some fundamental manner. The results of our studies and their implications are summarized in the following sections.

A Macrophage-Modulating Factor Produced by Cancer Cells

Since cancer cells seem to have the ability to impair macrophage function and the inflammatory response, we investigated the possibility that these cells produce factors capable of impairing macrophages in such a manner that the impairment would result in altered properties. Mouse peritoneal macrophages and their *in vitro* properties, such as migration, attachment to substratum, and spreading, were chosen for this study. Because of the possibility that any factor produced by tumor cells may be present in circulation *in vivo* or in culture supernatant *in vitro* in such small amounts that it may escape detection, *in vivo*–grown tumor tissue was used to look for such a factor. The mouse tumors used were mKS-A TU-5 (mKSA), an SV40-induced fibrosarcoma (19) obtained from Dr. Joyce Zarling; Lewis Lung Carcinoma (LLC), a spontaneous lung carcinoma obtained from the National Cancer Institute; B16, a spontaneous melanoma obtained from Jackson Laboratories; and Meth 1A, a methylcholanthrene-induced fibrosarcoma obtained from the National Cancer Institute. They were maintained in the corresponding syngeneic hosts, BALB/c for mKSA and Meth 1A and C57 B l/10 for LLC and B16. Liver, kidney, and heart were used as normal tissue controls.

The tissue was homogenized in 5 volumes of phosphate-buffered saline (PBS); the homogenate was sonicated twice for 30 seconds each and centrifuged at 2000 G for 10 minutes. The supernatant was further centrifuged at 100,000 G for 1 hour. The supernatant was dialyzed against 2 volumes of PBS for 48 hours at 5°. The dialysates were tested for the presence of activity capable of modulating macrophage properties. Dialysates were usually stored at 5°.

The dialysates containing molecules of less than 12,000 Daltons were tested for their effect on the migration of mouse peritoneal macrophages out of capillary tubes in a Sykes-Moore chamber (14). Peritoneal exudate cells were obtained from male C57B l/6 mice (6 to 10 weeks of age) which had been injected with 0.2 ml of Complete Freund's adjuvant intraperitoneally 36 hours previously. After washing with medium (Dulbecco's Modified Eagle Medium) containing 10% fetal calf serum (FCS) the cells were suspended in the same medium at a density of 4×10^7 cells per ml. The peritoneal exudate cells contained approximately 50% macrophages, 45% lymphocytes, and less than 5% polymorphonuclear leukocytes as determined by Hemal Stain (Hemal Stain Co., Inc., Danbury, Connecticut). Approximately 2×10^6 cells were drawn into sterile 15×100 mm siliconized glass capillary tubes and sealed at one end with 40:60 mixture of paraffin and vaseline. The capillaries were centrifuged (200 G for 7 min) and were cut at the cell-fluid interface. The stubs were placed in a Sykes-Moore chamber (Belco Glass, Inc., Vineland, N.J.) and secured with a drop of vaseline. The chambers were filled with approximately 1 ml of medium containing 10% FCS and the tumor or normal tissue dialysate and incubated at 37° in 10% CO_2 in air for 24 hours. Migration areas were projected onto a paper, traced, cut out, and weighed or the projected areas measured using a planimeter.

Figure 1 shows the migration patterns obtained in the presence of dialysates derived from liver (Fig. 1a) and Lewis Lung Carcinoma (Fig. 1b). Migration pattern obtained in the presence of medium alone (control) was similar to the one shown in Figure 1a. The dialysate derived from LLC enhances substantially the migration of macrophages, as measured in migration area, whereas the dialysate derived from the liver tissue has no measurable effect. Figure 2 illustrates the effect on macrophage migration of various concentrations of the dialysate derived from LLC. At the optimal concentration, this dialysate enhanced migration (measured in migration area) approximately 300%. Similar results were obtained with dialysates derived from all four tumors as shown in Table 1. In contrast,

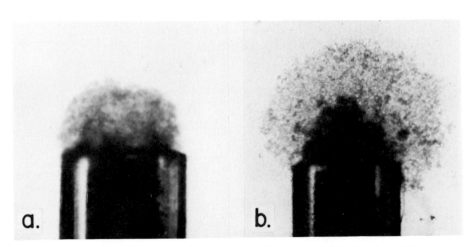

Fig. 1. Effect of tumor dialysate on peritoneal exudate cell migration. The experiment was performed as described in the text.

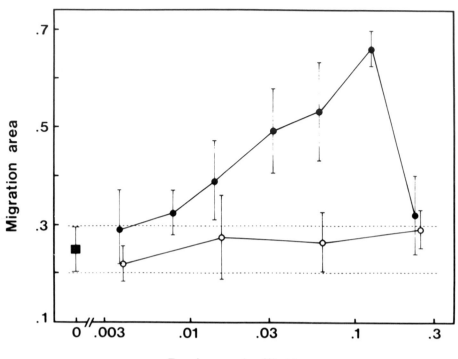

Fig. 2.   Effect of tumor dialysate on peritoneal exudate cell migration. Random migration areas in the presence of dialysates derived from the tumor, LLC (●) and liver (○) and medium control (■) are shown. The concentration of the dialysate is expressed in reciprocal dilution. Each point is the mean of four determinations ± S.D. Results are expressed as arbitrary units of migration area.

dialysates derived from liver, kidney, and heart at equivalent and higher concentrations did not have any measurable effect on the migration. The factor present in the dialysate which enhances macrophage migration is thus derived from tumors and not from these normal tissues. This factor could also be extracted from mKSA cells after two passages *in vitro* (Table 1) suggesting that the appearance of the factor is a property of malignant cells.

Peritoneal exudate cells used in the migration assay were largely macrophages and lymphocytes with a few polymorphonuclear leukocytes. To establish the nature of the cells which were affected in the migration assay, the cells that migrated out of the capillary onto the glass cover slip were fixed, stained with Hemal Stain and examined. Cells in the

Table 1.   Effect of various tumor dialysates on the migration of peritoneal exudate cells

Source of Dialysate	Migration Area ± S.D. in the Presence of		% Enhancement of Migration
	Medium Alone (Control)	Tumor Dialysate	
LLC tumor	0.16 ± 0.05	0.51 ± 0.08	219
mKSA tumor	0.13 ± 0.02	0.49 ± 0.07	280
B16 tumor	0.26 ± 0.01	0.47 ± 0.07	80
Meth 1A tumor	0.07 ± 0.02	0.26 ± 0.07	271
mKSA cells cultured in vitro	0.13 ± 0.06	0.37 ± 0.08	185

periphery of the migration area and those identifiable cells in the more crowded interior areas were all macrophages. However, it is not known whether the tumor factor acts directly on macrophages or through some other cell type.

Cells migrating in the absence of factor or in the presence of dialysate derived from liver had a spread morphology with pseudopod-like structures. Cells migrating in the presence of dialysates derived from tumors, in contrast, had a more rounded morphology. This morphological difference could be related to the enhancement of migration observed in the presence of the tumor factor since migration and the ability of cells to attach to substratum and spread are related properties in that they all depend on the function of the cytoskeletal structures, microtubules, and microfilaments (2, 17, 25).

The ability of the tumor factor to act directly on the macrophages and affect their attachment to substratum and spreading was also investigated. Monolayers of mouse peritoneal macrophages were prepared as follows. Peritoneal exudate cells were obtained as described before and in a typical experiment (Table 2) 5.28 × 10⁶ cells in 2 ml of medium containing 10% FCS were incubated for 2 hours in a 35 × 10 mm falcon tissue culture dish. Nonadherent cells were removed and the adherent monolayer was washed once with 1.0 ml PBS. The nonadherent fraction contained on an average 2.53 × 10⁶ cells. The adherent cells (> 95% macrophages as judged by their ability to phagocytose latex particles) were incubated with the indicated preparation diluted fourfold with medium containing 10% FCS. After 24 hours the cells in the nonadherent fraction were removed and counted. Cells remaining attached were lysed with 0.25% Triton

Table 2.   Effect of tumor dialysate on the adhesion of peritoneal macrophages

Treatment	No. of Cells in Nonadherent Fraction ($\times 10^{-5}$)	Total Protein in Adherent Fraction (μ g)
PBS (control)	3.7 ± 0.48	88.5 ± 7.04
Liver dialysate	4.2 ± 0.27	77.3 ± 4.20
mKSA dialysate	8.1 ± 1.10	56.2 ± 6.60
LLC dialysate	7.8 ± 0.81	54.9 ± 4.40

X-100 and the total protein in the lysate was determined. Cells in both the adherent and nonadherent fractions were mostly viable. As shown in Table 2, significantly more cells were present in the nonadherent fraction in the presence of tumor factor; proportionately reduced numbers of cells were found attached as compared to the control indicating the ability of this factor to inhibit adhesion of macrophages to substratum. In contrast, the dialysates derived from normal tissues showed no significant difference from the control. (Data shown are means of triplicates, plus or minus the standard deviation.)

Figure 3 shows the effect of the tumor factor on macrophage spreading. Monolayers of mouse peritoneal macrophages prepared as described before were cultured for 24 hours, at which time they had begun to spread. Those cells not attached were removed and the adherent spread macrophages were treated with tumor dialysate. As shown in Figure 3b the factor derived from LLC causes the cells to round up. Similar effects were observed with dialysates derived from the B16 and mKSA tumors; Meth 1A was not tested. In contrast, in the presence of dialysate derived from liver or kidney tissue the cells had a spread morphology similar to the control cells (Figure 3a). In all cases no cytotoxicity of macrophages by the tumor factor was observed.

These data clearly demonstrate that the dialysates derived from tumors contain one or several factors of molecular weight less than 12,000 Daltons capable of modulating three properties of macrophages studied *in vitro*. However, these data do not show whether the same factor mediates the different effects observed.

In order to gain further understanding of tumor factors capable of modulating macrophage properties, the tumor extracts were separated into fractions of different molecular weight ranges using a combination of Amicon ultrafiltration membranes XM-50 and UM2 which allow the filtration of molecules of 50,000 Daltons and 1000 Daltons respectively and

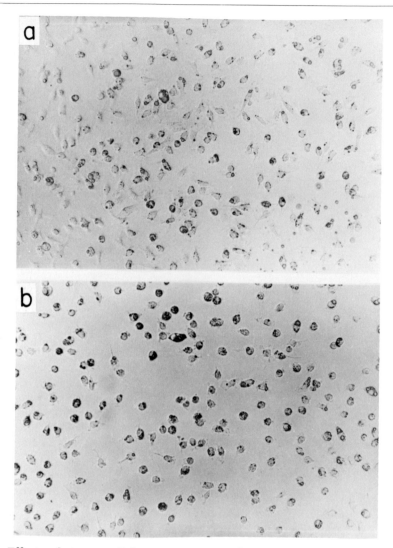

Fig. 3. Effect of tumor dialysate on macrophage spreading. Macrophage monolayers were incubated for 24 hours with liver dialysate (a) or LLC dialysate (b) and photographed. (See text for details.)

dialysis tubings which allow the passage of molecules of 12,000 Daltons and 3500 Daltons respectively. The different fractions were tested for their effect on macrophage migration. As shown in Table 3, the activity capable of enhancing macrophage migration is present only in fractions of molecular weight less than 12,000 Daltons and 3500 Daltons respectively.

Table 3. Enhancement of peritoneal exudate cell migration by various fractions of tumor extracts

	Molecular Weight Range of Fractions (Daltons)			
Tumor	50,000 to 12,000	< 12,000	< 3,500	< 1,000
LLC	−	+	+	−
mKSA	−	+	+	+−[a]
B16	+	+	+	−
Meth 1A	ND	+	ND	ND

a. Enhancement was observed in two experiments and no enhancement was observed in two other experiments.
ND: No data.

It is not established whether there is any activity in the molecular weight range 3,500 Daltons to 12,00 Daltons. The fraction of molecular weight less than 3500 Daltons not only enhances macrophage migration but also inhibits their ability to attach to substratum and spread (data not shown). The fraction of molecular weight less than 3500 Daltons was further fractionated by gel filtration on sephadex G-25 into several peaks showing absorption at 260 nm. One of the peaks retains the ability to enhance the

Table 4. Sensitivity of the LLC tumor factor to various treatments

	Migration Area $\pm$ S.D. in Presence of		
Treatment	Medium Alone (Control)	Untreated Factor	Treated Factor
At 100°C, 30 min.	9.56 ± 0.89	20.0 ± 2.1	18.2 ± 2.1
At pH 2.0 at 20°C for 30 min.	17.6 ± 2.5	33.4 ± 4.2	31.2 ± 0.7
At pH 11.0 at 20° C for 30 min.	17.6 ± 2.5	33.4 ± 4.2	32.06 ± 1.3
With Pronase bound to Sepharose	12.8 ± 0.9	28.73 ± 0.8	29.2 ± 1.4
With a mixture of bovine spleen phosphodiesterase II, E. Coli alkaline phosphatase, and pancreatic ribonuclease	12.0 ± 1.5	18.76 ± 0.8	17.32 ± 1.8

migration of macrophages and inhibit their ability to spread (data not shown). This preliminary finding suggests that either the same factor causes enhancement of macrophage migration and inhibition of their attachment and spreading or these effects are caused by different factors which behave similarly in gel filtration. Since migration, attachment and spreading are related properties as described before and since all these are affected by the same peak it is very likely that there is only one tumor factor responsible for the modulation of macrophage properties observed.

The tumor factor is stable at 5° for more than 14 days. Also, as shown in Table 4, it is not inactivated by exposure for 30 minutes at 100°, at pH of 2.0 or at pH of 11.0. It is insensitive to pronase bound to sepharose or to a mixture of bovine spleen phosphodiesterase II, E. coli alkaline phosphatase and pancreatic ribonuclease.

Inhibition of In Vitro Immune Response By The Tumor Factor

In order to test whether this tumor factor also has an effect on the immune response, the in vitro mixed leukocyte culture (MLC) reaction was used as the test system. In an MLC reaction spleen cells of one strain

Table 5. Effect of LLC tumor factor (fraction of less than 3,500 Daltons)[a] on the proliferative response and the generation of cytotoxic lymphocytes in a mixed leukocyte culture reaction

Responder-Stimulator Combination+ Addition	Thymidine Incorporation on 4th day, CPM ± S.D.	Percent Cytotoxicity ± S.D.	
		C57BL/6 target	BALB/c target
AA$_x$ + none	2,240 ± 452	−7.97 ± 12.1	− 3.59 ± 6.38
AB$_x$ + none	45,366 ± 1,903	−2.68 ± 10.68	46.22 ± 7.5
AB$_x$ + LLC factor, 100%	5,472 ± 159	−0.86 ± 12.47	5.60 ± 5.78
AB$_x$ + LLC factor, 25%	15,047 ± 1,024	−2.9 ± 10.99	11.60 ± 4.11
AB$_x$ + LLC factor, 12.5%	18,954 ± 1,296	−6.80 ± 11.01	12.97 ± 7.66
AB$_x$ + LLC factor, 3.1%	24,264 ± 1,037	−2.29 ± 3.37	19.24 ± 4.6
AB$_x$ + Liver dialysate, 25%	67,098 ± 2,628	−6.06 ± 11.91	45.37 ± 21.64

a. LLC factor was prepared in tissue culture medium and used directly to obtain the concentration of 100%. Appropriate dilutions were made to obtain the other concentrations. A = C57BL/6, responder. B = BALB/c, stimulator.

of mouse (responder cells) are cultured in the presence of X-irradiated allogeneic spleen cells (stimulating cells). The responder lymphocytes respond to the histocompatibility antigens of the stimulating cells and are induced to proliferate and generate specific cytotoxic T lymphocytes (CTL) capable of killing target cells which are either isogeneic to the stimulator cells or share the stimulating antigens (3). The degree of proliferation is determined by measuring the incorporation of ^{3}H-thymidine and the CTL generation is measured by the cell-mediated lympholysis (CML) assay (3). Spleen cells from C57B l/6 mice and X-irradiated spleen cells from BALB/c mice were used as responding and stimulating cells respectively. The effect of the tumor factor (fraction of molecular weight less than 3500 Daltons) at various concentrations on the ^{3}H-thymidine incorporation (proliferative response) and CTL generation was tested and the results are summarized in Table 5. The data show that the tumor factor inhibits markedly both the proliferative response and the generation of CTLs. In all combinations shown in Table 5, viable cells were present on the fifth day of culture showing that inhibition of the response is not due to any cytotoxic effect of the factor.

Role of Cytoskeletal Structures In The Control Of Macrophage Migration, Adhesion, and Spreading

As discussed before, migration, adhesion, and spreading of macrophages are related properties and at least in part are controlled by the cytoskeletal structures, microtubules, and microfilaments. These structures can be disrupted by treating the cells with the drugs colchicine and cytochalasin B, respectively. In order to understand how small changes induced in these structures would affect macrophage properties such as migration, adhesion, and spreading, the effects of colchicine and cytochalasin B on these properties at various concentrations were investigated. The areas of migration of peritoneal macrophages obtained in the presence of various concentrations of colchicine are summarized in Figure 4. There is clearly an enhancement in migration caused by colchicine in the concentration range of 10^{-12}M to 10^{-3}M. Maximum enhancement is observed in the concentration range of 10^{-6}M to 10^{-4}M. At a higher concentration of 10^{-2}M, colchicine clearly inhibits migration. The ability of macrophages to spread on the substratum in the presence of the same concentrations of colchicine was also investigated. The results summarized in Table 6 show that at all the concentrations tested colchicine inhibits the spreading of macrophages.

These results, shown in Figure 4 and Table 6, indicate the following: When the microtubules are disrupted maximally by using high concentration (10^{-2}M) of colchicine the macrophages are unable to spread and their

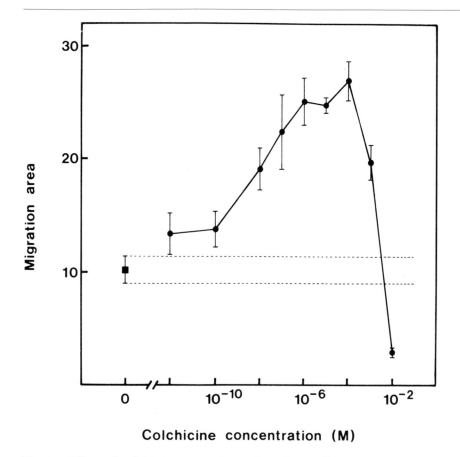

Fig. 4. Effect of colchicine on peritoneal exudate cell migration. (See Figure 2 legend and text for details.)

ability to migrate is markedly impaired. However, when the microtubules are disrupted moderately by treatment with moderate concentrations (10^{-8}M to 10^{-3}M) of colchicine the spreading is inhibited to a lesser degree and at the same time migration is enhanced quite markedly. The migration of macrophages on a surface may involve attachment and spreading, and a modulation of attachment and spreading may result in the modulation of migration. The relation between the two may be such that when the attachment and spreading are intense, the migration is minimal, and when they are moderately inhibited the tendency of the cells is to migrate faster. When the ability of the cells to attach and spread is impaired more severely their migration is inhibited markedly. Finally,

Table 6. Effect of colchicine on the spreading of peritoneal macrophages

Colchicine Concentration (M)	% Macrophages Spread
0 (control)	90
10^{-12}	30
10^{-10}	30
10^{-8}	15
10^{-7}	10
10^{-6}	10
10^{-5}	10
10^{-4}	5
10^{-3}	0
10^{-2}	0

microtubules may be very important in controlling the delicate dependence of migration on adhesion and spreading.

The areas of migration of macrophages in the presence of various concentrations of cytochalasin B are shown in Table 7. This table also shows the data on the effect of cytochalasin B on the spreading of macrophages. It is quite clear from these data that cytochalasin B inhibits spreading and at the higher concentrations tested there is a marked inhibition of migration. At lower concentrations, which inhibit spreading, no

Table 7. Effect of cytochalasin B on the migration and spreading of peritoneal macrophages

Cytochalasin B Concentration (μg/ml)	Migration Area $\pm$ S.D.	%Macrophages Spread
0 (control)	2.18 $\pm$ 0.64	70
0.00005	1.71 $\pm$ 0.13	80
0.0005	2.94 $\pm$ 0.69	60
0.005	2.49 $\pm$ 0.34	40
0.05	1.63 $\pm$ 0.68	30
0.5	1.40 $\pm$ 0.44	15
5.0	0.52 $\pm$ 0.35	2

significant enhancement in migration is observed. In this respect the effect of cytochalasin B is distinct from that of colchicine. It can be argued from these data that microfilaments also control the adhesion, spreading, and migration of cells but the manner in which it controls these properties is different from that of microtubules. It can also be suggested that microtubules and microfilaments act in a coordinate fashion but microtubules have a more profound direct effect on the migration of cells.

Discussion

We have presented evidence indicating that mouse tumors possess a low molecular weight (less than 3500 Daltons) factor or factors affecting peritoneal macrophages in vitro, resulting in the modulation of their properties. This factor causes an enhancement in macrophage migration and inhibits their ability to attach to substratum and spread. It is not known whether the modulation of these different properties is brought about by the same factor or different factors. However, upon fractionation by gel filtration on sephadex G-25 the activities capable of enhancing macrophage migration and inhibiting spreading appeared in the same peak. The chemical nature of this factor remains to be established.

Tumor tissues are known to contain host cells and also degradative events might be occurring in the vicinity of tumors. For these reasons it would be important to know whether the macrophage modulating factor extracted from tumors is indeed derived from the tumor cells. The fact that this factor could be extracted from mKSA cells after two passages in vitro strongly suggests that its presence is a property of malignant cells. Our preliminary studies also indicate that the factor is released into the culture medium by at least one of the tumor cell lines tested.

In a related study Snyderman and Pike established that mouse neoplasms possess a factor of molecular weight between 6,000 and 10,000 Daltons capable of inhibiting macrophage chemotaxis in vitro (27). Fauve et al. showed that mouse tumor cells in culture produce into the medium a factor of molecular weight between 1,000 and 10,000 Daltons with anti-inflammatory activity when injected in vivo (12). Holmberg obtained from tumor fluids a polypeptide with a molecular weight of approximately 2000 Daltons, capable of inhibiting adhesion and pseudopodia formation by L cells (18). It is not known at this time whether any or all of these factors have identity with the macrophage modulating factor we have described.

It is not known how this tumor factor affects the different properties of macrophages. Our observations, however, may be an indication of the modulation of cytoskeletal structures caused by the tumor factor. This notion is further strengthened by our finding (Fig. 4) that colchicine, an inhibitor of microtubule assembly, in the concentration range of $10^{-8}M$ to $10^{-3}M$ enhances migration of mouse peritoneal exudate cells; at the optimal concentration of $10^{-4}M$ the enhancement in migration area is 270%. In fact it is possible that the presence of this factor in tumor cells is related to the diminished assembly of microtubules and microfilaments observed in these cells as compared to normal cells (10, 24).

Depressed immune response has been observed in tumor bearing animals (13, 23). In addition, it has been observed that tumor cell culture supernatants have the capacity to inhibit immune response *in vitro*. Our results show that the same fraction of molecular weight less than 3500 Daltons derived from tumors which modulates macrophage properties also inhibits *in vitro* immune response to foreign histocompatibility antigens on allogeneic cells; inhibition of both the proliferative response and the generation of cytotoxic T lymphocytes is brought about by the tumor factor (Table 5). It may be that the same factor has both macrophage modulating activity and immunosuppressive activity. However, this remains to be established.

The modulation of macrophage properties and depression of immune response observed *in vitro* could be an indication of the ability of tumor cells to subvert the host defense mechanisms through the factor described here. The role of this factor, if any, in tumor-host relationships is a subject for further investigation. It would be of considerable value to test whether it appears in detectable amounts in the serum or urine or both of tumor bearers. If it is present in any of these fluids, it may provide an approach for early detection of cancer. Also deliberate immunization against this factor could be beneficial for the host in its defense against cancer.

ACKNOWLEDGMENTS

We wish to acknowledge gratefully the support and encouragement received from Dr. Fritz H. Bach of the Immunobiology Research Center during the progress of this study. This work was aided by Grant DRG 1283 from the Damon Runyon Memorial Fund for Cancer Reserach, Inc. and other grants, 1P01 CA16836 and 1F32 CA05596 awarded by the National Cancer Institute, DHEW. This is paper number 119 from the Immunobiology Research Center, University of Wisconsin.

REFERENCES

1. Alexander, P., Eccles, S. A., and Gauci, C. L. L. 1976. The significance of macrophages in human and experimental tumors. *Ann. N.Y. Acad. Sci.* 276: 124–133.

2. Allison, A. C. 1973. The role of microfilaments and microtubules in cell

movement, endocytosis and exocytosis. In *Locomotion of Tissue Cells*, Ciba Foundation Symposium. 14: 109–148.

3. Bach, F. H., Bach, M. L., and Sondel, P. M. 1976. Differential function of major histocompatibility complex antigens in T-lymphocyte activation. *Nature* 259: 273–281.

4. Berg, J. W. 1959. Inflammation and prognosis in breast cancer. A search for host resistance. *Cancer* 12: 714–720.

5. Black, M. M., Opler, S. R., and Speer, F. D. 1954. Microscopic structure of gastric carcinomas and their regional lymph nodes in relation to survival. *Surg. Gynecol. Obstet.* 98: 725–734.

6. Boetcher, D., and Leonard, E. J. 1974. Abnormal monocyte chemotactic response in cancer patients. *J. Natl. Cancer Inst.* 52: 1091–1099.

7. Bruley-Rosset, M., Florentin, I., Khalil, A. M., and Mathé, G. 1976. Nonspecific macrophage activation by systemic adjuvants. Evaluation by lysosomal enzyme and *in vitro* tumoricidal activities. *Int. Arch. Allergy Appl. Immun.* 51: 594–607.

8. Currie, G. 1976. Immunological aspects of host resistance to the development and growth of cancer. *Biochim. Biophys. Acta* 458: 135–165.

9. Eccles, S. A., and Alexander, P. 1974. Macrophage content of tumors in relation to metastatic spread and host-immune reaction. *Nature* 250: 667–669.

10. Edelman, G. M., and Yahara, I. 1976. Temperature-sensitive changes in surface modulating assemblies of fibroblasts transformed by mutants of Rous sarcoma virus. *Proc. Natl. Acad. Sci. USA* 73: 2047–2051.

11. Evans, R. 1973. Macrophage and the tumor-bearing host. *Brit. J. Cancer* 28 Suppl. 1: 19–25.

12. Fauve, R. M., Hevin, B., Jacob, H., Gaillard, J. A., and Jacob, F. 1974. Anti-inflammatory effects of murine malignant cells. *Proc. Natl. Acad. Sci. USA* 71: 4052–4056.

13. Friedman, H., Spector, S., Kamo, I., and Kateley, J. 1976. Tumor-associated immunosuppressive factors. *Ann. N.Y. Acad. Sci.* 276: 417–430.

14. Gorczynski, R. M., Miller, R. G., and Phillips, R. A. 1973. Reconstitution of T cell-depleted spleen cell populations by factors derived from T cells. I. Conditions for the production of active T cell supernatants. *J. Immunol.* 110: 968–983.

15. Hibbs, J. B., Jr. 1973. Macrophage nonimmunologic recognition: Target cell factors related to contact inhibition. *Science* 180: 868–870.

16. Hibbs, J. B., Jr. 1976. Role of activated macrophages in nonspecific resistance to neoplasia. *J. Reticuloendothel. Soc.* 20: 223–231.

17. Helentjaris, T. G., Lombardi, P. S., and Glasgow, L. A. 1976. Effect of cytochalasin B on the adhesion of mouse peritoneal macrophages. *J. Cell. Biol.* 69: 407–414.

18. Holmberg, B. 1962. Inhibition of cellular adhesion and pseudopodia formation by a dialysable factor from tumor fluids. *Nature* 195: 45–47.

19. Kit, S., Kurimura, T., and Dubbs, D. R. 1969. Transplantable mouse tumor line induced by injection of SV40 transformed mouse kidney cells. *Int. J. Cancer* 4: 384–392.

20. North, R. J., Kirstein, D. P., and Tuttle, R. L. 1976. Subversion of host defense mechanisms by murine tumors I. A circulating factor that suppresses

macrophage mediated resistance to infection. *J. Exp. Med.* 143: 559–573.

21. North, R. J., Kirstein, D. P., and Tuttle, R. L. 1976. Subversion of host defense mechanisms by murine tumors. II. Counter influence of concomitant antitumor immunity. *J. Exp. Med.* 143: 574–584.

22. Pike, M. C., and Snyderman, R. 1976. Depression of macrophage function by a factor produced by neoplasms: A mechanism for abrogation of immune surveillance. *J. Immunol.* 117: 1243–1249.

23. Plescia, O. J., Grinwich, K., and Plescia, A. M. 1976. Subversive activity of syngeneic tumor cells as an escape mechanism from immune surveillance and the role of prostaglandins. *Ann. N.Y. Acad. Sci.* 276: 455–465.

24. Pollack, R., Osborn, M., and Weber, K. 1975. Patterns of organization of actin and myosin in normal and transformed cultured cells. *Proc. Natl. Acad. Sci. USA* 72: 994–998.

25. Rydgren, L., Simmingskold, G., Bandmann, U., and Norberg, B. 1976. The role of cytoplasmic microtubules in polymorphonuclear leukocyte chemotaxis. Evidence for the release hypothesis by means of time-lapse analysis of PMN movement relative to dot-like attractants. *Exp. Cell Res.* 99: 207–220.

26. Snyderman, R., Pike, M. C., Meadows, L., Hemstreet, G., and Wells, S. 1975. Depression of monocyte chemotaxis by neoplasms. *Clin. Res.* 23: 297a.

27. Snyderman, R., and Pike, M. C. 1976. An inhibitor of macrophage chemotaxis produced by neoplasms. *Science* 192: 370–372.

28. Snyderman, R., Pike, M. C., Blaylock, B. L., and Weinstein, P. 1976. Effects of neoplasms on inflammation: Depression of macrophage accumulation after tumor implantation. *J. Immunol.* 116: 585–589.

CHAPTER 8

IMMUNOLOGICAL MECHANISMS FOR ALLOGENEIC TUMOR ACCEPTANCE

Richard C. Parks

American Cancer
Research Center and Hospital
Lakewood, Colorado 80214

Experimental findings are presented concerning the growth of strain specific tumors across strong histoincompatibility barriers and the possible mechanisms involved.

Tumor cells have been shown to possess antigens on their surfaces, which are recognized by the host in which the tumors arise (14, 17, 26). Under certain conditions these antigens can provoke immune responses which inhibit tumor growth, while in others, the tumors may thrive and progress in spite of the existence of foreign transplantation antigens on their surface. Consequently, a number of mechanisms have been proposed to explain the ability of antigenic tumors to overcome host immune responses (1, 5, 6, 8, 10, 13, 18, 20, 22, 24). However, it is not the intent of this author to reiterate that which has been adequately presented by others.

Normally strain-specific transplantable murine tumors will not survive in histoincompatible recipients due to the transplantation antigens expressed on their surface (14). Yet, by modifying the host's immune competence (20), or the allograft's immunogenicity (7, 8) progressive growth of strain-specific tumors across strong histoincompatible lines can be achieved. Novel techniques such as implanting together both tumor and sterile flannel fibers (9) or tumor within a lucite cylinder (23) have demonstrated the promotion of allogeneic tumor growth. Allogeneic tumor growth also has been demonstrated with strain-specific tumors wrapped in muscle syngeneic to the prospective allogeneic recipient (19). This technique is unique in that it uses normal syngeneic tissue as a promotor of allogeneic tumors in immunologically competent animals.

The Allogeneic Tumor–Syngeneic Muscle Model

The procedure employed for the preparation of the tumor allograft of the allogeneic tumor–syngeneic muscle model has been described in detail elsewhere (19). Essentially, a prospective strain-specific tumor is cut into trocar-size fragments (1–2 mm) and inserted between the abdominal muscle layers of a killed allogeneic host. The abdominal muscle surrounding and including the allogeneic tumor implant is excised and grafted subcutaneously to the flank of an immunologically competent host syngeneic to the muscle. The allogeneic tumor–syngeneic muscle sandwich (TMS) graft in toto is approximately 10 mm across.

Growth of the TMS tumor is not peculiar to muscle alone. Other tissues such as liver and kidney when used as a substitute for muscle facilitated growth of the tumor allograft (Table 1). Splenic tissue inhibited growth of the sandwiched allogeneic tumor. The appropriate sandwich-

Table 1.   Incidence of TMS tumor using different sandwiching tissues

Graft Recipients	Tumor	Sandwiching Tissue	Mice with Tumors	Percent
BALB/c $(H\text{-}2^d)$	S91 $(H\text{-}2^q)$	Muscle	4/7	57
BALB/c $(H\text{-}2^d)$	S91 $(H\text{-}2^q)$	Liver	3/7	43
BALB/c $(H\text{-}2^d)$	S91 $(H\text{-}2^q)$	Kidney	3/7	43
BALB/c $(H\text{-}2^d)$	S91 $(H\text{-}2^q)$	Spleen	0/7	0
BALB/c $(H\text{-}2^d)$	S91 $(H\text{-}2^q)$	——	0/7	0
DBA/1 $(H\text{-}2^q)$	S91 $(H\text{-}2^q)$	——	6/6	100

ing tissue probably acts as an immunological barrier which protects the allograft from the host's immune responses much in the same manner as that of the artificially created alymphatic skin pedicles (2).

The strain-specific tumors used in preparing TMS grafts have been the C57B1/6 $(H\text{-}2^b)$ melanoma—B16, A/J $(H\text{-}2^a)$ neuroblastoma—C1300, DBA/1 $(H\text{-}2^q)$ melanoma—S91, BALB/c $(H\text{-}2^d)$ Leydig cell tumor—C4092, and BALB/c methylcholanthrene-induced tumor—MCA (Table 2). Except for the MCA tumor, which has only been carried for 2 generations in its syngeneic BALB/c host, the rest of the described tumors have been serially transplanted in their appropriate syngeneic host for at least 30 generations. The B16, MCA, C1300, and S91 tumors are palpable in their host strain between 10–15 days. The C4092 is usually palpable after 30 days. When the B16 and the S91 tumors were sandwiched in either syngeneic or allogeneic muscle and grafted to the appropriate corresponding recipients, the tumor was palpable at about the same time in both recipients.

Old et al. (18) have demonstrated that small numbers of highly antigenic tumor cells can "sneak through" the immune system while large numbers are inhibited. Presumably the small number of tumor cells were not strong immunogens; thus they were able to proliferate unhindered by the immune apparatus and literally out run its development. The successful number of TMS tumor takes may in part depend on a similar mechanism.

It is not clear what the relationship is between immune responsiveness of the host and the growth or promotion of the TMS tumor. Histologically, the TMS graft appears to envolve a foreign body-like reaction and frequently foci of viable tumor are observed in close proximity to the reaction. It should be noted that although immediately after TMS graft implantation the tumor in residence appears dead (17), in actuality, it is

Table 2. Incidence of TMS tumor growth

Group	Graft Recipient	Tumor	Muscle Donor	Mice with Tumor	Percent
I	C57B1/6	B16	C57B1/6	6/6	100
	BALB/c	B16	BALB/c	21/24	88
	BALB/c	B16	———	0/13	0
	DBA/1	B16	DBA/1	10/10	100
	DBA/1	B16	———	0/6	0
II	DBA/1	S91	DBA/1	21/22	95
	BALB/c	S91	BALB/c	109/156	70
	BALB/c	S91	———	0/40	0
III	A/J	C1300	———	6/6	100
	BALB/c	C1300	BALB/c	5/6	83
	BALB/c	C1300	———	0/6	0
	DBA/1	C1300	DBA/1	3/6	50
	DBA/1	C1300	———	0/6	0
IV	BALB/c	C4092	———	6/6	100
	DBA/1	C4092	DBA/1	1/6	17
	DBA/1	C4092	———	0/6	0
V	BALB/c	MCA	BALB/c	6/6	100
	DBA/1	MCA	DBA/1	4/7	57
	DBA/1	MCA	———	0/7	0
	C57B1/6	MCA	C57B1/6	3/6	50
	C57B1/6	MCA	———	0/14	0

probably dormant. Tumor growth promoted by immune cellular reactions has been reported in several systems. Prehn (21) demonstrated with methylcholanthrene-induced tumors that an immune response to an antigenic neoplasm could be biphasic, i.e., a weak response would stimulate growth while a strong response would inhibit growth. Brand et al. (30) reported with foreign body tumorigenesis that the type and course of the reaction evoked influences growth.

Are the TMS Tumors Antigenic?

It has been previously reported that progressively growing TMS tumors as well as metastatic lesions that occasionally occurred will not grow when transplanted within the new host strain, but that uniform transplantation behavior occurred when transferred back to the strain of origin indicating that the established TMS tumor was incompatible within the new strain (19). Since it was observed that shortly after implantation of the TMS graft the tumor in residence undergoes cellular degradation, experiments were planned to examine potential changes in antigenicity of the TMS tumor during different periods of development. Single-cell suspensions of S91 tumor were prepared from TMS grafts implanted in BALB/c mice at different periods of time. These suspensions of cells (2.7 $\times$ 10^5 in 0.05 mls of medium-199) were injected into the left hind foot-pads of C57B1/6 mice specifically immunized against DBA/1 mice. The right hind foot-pad was injected with an equal amount of media. The experimental mice were subsequently injected with 2 μCi of ^{125}I-iodo-deoxyuridine (Amersham/Searle) according to the method of Miller et al. (15) and assessed after 36 hours for a delayed-type hypersensitivity reaction (DHR). The DHR was expressed as a ratio of cpm of left foot to cpm of right foot (foot-pad ratio). The information gained (Table 3) demonstrated that there was no significant reduction in the antigenicity during TMS-

Table 3. Induction of DHR in DBA/1-sensitized C57B1/6 mice with S91 tumor cells from a TMS graft

Stage of TMS Graft	Number of Mice	Mean Foot-Pad Ratio $\pm$ SE
0[a]	6	1.64 $\pm$ .24[b]
7	6	1.55 $\pm$ .17
14	6	2.37 $\pm$ .35
21	6	2.20 $\pm$ .29
28	6	1.88 $\pm$ .16
Control[c]	6	1.01 $\pm$ .10

a. Number of days the TMS graft was implanted in BALB/c recipients.

b. Foot-pad ratio greater than 1.2 was deemed a significant DHR.

c. Control syngeneic spleen cells.

tumor development. Thus success of the TMS-tumor in their allogeneic recipients may partly be dependent on host adaptation (8, 27).

Are TMS-Tumor-Bearing Mice Immunologically Impaired?

It has been reported (19) that: (1) animals in which TMS grafts failed to develop or animals specifically sensitized against the TMS-tumor graft do not support growth of a similar TMS challenge; (2) mice challenged concurrently with tumor or skin syngeneic to the TMS-tumor graft prevent tumor growth; (3) animals challenged with skin grafts syngeneic to the TMS tumor several weeks after TMS implantation develop TMS tumors; and (4) mice bearing TMS implants demonstrate a primary rejection of skin syngeneic to the tumor allograft throughout the development of the tumor. With regards to these observations, experiments were designed to test the potential existence of an immunological impairment.

Spleen and lymph node lymphoid cells from BALB/c mice bearing progressively growing S91-TMS implants were adoptively transferred to naive adult BALB/c recipients. Similar transfers of lymphocytes from BALB/c mice immunized with a single implant of S91 tumor and from naive BALB/c donors were performed. Each animal received intraperitoneally the equivalent of one spleen. Within three days following the lymphoid cell transfer, the recipients were grafted with DBA/1 skin (Table 4). The median survival time (MST) for the DBA/1 skin grafts was 10.5 ± 1.1 days for the TMS group, 9.5 ± 1.0 days for the naive group, and 7.2 ± 1.0 days for the immunized group. There was a significant difference (P <.05) between the MST of the immunized and naive mice and no difference between the TMS and naive mice. The immunized group

Table 4. Effect of adoptively transferred lymphocytes from TMS tumor-bearing mice on primary allogeneic skin grafts syngeneic to the TMS tumor

Lymphocyte Donor	Number of Mice	MST ± S.D. (days)	Range (days)	P
TMS-Bearer	10	10.5 ± 1.1	9–13	—
S91-Immunized	12	7.2 ± 1.0	5–8	S[a]
Naive	12	9.5 ± 1.0	9–12	—

a. Significantly different from naive control (P < .05).

Table 5. Effect of adoptively transferred lymphocytes from TMS tumor-bearing mice on second set
allogeneic skin grafts syngeneic to TMS tumor

Lymphocyte Donor	Number of Mice	MST ± S.D. (days)	Range (days)
TMS-bearer	6	9.0 ± 1.0	8–10
S91-immunized	6	4.6 ± 1.1	4–6
Immune naive[a]	6	4.6 ± 1.1	4–6
Naive control[b]	6	9.3 ± 1.1	8–11

a. Control mice from primary skin rejection study (Table 4).
b. Naive control mice for second set rejection.

demonstrated a weak, but definite, second set reaction. The reason for the
weak response was attributed to the manner in which the mice were
immunized (a single implant of S91 tumor).

Several weeks after the primary skin graft rejection, a random portion
of the experimental mice were re-challenged with a second set of DBA/1
skin (Table 5). Naive control mice were used to establish the MST of the
primary response. As with the naive control, the MST of the second set
challenge for the TMS group was essentially the same (MST = 9.3 ± 1.1
days and 9.0 ± 1.0 days, respectively). The S91 immunized group and the
immunized naive mice both expressed a strong second set rejection of
DBA/1 skin (MST = 4.6 ± 1.1 days for both groups).

The adoptive transfer of lymphocytes from tumor bearing mice demonstrates a lack of immune recognition in response to H-2 antigens associated with the TMS tumor. This inability to respond may be attributed
to several possible conditions. First, the TMS tumor may be antigenically
inert. However, this has been shown not to be the case (Table 3). Second,
the lymphocytes of the TMS-tumor-bearing mice have not been
adequately programmed against the antigenic TMS tumor, indicating a
possible afferent blockade. This could be accomplished by humoral
mediators produced by the tumor which specifically inhibits
macrophage-mediated resistance (16) and blast-transformation (25).
Thirdly, the adoptively transferred lymphocytes are immunologically
suppressed. The inability of the lymphocytes from TMS-tumor-bearing
mice to evoke a second set rejection response to the primary H-2 antigen
challenge suggested an absence of immune recognition. However, the
inability to demonstrate second-set response to a second antigenic challenge suggests that a cell-mediated suppressor possibly specific for the

anamnestic response was transferred. It is now accepted that thymus-derived lymphocytes (T cells) which effect cell-mediated immune responses (4) produce specific and nonspecific immune suppression (11, 13).

Summary and Conclusions

Of the described TMS tumor model it could be concluded that:

1. The TMS tumor retains its strain specificity throughout its development in the allogeneic host, and that acceptance is probably a host adaptation phenomenon (10, 22).
2. The sandwiching tissues of the TMS graft probably are a temporary immunological barrier which gives the antigenic allograft a slight edge over the emerging immune response—"sneaking through" (12).
3. The sandwiching tissue evokes a foreign body-like reaction which may benefit tumorigenesis by either directly stimulating incipient tumor growth (8, 19) or indirectly stimulating growth through suppression of cell-mediated immunity (4, 11, 26, 27).
4. Lymphoid cells from TMS-bearing mice are immunologically unresponsive to H-2 antigens associated with the TMS tumor upon adoptive transfer to a naive host. It is suggested that this lack of antigen recognition is cellularly-mediated and possibly a specific suppression of the anamnestic immune response.

Studies are in progress to further elucidate these observations.

ACKNOWLEDGMENT

This investigation was supported by Grant Number CA18923-01, awarded by the National Cancer Institute, DHEW.

REFERENCES

1. Baldwin, R. W., and Robins, R. A. 1975. Humoral factors abrogating cell-mediated immunity in the tumor bearing host. Current Topics Microbiol. Immunol. 72: 21–53.

2. Barker, C. F., and Billingham, R. E. 1968. An artificial immunologically privileged site. In J. Dausset, J. Hamburger, G. Mathe (eds.), Advances in Transplantation 1968, pp. 25–30. Baltimore, Williams and Wilkins.

3. Brand, K. G., Buoen, L. C., Johnson, K. H., and Brand, I. 1975. Etiological factors, stages and the role of the foreign body tumorigenesis: A review. Cancer Res. 35: 279–286.

4. Brunner, K. T., Nordin, A. A., and Cerottini, J. C. 1970. *In vitro* studies of sensitized lymphocytes and alloantibody-forming cells in mouse allograft immunity. *In* S. Cohen, G. Cudowicz and R. T. McCluskey (eds.), *Cellular interactions in the immune response, 1970,* pp. 220–230. Kauger, Basel.

5. Cruse, J. M., Lewis, G. K., Whitten, H. D., Watson, E. S., Fields, J. F., Adams, S. T., Jr., Harvey, G. F., III, Paslay, J. W., and Porter, M. 1974. Mechanisms of immunological enhancement. *Progr. Exp. Tumor Res.* 19: 110–156.

6. Gershwin, M. E., and Steinberg, A. D. 1973. Loss of suppressor function as a cause of lymphoid malignancy. *Lancet* 2: 1174–1176.

7. Jacobs, B. B., and Huseby, R. A. 1967. Growth of tumors in allogeneic hosts following organ culture explanation. *Transplantation* 5: 410–419.

8. Jacobs, B. B., and Uphoff, D. E. 1974. Immunologic modification: A basic survival mechanism. *Science* 185: 582–587.

9. Jones, E. 1926. The breakdown of hereditary immunity to a transplantable tumor by the introduction of an irritating agent. *Amer. J. Cancer* 10: 435–449.

10. Kaliss, N. 1958. Immunological enhancement of tumor homografts in mice. A review. *Cancer Res.* 18: 992–1003.

11. Katz, D. H., and Benacerraf, B. 1972. The regulatory influence of activated T cells on B cell responses to antigen. *Adv. Immunol.* 15: 1–94.

12. Kirchner, H., Muchmore, A. V., Chaused, T. M., Holden, H. T., and Herberman, R. B. 1975. Inhibition of proliferation of lymphoma cells and T lymphocytes by suppressor cells from spleen of tumor bearing mice. *J. Immunol.* 114: 206–210.

13. Kirkwood, J. M., and Gershon, R. K. 1974. A role for suppressor T cells in immunological enhancement of tumor growth. *Prog. Exp. Tumor Res.* 19: 157–164.

14. Klein, G. 1966. Tumor antigens. *Ann. Rev. Microbiol.* 20: 223–252.

15. Miller, J. F. A. P., Vadas, M. A., Whitelaw, A., and Gamble, J. 1975. H-2 gene complex restricts transfer of delayed-type hypersensitivity in mice. *Immunology* 72: 5095–5098.

16. North, R. J., Kirstein, D. P., and Tuttle, R. L. 1976. Subversion of host defense mechanisms by murine tumors. I. A circulating factor that suppresses machrophage-mediated resistance to infection. *J. Exp. Med.* 134: 559–573.

17. Old, L. J., and Boyse, E. A. 1964. Immunology of experimental tumors. *Ann. Rev. Med.* 15: 167–186.

18. Old, L. J., Boyse, E. A., Clarke, D. A., and Carswell, E. A. 1962. Antigenic properties of chemically induced tumors. *Ann. N.Y. Acad. Sci.* 101: 80–106.

19. Parks, R. C. 1976. Allogeneic tumor-syngeneic muscle sandwich grafts: A method for promoting non-specific growth. *J. Natl. Cancer Inst.* 56: 1281–1284.

20. Parks, R. C., and Jacobs, B. B. 1975. Transplantation behavior of allotransplantable tumor lines derived from immunologically modified hosts. *J. Natl. Cancer Inst.* 54: 1079–1083.

21. Prehn, R. T. 1972. The immune reaction as a stimulator of tumor growth. *Science* 176: 170–171.

22. Prehn, R. T., and Lappe, M. A. 1971. Immunostimulation theory of tumor development. *Transplant. Rev.* 7: 26–54.

23. Saal, F., Colmerauer, M. E., Braylan, R. C., and Pasqualini, C. D. 1972.

Tumor growth in allogeneic mice bearing a lucite cylinder. *J. Natl. Cancer Inst.* 49: 451–456.

24. Schwartz, R. S. 1972. Immunoregulation, oncogenic viruses, and malignant lymphomas. *Lancet* I: 1226–1269.

25. Silk, M. 1967. Effect of plasma from patients with carcinoma on *in vitro* lymphocyte transformation. *Cancer* 20: 2088–2089.

26. Smith, R. T. 1968. Tumor-specific immune mechanisms. *N. Engl. J. Med.* 278: 1207–1214, 1268–1275, 1326–1331.

27. Warden, G. D., Reemtsma, K., and Steinmuller, D. 1973. The phenomenon of adaptation: graft or host? *Transplant. Proc.* 5: 635–639.

INDEX